AF334141

Private Practice
in
Communication Disorders

PRIVATE PRACTICE
IN
COMMUNICATION
DISORDERS

Mary Lovey Wood, PhD

CCC Speech-Language Pathology

Singular Publishing Group, Inc.
San Diego, California

Singular Publishing Group, Inc.
4284 41st Street
San Diego, California 92105

Library of Congress Cataloging-in-Publication Data
Main entry under title:
Wood, Mary Lovey.
    Private practice in communication disorders.

    Includes bibliographies and index.
    1. Speech therapy—Practice. 1. Title.
[DNLM: 1. Communicative Disorders. 2. Private
Practice—organization and administration. W 89 W877p]
RC428.5. W66 1986 616.85'5'0068 86-9731.

ISBN 1-879105-30-6

Printed in the United States of America

*To my dear parents, Florella and David Wood,
who have always encouraged me to
keep on practicing until I get it right*

CONTENTS

PREFACE

This book is not intended to define speech, language or hearing disorders; nor is it designed to describe approaches to diagnosis or intervention. The book is intended to be a practical resource for those who are already in private practice and wish to expand or change their practices, as well as for those who are considering beginning a practice. Parts of the book are applicable for any job setting as a vehicle for analyzing the tasks, efficiency of services, and options for change. Some content is easily adaptable to other professions in which services are exchanged for fees.

Material for the book was drawn from current issues in the profession and the economy; changing laws and regulations may require adaptation by the reader. Most of the content comes from personal experiences and opinions derived from those experiences; several sections provide technical information with documentation for additional research by the reader.

The book does not have to be read from cover to cover to be useful. The chapters, although related, are neither interdependent nor sequential. The reader may choose a topic, turn to that section and find opinion, advice, technical information, and appended examples. The annotated bibliography can be used without reference to the text.

Information relating to taxes, bookkeeping, and the law are not intended to replace the use of consultants nor to substitute for a working knowledge of the profession's code of ethics. Terminology and issues are included to acquaint the reader with some of the considerations that affect our practice.

The sharing of experiences, information, and opinions contained in this book is to assist the professional in the most exciting of all endeavors—learning how to take care of oneself while caring for others.

ACKNOWLEDGMENTS

This book represents an effort to describe lessons learned from mistakes made in the course of nearly 20 years of private practice—and to pass on to others some of the help that has been given to me.

Family, friends, colleagues, consultants, and clients have formed a powerful force to keep me from too much harm. To those people, I attribute any success I might have in my practice and any help this book might provide someone else.

Several practitioners in my own profession and in allied professions have contributed to this book. These people are mentioned in the Bibliography, but a few must be highlighted: Richard Flower and his book on delivery of services; Mary Marshall and her colleagues with their specific items of organization and planning; Jay Foonberg, an attorney with the eye of a businessman; Paul Knight and Wallace Goates, who insisted that private practice in speech-language pathology was honorable when it was not fashionable.

Particular thanks is extended to Dr. M. Marjorie Menefee, a highly successful practitioner in psychology, whose ideas for the content of this book were enormously helpful. Dr. Menefee also spent many hours editing the writing style and form of this manuscript and is responsible for any proper punctuation and complete sentences found within.

And for comic relief, my gratitude is extended to Clover and his 26 grandchildren.

Chapter 1

Introduction

It is presumed that before considering independent practice, one is secure in the belief that he or she provides the highest quality of professional care and that that care is worth a fee.

It is also presumed that anyone who is, or aspires to be, a private practitioner maintains clinical skills that are appropriately current for the delivery of services to the communicatively impaired.

If these presumptions do not fit, please consider another avenue of professional endeavor.

If these presumptions do fit, please continue.

Private practice is not a description of a work setting; it is a philosophy. Private practice is a form of service delivery set within an arena of private enterprise that carries the opportunity to fail. Without failure, there is no lure to succeed. Without the fear of failure, there is no competition, hence the loss of the natural selection process that is so important to the profession and, of course, to the consumer. Professional success, which is achieved by minimizing or resolving communication problems, can be achieved without financial success. Financial success, which is making more money than one spends, cannot be achieved for very long in professional private practice without professional success.

A majority of private enterprise ventures fail in the first year or two; the most frequent cause is related to financial planning and management. The Small Business Administration (1983), responding to questions regarding the failure rate of small businesses, cited the following as the primary reasons (parenthetical comments by this author):

1. poor financial planning (overspending, under capitalization, inappropriate spending);
2. poor market analysis (finding a place and population where the professional's unique services are needed and can be afforded);

3. poor general administration (poor management of money, time, and personnel).

Macfarlane (1977) studied 30 minority-owned small businesses, half of which had failed, and asked the owners what they wished they had known prior to opening for business. Respondents indicated a need for more knowledge of

1. management skills required;
2. the specific business (the variations of service delivery that are possible);
3. interactions with lenders and investors (i.e., lenders' influence or restrictions or both on the use of business assets, limits on future borrowing, retaining control of the corporate board, and so forth);
4. accounting (keeping business books and understanding the management information which they can provide);
5. location of the business (site selection);
6. selection of business partner (did not realize before beginning that the partner or partners did not agree with their own ideas of goals, policies, strategies, and so on);
7. amount of initial financing required (underestimated financial needs at start-up, resulting in an undercapitalized venture that produced persistent, unsolvable difficulties);
8. governmental regulations and requirements (e.g., withholding taxes, employee taxes, social security deductions, business licenses, local regulations);
9. demands of self-employment on themselves and their families (had they known the heavy work commitment required and the resulting stress on their families, some would have forewarned their families that they would need the family's support and resources; others would have chosen not to enter the venture).

Delivering professional services for fees on the open market is more hazardous than in any other service delivery system. The private enterprise system imposes many more contingencies that are crucial to success. In private practice, not only must the quality of professional services be assured, but the factors of management, money, marketing, and professional morality must be juggled.

MANAGEMENT, MONEY, MARKETING, AND MORALITY

The life span of a private practice will survive the errors one makes in management and marketing as long as those errors are made in the honest pursuit of good clinical care for each client—that is, as long as morality is consistently present. It is fatal, of course, to practice and not attend intelligently to the money, management, and marketing of one's practice. One must organize the operations of a practice, pay attention, and collect fees.

Management

The management principle of a practice is simply stated: ''Revenue must exceed expenditures.'' In everyday decision-making, this means that fees must cover expenses; overhead must be contained while revenue increases; a line of credit must be available at the bank; and decisions must be made with regard to personnel, salaries, and office priorities and policies. Management is more than money, but money is an ever-present concern.

Money

If you feel that charging money as direct compensation for services is indecent, then you should not be in private practice. There are programs and agencies designed to serve those who cannot pay. Those agencies, and our colleagues who work there, survive by obtaining money from grants reserved for those who cannot pay for services *and* reserved for those agencies that serve only the financially needy. Public monies and federal and state grants are rarely granted to private enterprise, even when private enterprise serves clients who are financially needy.

Making money is not only decent; it is an absolute necessity. When your practice has reached the point where it can pay for itself, other than overhead and owner compensation, then you may want to consider a sliding fee schedule or a drastic fee reduction for a certain number of your clients. Beware, however, that you do not create a philanthropic noose for yourself. If your revenue drops, and your landlord and creditors press you because you are behind on your payments, professional morality still demands that you continue to donate the time to your no-fee clients. If collections remain lower than overhead, you will note sooner or later the lack of sympathy extended to you by your creditors. Ultimately your inability to meet the demands of your creditors will lead to the demise of your practice. You will be looking for employment, and the clients for whom you did the financial favor will find someone else to help them; ironically, they may not even remember your name or that you reduced their fees.

Marketing

There are at least two parts of marketing—convincing yourself and convincing others. First of all, you must be convinced that what you do with your patients is valuable, worth the time, effort, and money. If you are not *absolutely convinced* that your best efforts on behalf of your patients are efforts worth making, then you will not be able to sustain a practice. Your uncertainty will transmit to your patients, their families, your colleagues, your referral sources, and to your bank account. The real shame in professional services is not in the charging of money for services; it is in charging for efforts that you think are worthless.

But it is not enough to be convinced and charge money for your services. You must have a constant supply of patients; thus, you must convince a lot of other people that your services are available and worth the money.

Morality

You must improve the communicative abilities of your patients. Good management, good location, sufficient capitalization, and good intentions will not support your practice. Your survival also depends on your professional competence. If you do not have expertise, if you are not good enough to make a 'difference,' your practice will not survive. Working hard to find a way to help your patients improve their communicative abilities will be the best basis for a practice. You will make many mistakes—out of ignorance and/or misjudgment—but usually these will not kill your practice. Not caring enough or working hard enough to improve the communicative abilities of your clients will. Whether starting or maintaining a practice, the practitioner must sincerely want to help the person with communicative difficulties. If one regards private practice merely as a means of generating money, the practice is doomed before it is begun. But with quality services and proper management, economic success usually will follow. In every endeavor there are elements beyond our ability to know and/or control. Should these result in the failure of your practice, at least you will have learned valuable lessons. These will help you to be a better business person and quite possibly a better practitioner. Certainly the profession benefits from sincere efforts of private practitioners.

THE PROFESSION AND PRIVATE PRACTICE

Cooper (1982) supports the premise that one may judge how highly professional service is valued by society by the extent to which that service is carried on by private practitioners. Cooper (1982) and several others (Chapey, Chwat, Curlans, Pieras, 1981; Feldman, 1981; Fox, 1971; Marshall, Johnston and Lord, 1982) hold that private practice represents a focus of all the skills of the profession. The practitioner deals with clinical issues, administrative concerns, income and expenditures, public relations, peer interaction, and personnel problems that do not usually face the salaried clinician in the same simultaneous fashion. Dependence of the practitioner upon fees-for-services adds another dimension to factors such as vacation, professional association volunteerism, and continuing education. To leave the office is to pay twice: once for the time without income, and again for travel and cost of the event.

The practitioner faces the open marketplace with all its advantages and disadvantages. No one takes care of the practitioner. There are few kindly ears and fewer kindly sources of income. Sick leave is nonexistent. Competition with one's own colleagues abounds. Such competition usually serves to improve services to the communicatively impaired, but can be a wash of cold water to the hungry practitioner. There is no automatic referral system for clients, and the realities of overhead are ever present.

One way of measuring the public image of a profession is the regard with which consumers hold the profession's services and the amount of money they are willing to pay. Only in private practice is such a measurement possible because only in private practice is the profession's identity separate from the job setting and from the identity of the host institution, and only in private practice is professional competence tied directly to income.

The profession is defined best not by specialty or discipline, but rather by the form of service delivery. The form of delivery differentiates one professional from another because of the many features related to the service delivery system, including autonomy, money expectancies, public image, job security or risk, standards, and immediacy of punishment or reward.

THE PROFESSIONAL AND PRIVATE PRACTICE

It is likely that the person who is drawn to private practice, and indeed the person who stays in private practice, is attracted primarily by the opportunity to be self-governed. It is this feature that heavily outweighs any other in luring the professional into private practice. Even the love of money, often attributed to the private practitioner, is overshadowed by the overwhelming desire to be one's own boss. Anyone who has been employed in a position of responsibility without commensurate authority already has empathy for the need to make a decision and act on it, right or wrong! It is not accurate to describe private practitioners as being free spirits; nor is it accurate for professionals to assume that they will enjoy more professional freedom in private delivery of services. A much more realistic description focuses on self-control and independence. Consider some fantasies and realities that surround the private form of service delivery and the professional who provides it.

Fantasy	Reality
The private practitioner has personal and professional freedom.	While the private practitioner can exercise a great deal of independence and autonomy, legal and ethical restrictions are rigorous and the demands for self-control are great.
The private practitioner makes a lot of money.	With hard work and good management, the private practitioner has the potential for making more money than a salaried professional. Initial debt and continuing financial risks are large, and the ever-present possibility of financial failure blurs any thoughts of job security.
The private practitioner can work when he/she chooses and can take time off at will.	That is true if one is independently wealthy, can afford not to work, and is not concerned about losing current clients and/or missing new referrals. It is not a valid assumption when considering the professional's on-going obligations to clients. The obligation not to desert clients is just as great in private practice as it is in any other form of service delivery.
The private practitioner can take a tax write-off on all business expenses.	So can any other practitioner. But one has to have income before a tax write-off has any value, and professionals who are employed have many business expenses paid by their employers, resulting in fewer out-of-pocket expenses to write off.
The private practitioner does not have to answer to anybody, because there's nobody to boss him/her around.	That's right, unless one considers the clients who might not pay if they don't like the services. (Of course, there's always the IRS, licensing regulations, and one's own ethics.)

The private practitioner by definition is self-employed.	Not necessarily. The private practitioner may work on contract to a hospital, or nursing home, or other agency; may serve as a school district consultant; or may contract through third-party payers (e.g., Vocational Rehabilitation, Champus). In such instances, the practitioner has sold his services to someone, other than the client, who is responsible for payment.
Private practitioners are fiercely competitive.	There is no more competition in private practice than in any other setting. Most professionals will refer to each other as needed and complement other professionals. This is particularly true if a practitioner has a recognized specialty.
Private practitioners often work in isolation.	Independence and autonomy do not mean isolation. Should a private practitioner begin a practice with the intent of separating himself/herself from professional interaction, that intention quickly changes. All practitioners need contact with colleagues and professional exchanges.
The private practitioner has greater professional autonomy than employed professionals.	That is probably true if the private practitioner works in a sole proprietorship and does not accept third-party payment.

The professional seeking self-governance and diversity should find satisfaction in private practice. The wide range of activities and responsibilities in private practice requires consistent focal attention from the practitioner and can create an emotional and physical energy drain. If the practice meets the individual's personal and professional goals, then energy will surface. The professional who really wants to ''make a difference'' has a chance to do so within the purview of private practice. The chance to excel, however, must be met with goals that allow for excellence; rarely does one exceed his/her goals.

CLINICAL SKILLS AND SUCCESS

If you don't have anything to market, stay out of the marketplace—in other words, expertise and/or specialization in clinical skills are absolutely necessary to the success of a practice. The general public is not as naive about utilizing professional services as it once was. Even if someone found you by throwing darts at the Yellow Pages, the client won't stay with you unless you produce. For the sake of your practice, it is impossible to be too blunt with yourself when assessing your clinical skills and professional expertise. If you over-estimate your own worth, your practice will be affected negatively. Your entire practice will be a reflection of your clinical skills and your well-founded confidence in your expertise.

If, as owner/practitioner, your own clinical successes are the basis of your successful practice, take care to protect that reputation as you expand by hiring clinicians. Do not be too quick to ''give away'' a newly referred client to an employee. Assess the source of referral and its basis. When you transfer a referral to an employee, you may be violating the trust and expectations of the referral source, hence damaging a hard-earned professional relationship.

HEAD FIRST OR TOE FIRST?

Everyone who has ever considered entering private practice has faced the dilemma of the early commitment. If a professional believes that private practice is compatible with professional goals and personal life style, then the decision of leaving the employment nest must be confronted. How much? How soon? The final decision is very personal, and you may never know for sure if the way you entered private practice was the best way for you. Moonlighting provides no information about private practice as a career. Moonlighting is a way to supplement income, perhaps expand one's professional experiences, and make an occasional contact with a potential referral source.

In private practice, you won't know if you have succeeded until you have, and referrals are hard to get until you succeed. It is true to some extent that potential referral sources will wait until you have some kind of track record in service delivery at the private level. Of course, you cannot have much of a track record without referrals.

Be wary of entering private practice on a part-time or half-time basis while you maintain another position of employment. Part-time is part-effort; the part-time salary and work from another position will dilute your desire to pay the necessary attention to your practice. If you are going to enter private practice, give thorough consideration to the nature and areas of your own expertise, the need for your skills, sources of payment for your services, and your own temperament. Make your decision to try totally, or not to try at all. Foonberg (1984) suggests that one work an extra year or two in a secure job position, for the purpose of saving money to enter private practice full time rather than develop a practice piecemeal. In some ways, the consideration of how to begin a private practice is analogous to that of approaching a bank for a loan—don't ask for money until you can look like you don't need it. In other words, don't begin your own practice until you can afford the many demands.

In deciding to enter—or stay in—a private practice setting, there are at least three crucial considerations: *personal goals*, *professional goals*, and the *waiting clients*. These considerations are never obsolete when making, remaking, and executing the commitment to private practice. Suggested features of each consideration follow; modify them as they may apply to your own decision.

- **The First Consideration**
    - You As a Person
        - Personal goals
        - Time
        - Energy
        - Family
        - Money (credit)
        - Interpersonal resources

- **The Second Consideration**
    - You As a Professional
        - Professional goals
        - Skills/specialty
        - Contacts
        - Reputation

- **The Third Consideration**
    - The Waiting Clients
        - How many are there?
        - How many will come?
        - How many will pay?
        - Who else is there to serve them?

Appendices

APPENDIX 1–1
SUMMARY LIST OF CONSIDERATIONS FOR PRIVATE PRACTICE

Reasons for Professionals to Consider Private Practice

self-governance (autonomy)
service provisions with maximum flexibility
money
diversity

Necessary Characteristics

physical health and stamina
emotional stability
persistence
professional confidence and prominence in community
enjoyment of direct delivery of services
ability to assume responsibility
tolerance for unpredictability
fiscal responsibility

Clinical Skills

clinical expertise
specialization within the profession (age, type of disorder)
interpersonal skills
professional activity (keeping abreast of professional changes and developments; maintaining contact with colleagues)

Other Considerations

need for services in the community or region
local respect for the profession
professional career goals
personal goals (income, lifestyle, environment)

APPENDIX 1–2
CONSIDERATIONS FOR INDEPENDENT PRACTICE: A CHECKLIST*

Decisions to Be Made	Yes	Not a Problem	Needs Attention
1. Am I professionally prepared for independent practice?	☐	☐	☐
2. Am I financially prepared for the personal and family financial transition (8 to 18 months with little or no income from the practice)?	☐	☐	☐
3. Is my family prepared to support and tolerate a time-consuming, stressful transition?	☐	☐	☐
4. Do I have adequate financial resources to open an office? Loan or savings for			
Office rent and add-on fees	☐	☐	☐
Office modification, decoration	☐	☐	☐
Furniture and equipment	☐	☐	☐
Secretarial services	☐	☐	☐
Stationery, forms, testing supplies	☐	☐	☐
Telephone services	☐	☐	☐
State, county, city licenses	☐	☐	☐
Office fire, theft, accident insurance	☐	☐	☐
Disability insurance	☐	☐	☐
Bookkeeping/accounting/tax service	☐	☐	☐
5. Can the community support my practice?	☐	☐	☐
6. Do I have, or can I get, enough referral sources?	☐	☐	☐
7. Should I begin practice in association with colleagues?	☐	☐	☐
8. Would I enjoy working independently?	☐	☐	☐
9. Could I purchase an established practice?	☐	☐	☐
10. Do I have the organizational skills to manage an independent practice?	☐	☐	☐
11. Have colleagues and potential referral sources given me feedback that supports my going into independent practice?	☐	☐	☐

---

*Checklist adapted from Peter Keller and Lawrence Ritt, 1983. Independent Practice: Checklist and Resources Guide. From *Innovations in Clinical Practice: A Source Book*, Vol. 2 (cited in References). Copyrighted 1983 and reprinted with permission of The Professional Resource Exchange, Inc.

Planning

12. Are my areas of professional competence clearly defined for the public and for referral sources? (i.e., Do they know how I can be of service?) ☐ ☐ ☐

13. Is there any reason to incorporate? ☐ ☐ ☐

14. Do I know effective ways of letting people know about my practice?

    Yellow Page listings ☐ ☐ ☐
    Formal announcements for mailings ☐ ☐ ☐
    Newspaper articles/announcements ☐ ☐ ☐
    Personal letters to key sources ☐ ☐ ☐
    Speaking engagements ☐ ☐ ☐
    Other ☐ ☐ ☐

15. Do I have office space that is conducive to a successful practice?

    Accessible location in community ☐ ☐ ☐
    Location in appropriate professional building ☐ ☐ ☐
    Security and/or alarm system ☐ ☐ ☐
    Adheres to zoning regulations ☐ ☐ ☐
    Adequate space and design ☐ ☐ ☐
    Soundproofing ☐ ☐ ☐
    Desirable lease negotiated ☐ ☐ ☐
    Storage space ☐ ☐ ☐
    Janitorial ☐ ☐ ☐
    Utilities ☐ ☐ ☐
    Grounds maintenance ☐ ☐ ☐
    Lighting ☐ ☐ ☐
    Others ☐ ☐ ☐

16. Do I have appropriate licenses/registration/certification?

    State (including professional licenses) ☐ ☐ ☐
    City and county ☐ ☐ ☐

17. Is my insurance adequate?
    Professional liability ☐ ☐ ☐
    Term insurance for loans ☐ ☐ ☐
    Office fire, theft, accident ☐ ☐ ☐
    Furniture and equipment ☐ ☐ ☐
    Disability income (income protection) ☐ ☐ ☐
    Medical ☐ ☐ ☐
    Life ☐ ☐ ☐

18. Do I know what telephone service I will need?
    Adequate number of phones ☐ ☐ ☐
    Adequate number of lines ☐ ☐ ☐
    Answering service or machine ☐ ☐ ☐
    Intercom system ☐ ☐ ☐
    Own or lease system ☐ ☐ ☐

Planning *(Continued)*

	Yes	Not a Problem	Needs Attention
19. Do I know what office equipment I will need for office personnel and for clients?			
Typewriter	☐	☐	☐
Copier	☐	☐	☐
Microcomputer system	☐	☐	☐
Dictation system	☐	☐	☐
Audio recording equipment	☐	☐	☐
Video recording equipment	☐	☐	☐
Other	☐	☐	☐
20. Do I know what office furnishings I will need?			
Waiting room tables, chairs	☐	☐	☐
Secretarial desk, chairs, tables	☐	☐	☐
Filing cabinets (locking/fireproof)	☐	☐	☐
Small refrigerator	☐	☐	☐
Coffee maker	☐	☐	☐
Desk and table lamps	☐	☐	☐
Table and chairs for testing room	☐	☐	☐
Professional desk and chairs	☐	☐	☐
Book cases	☐	☐	☐
Storage cases	☐	☐	☐
Client seating	☐	☐	☐
Reclining chair	☐	☐	☐
Art work	☐	☐	☐
Other	☐	☐	☐
21. Do I know what professional supplies I will need and do I know where to purchase them?			
Toys for therapy	☐	☐	☐
Books	☐	☐	☐
Pictures	☐	☐	☐
Testing supplies	☐	☐	☐
Therapy supplies (list)	☐	☐	☐
22. Do I know what professional equipment I will need?	☐	☐	☐

Managing

	Yes	Not a Problem	Needs Attention
23. Are my practices and policies consistent with the established standards for service providers in my profession?	☐	☐	☐
24. Do I know what financial procedures and forms I will use?			
Accounting system	☐	☐	☐
Billing system	☐	☐	☐
Insurance claims procedures	☐	☐	☐
Pegboard (one-write) system	☐	☐	☐
Computer	☐	☐	☐
Other	☐	☐	☐

Managing *(Continued)*	Yes	Not a Problem	Needs Attention
25. Will I need the help of consultants?			
Accountant	☐	☐	☐
Bookkeeper	☐	☐	☐
Attorney	☐	☐	☐
Insurance broker	☐	☐	☐
Investment broker	☐	☐	☐
Other	☐	☐	☐
26. Do I know what stationery and forms I will use?			
Public visibility			
Stationery	☐	☐	☐
Business cards	☐	☐	☐
History questionnaires	☐	☐	☐
Report forms	☐	☐	☐
Office use only			
Memos	☐	☐	☐
Assessment forms	☐	☐	☐
Progress summary forms	☐	☐	☐
Other	☐	☐	☐
27. Are my office personnel prepared for			
Routine office procedures	☐	☐	☐
Questions about office policy	☐	☐	☐
about bills	☐	☐	☐
about clients	☐	☐	☐
Difficult clients	☐	☐	☐
Dangerous clients	☐	☐	☐
Other emergencies	☐	☐	☐
Other	☐	☐	☐
28. Do I have consistent office management policies and systems to handle			
Billing	☐	☐	☐
Insurance reimbursement	☐	☐	☐
Collections	☐	☐	☐
Bookkeeping	☐	☐	☐
Security against thefts	☐	☐	☐
Other	☐	☐	☐
29. Do I have consistent clinical policies to handle			
Releasing information	☐	☐	☐
Allowing clients to see records	☐	☐	☐
Handling confidential information	☐	☐	☐
Managing/disposing of old records	☐	☐	☐
Informing clients about confidentiality	☐	☐	☐
Requesting confidential information	☐	☐	☐
Making referrals to other professionals	☐	☐	☐
Other	☐	☐	☐
30. Do I have a system for developing clinical records that include			
Development of a data base	☐	☐	☐

Managing *(Continued)*

	Yes	Not a Problem	Needs Attention
Mental status evaluation	☐	☐	☐
Physical status evaluation	☐	☐	☐
Information from previous treatment	☐	☐	☐
Level of functioning evaluation	☐	☐	☐
Clear problem definitions	☐	☐	☐
Diagnosis	☐	☐	☐
Long term goals	☐	☐	☐
Intermediate objectives	☐	☐	☐
Statement of available services	☐	☐	☐
Updated record of service contracts	☐	☐	☐
Evidence of regular review of problems, changes, and goals	☐	☐	☐
Appropriate release signatures	☐	☐	☐
Discharge summary	☐	☐	☐
Other	☐	☐	☐

31. Can I ensure that clinical records will be

	Yes	Not a Problem	Needs Attention
Easily used	☐	☐	☐
Accessible	☐	☐	☐
Legible	☐	☐	☐
Organized	☐	☐	☐

32. Do I have procedures/policies for keeping collections updated?

	Yes	Not a Problem	Needs Attention
Payment policies	☐	☐	☐
Overdue charges	☐	☐	☐
Collection policies	☐	☐	☐
Procedures for handling delinquent accounts	☐	☐	☐
Other	☐	☐	☐

33. Do I have a plan to keep financial records current and to meet all payment and tax deadlines? ☐ ☐ ☐

Maintaining and Growing

34. Will I consult with colleagues and obtain outside opinions as appropriate? ☐ ☐ ☐

35. Do I have plans/policies for updating my professional knowledge? For my staff? ☐ ☐ ☐

36. Will I evaluate the success of my ongoing practice? ☐ ☐ ☐

37. Am I aware of possible alternatives to my current form/structure of practice? ☐ ☐ ☐

38. Will I expand/change the nature of my practice? ☐ ☐ ☐

APPENDIX 1-3
QUESTIONS AND ANSWERS ON PRIVATE PRACTICE

Question 1:   What legal and professional frameworks define "private practice" as compared with other job environments?

In private practice there is a direct contract between the clinician and the client. Clients may be individuals and/or organizations (such as hospitals, nursing centers, schools). In private practice the clinician is responsible for every aspect of the service and sets his/her own goals, hours, and practice methods. In nonprivate practice situations there is a third person or agency contracting with the clients and the clinician, thereby arranging services. For tax purposes, the differentiation of "independent contractor" status from "employee status" is crucial because businesses (e.g., schools and hospitals) are required to pay income and social security taxes on employees. Retirement fund regulations are also affected by the classification.

Question 2:   How many speech-language pathologists and audiologists are presently engaged in full-time (30 hours per week or more) private practice? How many are engaged in part-time private practice?

The Official Count Report (July 1, 1980) from the ASHA Accounting Office shows that 1,583 members are engaged in private practice activities 30 hours or more per week and 6,397 members are engaged in private practice activities less than 30 hours per week. The total 7,981 members involved in some degree of private practice is an increase of 669 over the total of 7,313 as of 7/1/79. It should be noted that not all members of the profession are members of ASHA, so that the actual number of private practitioners may be greater.

Question 3:   What are the differences between private practitioners in audiology and in speech-language pathology?

There are two primary factors which differentiate practices in speech-language pathology and in audiology. The first is the cost of establishing private practice. The equipment needs of an audiologist are significant and very often preclude the audiologist from maintaining his/her own facilities. Many audiologists are associated with physicians to minimize the financial investment required. Secondly, audiologists may sell hearing aids. Third, reports and record-keeping for speech-language pathology intervention may be time-consuming, detailed endeavors that usually require substantial secretarial support.

Question 4:   What special, financial, educational, and/or experimental requirements are there for entering private practice?

There are no special requirements mandated by ASHA or by either federal or state laws. Many states require a professional license or certification to render speech-language and audiological services to the public. In many cases the requirements for licensure are equivalent to requirements for ASHA Certificate of Clinical Competence (CCC). The ASHA member speech-language pathologist and/or audiologist must have the CCC to work independently. The Committee feels strongly that the speech-language pathologist and audiologist must have a thorough and complete knowledge of their respective areas and a comprehensive complete clinical experience. The private practitioner needs to have his/her skills intact upon entry. In addition, courses in basic business, business law, and administration are extremely important and professionals are urged to acquire these courses prior to engaging in private practice activities.

Question 5:   How do I determine what to charge for my services?

In order to stay in business and ultimately earn a living, you must know what direct and indirect costs you will have and how much profit you hope to make to set fees accordingly. A publication available through ASHA, "Determining cost of speech and hearing services: A guide to developing costs analysis procedures," (ASHA, Feb. 1985), provides step-by-step procedures for doing this. In health care facilities in which a Certificate of Need is required before services can be rendered to the public, the Health Services Administration (HSA) may require that your fees be commensurate with rates at similar facilities in your area.

Question 6:   What form can advertisements and/or announcements have regarding provision of services?

(February 1981) The *ASHA Journal* details the guidelines for public announcements and public statements. An announcement of services is a statement "designed to inform the public about professional services or products related to the field," and in general should conform to "the type of announcement customarily used by other professionals including physicians, psychologists, and others." When a question is specific with regard to listings or announcements, such questions can be referred to the Committee on Private Practice and/or to the Ethical Practice Board.

Question 7:   As a private practitioner in speech-language pathology and/or audiology, can I directly bill Medicare, private insurance companies, and/or contract with Medicaid and Health and Human Services (HHS)?

Yes, in some situations. Medicare will directly reimburse services provided by speech-language pathologists whose practices can be certified as rehabilitation agencies, and hearing evaluations performed by audiologists in their own offices if requested by a physician for diagnostic purposes. Medicare does *not* pay for other services provided by independent, private practitioners. Both Medicaid and insurance payments are based on state requirements or individual policy constraints. In some states, Medicaid covers speech-language evaluations and treatment for children and adults while, in others, it may only provide coverage for children, and in some, no coverage whatever. Many insurance companies also pay for services and have their own regulations with respect to this coverage. Some considerations with respect to payments are the individual's ability to pay for private services and whether any type of physical plant or professional certification is required to provide the service. At this time, it is unrealistic to expect that a private practice in speech-language pathology or audiology could exist solely on the financial basis of third party support. More information on reimbursement is available from Steven White, Director, Reimbursement Policy Division at the National Office. A Medicare Supplement is also available from Accounting Services at a nominal cost.

Question 8:   How does Public Law 94-142 (the Education for All Handicapped Children Act) affect private practice?

Public Law 94-142 requires that all children who are identified as handicapped receive a free and appropriate education. The age ranges of children eligible for service are determined by the states in their compliance plans and, therefore, differ from state to state and from region to region depending on how the state has implemented the law in the schools. In some areas the law has had the effect of focusing attention on handicapping conditions, including alternatives to direct service in the public schools, such as private services. As the political climate changes, the interpretation of the law will also change. Ultimately, the parent and school special education team decides what services are "appropriate" for the child.

Question 9:   What kind of salary can I expect if I enter private practice?

Many given variables affect salary. These include number of private practitioners within a given geographic area, whether community or nonfee university clinics' services are available, and type and amount of overhead expenses. An individual entering full-time private practice should have sufficient resources available to cover expenses for approximately the first 1½ years. A private practice, just like any other small business, runs the same risk of failure or success.

Question 10:   What geographic influences affect the success of a private practice?

The variables that affect private practice in speech, language, and hearing are similar to those in the marketing of any service: density of population; economic characteristics of the community; availability of other services; public satisfaction with services; institutions, agencies, or businesses in the community with which contracts might be arranged; and health care/educational climate of the community. In rural areas, the clinician may have to travel to deliver services more frequently than in urban areas. Since a significant portion of referrals for speech, language, and hearing services comes from physicians, the attitude of the medical community toward the service is also important.

Question 11:   What type of liability insurance is available to me?

ASHA sponsors a professional liability insurance plan underwritten by the Chicago Insurance Company. All members of ASHA are eligible for such coverage, whether as a private practitioner or as an employee of another person, agency, or institution. Requests for information should be directed to ASHA National Office, 10801 Rockville Pike, Rockville, MD 20802.

Question 12:   Where do I begin?

Be sure to complete pre-entry steps. Get the courses you need in business and accounting. Use the Small Business Administration in your area as they often offer seminars and printed information. Attend the ASHA management, marketing, and private practice continuing education experiences. Investigate your geographic area and decide whether you will be comfortable working independently. When these preparations have been made, you can feel assured you are entering your career choice setting with adequate information.

For additional information regarding private practice, write to Professional Practices Division, ASHA National Office, 10801 Rockville Pike, Rockville, MD 20802.

Chapter 2

The Organizational Structure

A private practice can take any of several organizational structures, depending on the owner's wishes regarding legal definitions of the practice, tax implications, and liability responsibilities. The difficulty in determining one's wishes lies in understanding what the choices mean. It is hard to determine which is best for a given individual, until that individual has had the opportunity to *live* with his/her decision for some period of time. All of the choices include some paperwork and record keeping; all involve taxation. One does have an escape valve if the structure chosen proves to be inadequate or incompatible. There are procedures for terminating one organizational form and changing to another.

Organizational structures exist in many forms. Among them are the following:

Sole Proprietorship
Partnerships
      General
      Limited
Corporations
      For Profit
      Sub-Chapter S
      Not-For-Profit
Joint-Stock Company
Syndicates
Investment Trusts
Partner Associations
Pools
Joint Ventures

Don't try to figure out the differences among them by looking at labels, for you may be misled. Some structures listed above are not appropriate vehicles for professional practices. Generally, Joint-Stock Companies, Syndicates, Investment Trusts, Partner Associations, Pools, and Joint Ventures do not lend themselves to the structure of a private practice and will not be discussed here.

The structures most often used by professionals are Sole Proprietorship, Partnership, and Corporation. Descriptions of these structures include the following:

SOLE PROPRIETORSHIP

A *sole proprietorship* is a business operated by one person; the business (the practice) is the same entity as the owner. This is the simplest form of organization, requires the least red tape, and is subject to the fewest governmental restrictions.

Features

1. The organizational structure provides the greatest autonomy.
2. The owner has all the loss, all the debt, and all the income.
3. Since the practice is the same legal entity as the owner, a law suit against the practice is a law suit against the owner; thus, the owner and any personal holdings are liable.
4. If there are no money problems (either with capitalization or start-up funds); if the owner wants a fast start with the least fuss, already has other avenues of professional contact, and is a hard worker with no health problems, then this organizational structure may be the most suitable.
5. To open this form of practice, just open the doors; to end this form of practice, close the doors.
6. Paperwork and red tape are minimal.
7. The owner/practitioner has 100 percent control of services and operations.
8. The tax situation could become a problem. Everything earned in a sole proprietorship is considered personal income by the Internal Revenue Service and is taxed as personal income. In other words, the business itself does not pay any income taxes. The sole proprietor includes the profit or loss on his/her income tax return.
9. Proprietary interest ends when the owner dies or quits.
10. Whether assets are used in the business or are personally used and owned, the proprietor bears all risks of the business and taxation.
11. The sole proprietor is usually liable for self-employment tax (see IRS Pub. No. 533, Rev. Nov. 1983).
12. Sole proprietors can use their social security numbers as their business taxpayer identification numbers (but it is possible to obtain a separate taxpayer ID number for the practice).
13. The owner establishes a tax year when he/she files the first business income tax return. If, in a later year, the owner changes the business to a sole proprietorship, the same tax year must continue to be used unless permission from the IRS is obtained to change that year.

14. Sole proprietor structure is adequate for outpatient, independent office Medicare coverage.
15. The proprietorship is the only resource for raising capitalization funds.
16. The proprietor must pay quarterly tax estimates.
17. Fringe benefits are not always deductible to the self-employed.
18. The owner can spend time and money on anything he/she chooses, without explaining to a partner or shareholder.
19. The owner's schedule is his/her own; he/she may come and go without accounting to anyone.
20. The owner has all the administrative responsibility.
21. The owner has all the public relations responsibility.
22. A sole proprietor may lose some clients because he/she must refer when his/her own resources with certain types of clients are inadequate.
23. Some people feel a sole proprietorship lacks the knowledge or resources to manage certain clients. The professional's work and reputation are all the professional has to recommend the practice.
24. The owner does not have to work alone; employees, part-time or full-time, may be hired, or contracts may be developed with independent consultants to work on an as-needed basis with salary determined by a commission arrangement.
25. Unless the sole proprietor has hired or contracted with others to provide client services in his/her absence, the office overhead continues, but the income does not.

PARTNERSHIPS

A *general partnership* is not a taxable entity, although it has independent legal status. It is a relationship between two or more practitioners who join to carry out business (a practice). A partnership may exist without formal partnership agreement and without any legal declaration if each of the partners contributes, among other things, money, property, labor, and if each of the partners intends to share profits, debts, responsibility, and so forth.

Features

1. Each partner can develop expertise in a specific area, relying on the other partner to cover another area.
2. If both partners have the same skills/technical knowledge, they are competing for the same clientele.
3. The partners share debt, losses, income, and resources for capitalization.
4. The partners share control and authority.
5. The liability is unlimited, as in solo practice, since a partnership is not an incorporated entity.
6. One partner's reputation becomes attributed to the other, for good and ill.
7. Each partner must compromise on certain issues and live with disagreement on others.

8. Partners need to agree on the general philosophy of service delivery and on each partner's contributions to the practice.
9. Any number of persons can join together to form a partnership.
10. A partnership agreement may be modified for a particular tax year after the close of that tax year, but not later than the date for filing the partnership return.
11. A partnership may have greater financial strength than a sole proprietorship, because presumably both (all) partners contribute something that is more than one person can contribute.
12. Each partner is held liable for the debts of the business/practice.
13. Someone remains to earn money when one partner is sick or on vacation.
14. The overhead for each of two or three practitioners in a partnership *may* be less than for one practitioner.
15. Partnerships can become conflictual if individual goals change, resulting in partner-incompatibility.
16. To deal with the possibility of future partner incompatibility, partners should put in writing, at the initiation of the practice, the policies that will be followed should various contingencies occur (for example, define a buy–sell agreement).
17. A partnership is an adequate structure for outpatient, independent Medicare coverage.
18. A partnership must figure its profit or loss and file a return.

IRS Requirements for a Partnership

Important factors to the IRS in determining if parties intend to carry on a partnership include:

1. Conduct of each in carrying out the provisions of the partnership agreement;
2. The testimony of disinterested persons;
3. The relationship of the parties;
4. The abilities and contributions of each;
5. The control each has over the partnership income and the purpose for which the income is used.

A joint undertaking merely to share expenses is not a partnership. The partnership agreement may be written or oral and includes the original agreement and any other modifications agreed to by all the partners. Usually a partner's share of income, gain, loss, deductions, or credits is specified in the partnership agreement. Choices affecting income from a partnership are made by the partnership, not by individual partners.

A *general* partnership is a verbal or written agreement between two or more persons to work together and share income and expenses. Partners are taxed separately, and each partner is liable individually for *all* debts. Any change in the general partnership will change or terminate the existing partnership.

The distributive share of partnership income is income earned from self-employment. Guaranteed payments from a partnership should be included, along with the share of earnings, or minus the share of losses, when figuring net earnings from self-employment.

An inactive partner figures income from self-employment by including the distributive share of partnership income or loss and any guaranteed payments. A retired partner pays no self-employment tax on retirement income received from a partnership under a written plan.

CORPORATIONS

For-Profit Corporation

A *for-profit corporation* is a formal legal structure that is a separate entity from the individuals who create it. It is restricted to its own charter and has responsibilities and privileges of its own. The corporation can sue and be sued, invest money, and pay taxes separately from its owners.

Features

1. The corporation has close governmental regulations (and the records and reports to go with it).
2. Taxes and law suits are collectible only from the corporation and not from owners (personal assets may not be seized by creditors).
3. The corporation perpetuates until legally stopped, regardless of death of owners, stock transfers, and so forth.
4. Its charter is limited to the state in which it was issued.
5. It is usually expensive to form because of legal fees, filing fees, and so forth.
6. Ownership is easily transferable.
7. Stockholders and officers are liable only to the extent of the value of the stock they hold.
8. Managers of the corporation may or may not be stockholders.
9. Corporate structure is adaptable to both small and large practices.
10. Of all the structures possible for a practice, the corporate structure allows the most favorable tax planning because corporations are entitled to special deductions, although new tax laws may reduce or change these.
11. Corporate profits normally are taxed to the corporation. When profits are distributed as dividends, the dividends are taxed as ordinary income to the shareholders (a double tax on profits).
12. It is usually advisable, if not necessary, to hire an attorney who is familiar with the practice in the event that legal problems arise.
13. Stockholders can be employees of the corporation and receive salaries for specified duties.
14. Corporations are subject to special taxation.
15. A corporation, as a legal entity recognized by the state, is subject to many state and federal controls.

A *professional corporation* is required by some states if a professional wishes to incorporate his/her practice. The features of such corporations vary from state to state but usually require shareholders to be members of the same profession. Further, the corporate shield does not protect the professional from legal actions involving ethical or malpractice issues. One should consult an attorney with regard to special provisions that may be required by the state in which the practice is established. A professional practice must be both *organized* and *operated* as a corporation to be classified as one. All of the states and the District of Columbia have professional association acts.

Unincorporated organizations are organizations that have certain corporate characteristics, are classified as associations, and are taxed as corporations. These organizations must have associates and must be organized to carry on business and divide any gains. In addition, they must have a *majority* of the following characteristics:

1. continuity of life;
2. centralization of management;
3. limited liability; and
4. free transferability of interests.

Other factors may also be important in classifying an organization as an association. ''An organization will be treated as an association if its characteristics are such that it more nearly resembles a corporation than a partnership or trust. The facts in each case determine whether or not characteristics are present'' (IRS Pub. No. 344, Rev. Nov. 1983).

Sub-Chapter S Corporation

A *Sub-Chapter S corporation* is a special small business tax status, which may be elected, that gives small firms the advantages of corporate form, but provides tax advantages that are special to a small corporation and not available to larger corporations. The IRS code describing the Sub-Chapter S provisions limits the size of a corporation that may take advantage of special tax options. The shareholders of a Sub-Chapter S corporation include their share of corporate profits or losses in their gross income (much like a partnership). The primary requirements of a corporation to qualify for a Sub-Chapter S are

1. The Sub-Chapter S can have no more than ten stockholders, all of whom must be U.S. citizens.
2. No more than 20 percent of corporate income may be derived from investments.
3. At least 20 percent of corporate income must come from operations within the U.S.
4. The corporation can have only one class of stock to qualify for the Sub-Chapter S designation.

Taxation of the Sub-Chapter S, similar to that of a partnership, avoids the double taxation imposed on regular corporations. Corporate income is divided among shareholders as per agreement and reported in individual income tax returns. Although flexibility is somewhat limited, tax advantages make the Sub-Chapter S attractive for beginning practices until earnings reach a certain limit. A Sub-Chapter S election can be made every year; however, a Sub-Chapter S election, when refused, is not available again for 5 years to the shareholders. It is essential to have assistance from an accountant to predict potential earnings of the practice in order to consider alternative structures. Some practitioners feel that the regular corporate structure is appropriate for rehabilitation agencies and comprehensive outpatient rehabilitation facilities, because of certain corporate and fringe benefits that only apply to regular corporations (Marshall et al., 1982).

Not-For-Profit Corporation

Not-for-profit corporations are usually referred to by the term ''nonprofit.'' The labels ''profit'' and ''nonprofit,'' if interpreted literally, are misleading; the labels merely indicate the structure of the organization. A corporation organized for *profit* is one in which shareholders are also directors; control of the corporation is in the hands of shareholders. Shareholders may also be employees and receive wages, as well as their shareholder's profits from the corporation. A corporation organized as *not-for-profit* is one in which the incorporators are not always the policy-making body of the corporation; the board of directors is usually acquired from various interested public and professional persons who have money, power, time, or some expertise to contribute. Profit is returned to the operation of the corporation; the employees, who may or may not be the incorporators, receive salaries.

WHY INCORPORATE

Since 1982, when a new tax law was passed, the question of whether a new small business should incorporate or not has been the focus of some scrutiny. Prior to 1982, the corporation was clearly first choice because of tax shelters, fringe benefits, and minimum regulations (comparatively speaking). Now, tax benefits and other privileges previously allowed to corporations have been reduced, and almost yearly, regulations and restrictions become more stringent.

However, some advantages still exist:

1. *Use of a fiscal year:*　Income can be deferred to avoid coinciding with personal tax year.
2. *Capital accumulation:*　Capital can be accumulated at a faster rate in a corporate structure than in a nonincorporated one (subject to limits of undistributed earnings).
3. *Fringe benefits:* *　Deductible fringe benefits may be available to corporate employees but not necessarily to self-employed persons, such as sole proprietors and partnerships. Some of these include

   a. group-term insurance
   b. health and accident insurance
   c. disability coverage
   d. retirement plans
   e. profit-sharing plans
   f. medical expense reimbursement

---

*Fringe benefits are usually considered to be those non-salary benefits of employment that may be deductible by the employer and are not necessarily taxed as income to the employee.

    g. coverage for liabilities incurred or caused by employees
    h. stock purchase options

At the time of this writing, these benefits are still allowable, although their continued existence as nontaxable entities seems to be in jeopardy. It is critical that practitioners keep current regarding tax law or, at least, engage the services of a tax accountant who can provide updated tax information.

When incorporating, whether alone or with others, an individual may become an employee of the corporation. In that case, only salary is taxed as personal income and not the income of the corporation. Of course, the distribution of corporate profits that is passed on to stockholders is taxed as personal income. Corporate reimbursement for business-related expenses, such as eating meals on the premises for work purposes and expenses for business travel, is not considered employee income. Maintenance and repair of vehicles used for business-related activities usually are paid by the corporation, although great care must be exercised in the documentation of business use. These items, as well as others, that are paid from the corporate pocket help to reduce the practitioner's personally paid expenses and are not considered income.

Some professionals feel that their image as successful entrepreneurers is enhanced by a corporate structure and the addition of ''Inc.'' or ''P.C.'' to their letterhead. Incorporating merely for cosmetic reasons, however, is not a sound basis for selecting an organizational structure. A noncosmetic reason for incorporating that is often overlooked is one that seems very obvious to any person who has tried to terminate a partnership without having planned ahead. That reason is the corporate structure, whose regulations lend themselves to planning for a multiplicity of contingencies.

Many professionals who practice in partnerships or group arrangements of sole proprietorships put off the delineation of owner's rights, responsibilities, and worst-case situations. The departure of one partner or group practitioner, regardless of the reason for his/her departure, may lead to irreparable disagreement and conflict by all concerned. A corporation must have by-laws, employment contracts, and shareholders' agreements that guard against unforeseen problems in the future. The act of incorporating helps to produce guidelines for dealing with problems both within the organization and external to it. This protects us from our natural predilection to avoid discomfort and therefore to give only perfunctory attention to potential problems.

DESIGNING A STRUCTURE THAT FITS

In order to be realistic in predicting what the worst might be, it is necessary to be realistic about the best. Being realistic, however, is hard work and takes some of the fun out of planning. Do it anyway; it could save years of trouble for you and your practice. Some of the key issues to face realistically are:

1. Are you best suited for operating a practice completely alone?
2. Are you best suited for operating a practice in joint venture with others who will share the authority, responsibility, expenses, and income?

3. Are you best suited for having many employees, or for doing the service delivery alone?
4. If you employ professionals to help with the service delivery, are you best suited for being the only chief, or would you want to share the authority with a partner?

If you are certain that you are best suited personally and professionally for being the only owner and boss, you have an easier job than those who are not completely comfortable with lone ventures. You only have to decide how *you* want to organize your legal identity and tax structure and how *you* want to operate your practice.

If you are not completely certain of the best approach for you, you will need to give serious consideration to all potential sources of harmony and discord that can arise from working with others. In a partnership, or corporation, when more than one person is owner, each partner or owner has the potential for:

1. Applying a wider range of professional and personal resources to service delivery than either partner would have alone;
2. Saving on overhead with the sharing of office and supplies;
3. Benefiting from regular contact with a colleague;
4. Leaving someone who shares a similar concern for the practice to mind the store during the absence of the other.

A novice clinician who joins someone already in practice has an immediate source of referrals with the ''bugs'' already worked out of the office system. An established clinician who brings in an inexperienced partner benefits from having someone to take the overload, to provide substitute work, and possibly to become a ready-made buyer for the practice when and if desired.

As mentioned in the separate discussion of organizational structures, joining anyone for any venture has disadvantages by definition. No two people have exactly the same ideas of how to accomplish anything, particularly when each has an enormous personal and professional investment in the outcome of the practice. When you share ownership, you no longer have the privilege of independent decisions. There is not always time or energy for resolution of conflict through discussion and consensus. You are liable for the co-owner's mistakes, debts incurred in the name of the practice, and law suits. Before the advantages to sharing a practice become disadvantages, work out solutions to potential problems. If the problems never arise, then you are forearmed. If problems do arise in the course of a partnership or corporation, then you will have previously agreed upon solutions to apply rather than having to search for a resolution in the heat of battle.

Operating Agreements

Written operating agreements are essential when working in any format other than a sole proprietorship. To produce such an agreement, get the help of someone who has arranged agreements for other partnerships or corporations similar to the one you have, or intend to have. Such help might come from a management consultant, attorney, or accountant. If you decide that an attorney is the best source of help, choose an attorney that is neutral to all partners or stockholders. If problems arise later, the fact "*your* friend, the lawyer" wrote out the agreement may lead to accusations of unfairness or attorney bias. If all the partners or stockholders use a different attorney, the sparring over details could be quite expensive and time consuming. Regardless of the consultant or advisor, the partners must still decide the key issues for working together that might include:

1. Do the partners or co-owners have the same philosophy about service delivery?
2. Do the partners or co-owners have the same philosophy about long-term roles in the practice?
3. Do the partners or co-owners complement each other professionally and personally so that their partnership enhances the practice?

When these issues are clear, then specific arrangements can be approached, which should include the following:

1. *Initial Investment:*   The amount of cash and other contributions each partner will make to the practice should be specified. If one joins an existing practice, an outside appraiser or accountant can be consulted regarding the amount the new partner is required to pay or contribute.
2. *Financial Obligations:*   Determination should be made with regard to who will make deposits and withdrawals from the bank account; who will authorize payments for debts of the practice; how much each partner is allowed to debit from the practice account for business expenses; who can request loans on behalf of the practice; and who among the partners are responsible for the various financial obligations of the partnership.
3. *Time Devoted to the Practice:*   Determination should be made whether all professional income acquired by each partner is to be considered the property of the practice. Some practices include as income payable to the practice only assessment, conferences, and in-office intervention; other fees realized by the partners from writing, lectures, and consultations are not considered joint revenue to the practice.
4. *Dividing Income from the Practice:*   It is important to determine how the partners or owners divide income from the practice. If partners could pool their revenue in the practice account, pay bills and equally divide the remaining money, there would be no need to write this part of the operating agreement. If partners each brought in the same amount of revenue and spent the same amount in the name of the practice, division of income would be easy. This is not usually the way it works, however. Most partnerships must divide income according to some formula that takes into account income-generating potential, work habits, and the spending habits of the individuals involved. An experienced attorney, accountant, or management consultant can help develop a compensation package in the operating agreement.

With clinicians of approximately the same age, experience, and reputation, and where only two or three individuals are involved in income division, it is not difficult to track the income generated by each and divide partnership profits according to the percentage of gross income each generates and collects (Ridgewood Financial Institute, 1984). In some cases, it is also necessary to track expenses of each partner in order to realize equitability in terms of the drain on money in the account that is available for distribution.

In the case of a new clinician joining an established clinician, the established clinician receives a greater portion of income, with the new clinician's share resulting from a previously agreed upon formula. The portion of income that goes to each can be adjusted over time, to reflect the income-expense ratio generated by each.

5. *Fringe Benefits:*   Two clinicians who initiate a practice together usually have little difficulty determining parallel fringe benefits. However, one may have different goals in terms of retirement, insurance, or time off. A new clinician joining an established practice should take some care in developing a benefit plan that will grow to approximately the level and value of the others' benefits.

6. *Withdrawal* and *Buy–Sell:*   Probably the single greatest source of conflict in any partnership or corporation is withdrawal by one principal. This brings to the fore all the issues from past years that have been ignored, avoided, or never resolved. Without careful planning for termination of a partner or dissolution of the practice itself, such an event will often generate negative feelings on the part of all involved. A plan for termination should be part of the start-up policies of the practice.

7. *Death or Disability:*   Provisions should be made to handle death or disability of a partner or stockholder. Prior funding of insurance whose proceeds would be used by the remaining owner(s) to buy-out the estate of the deceased or disabled owner is a standard feature of good business practice. Terms of the insurance policy, method of payment, time schedule of the payment, and beneficiaries of the payment should be specified.

Provision should also be made for illness. Such provision for illness usually doesn't have to cover short absences of a week or two. But it should spell out what happens if a partner is incapacitated for a long period. Most partnership agreements also provide for extended disability. For example, usually after a full year of disability, partnership status ends completely.

Agreements should include retirement benefits with a provision for paying out each partner's share of assets, accounts receivable, and possibly some value for good will that is a measure of the partner's contribution to the overall success of the enterprise.

If a partner decides to leave the practice, that person may be entitled to a return of the original invested capital and a portion of accounts receivable based on his/her income generation. This should be managed so that no hardship is placed on remaining partners. Usually the withdrawing partner does not receive payment for the current value of the partnership. The obligations that accrue to the terminating partner for the debts of the practice should be determined and provided for prior to his/her termination, because such liability is usually terminated with the individual's termination.

If the corporation liquidates, or if a partner decides to leave the practice and begin a new practice, the issue of *competing proximity* may be a factor. Some professionals try to prohibit another professional from practicing in the same vicinity, because they feel the latter individual will compete for regional clientele. At the outset of the practice, the partners should agree on the issue of who may practice, where each may practice, and to whom the clients of the joint practice belong should the partners separate.

If one partner wishes to buy out the other, and the other wishes to sell his/her portion of the practice, a buy–sell agreement included in the initial corporate or partnership agreement should cover the contingencies. For example,

1. To whom must the first offer to sell be made? This is usually referred to as first ''Right of Refusal'' and is often given to the other partners in the practice.
2. Does first ''Right of Refusal'' have a time limit?
3. What restrictions are there on the potential buyer of the offered portion? Usually in a professional setting it is specified that potential buyers hold certain credentials, be experienced in the profession, and so forth.
4. What is to happen to the distribution of profits? Do the old partners divide it evenly? What if one partner generated all the current profits? What if another partner spent all the profits on expenses?
5. How will the value of the practice (and each partner's share of the practice) be determined? What formula will be used?

In some situations, modifications in original operating agreements are not adequate to eliminate major sources of disagreement among partners or owners. Just as people change and practitioners' goals change, so may the form of practice change. If the partnership or corporation cannot be modified sufficiently to accommodate the changes of all partners or owners, then the partnership must be terminated or the corporation dissolved. In such instances, it will be necessary to make decisions similar to those generated by one person leaving a practice. Just as with that situation, dissolution will be facilitated by spelling out policies for dissolution in the original operating agreement. In the event of dissolution (liquidation) of a practice, certain steps by the partners or owners will be necessary and/or desirable:

1. Review the original operating agreement for resolution of issues pertinent to the dissolution.
2. Agree on other issues that were not covered in the original operating agreement (see Appendix 2–1).
3. Compose letters to debtors, creditors, clients, referral sources, and staff members (see Appendix 2–2).
4. Have the accountant prepare information relevant to personal tax and/or income records (i.e., for preparing necessary forms for reporting the liquidation and losses on personal returns of each partner) that may include

   - unrealized receivables of the practice
   - taxable income that is passed through to stockholders (in addition to the amount ordinarily calculated for the year)
   - undistributed taxable income for the year ended (the year of liquidation); one may be able to take short-term capital loss for the bases of stock
5. Obtain the necessary forms for dissolution, change of name, and so forth from the secretary of state or other appropriate state official, complete, and return (see Appendix 2–11).

MAKING THE DECISION

After my own random pursuit of various forms of organization structures for professional purposes, it has occurred to me that there may be a sequential order for moving from one structure to another. A reasonable sequence is as follows:

1. *Shared Office Arrangement.*   An individual can remain a sole practitioner with the advantages of a partnership and a group practice by joining other practitioners in the same office or suite of offices and without enjoining them in a formal business structure. Office sharing may include only rent, utilities, and janitorial services, although sometimes it includes sharing a receptionist, general waiting room, library, and computer.

    This agreement is good for the beginning practitioner who wants the advantages of a partnership or group practice (contact with colleagues, sharing of expenses, and so forth) along with the advantages of being a sole practitioner. If office sharing is done with colleagues who have different specialties, but good reputations, and if guidelines for space sharing are carefully drawn, there are many advantages to all.

    In this situation, the sole practitioner can hire employees or independent consultants as would be done in any other office, as long as the office sharing agreement allows this arrangement.

2. *Expense Sharing.*   If one wants to establish an office name, share expenses with another practitioner, and not undertake the entire operation alone, the logical step is expense sharing. Expense sharing can include (in addition to office-space sharing) sharing of telephone, recording machine, secretary, bookkeeper, costs of public relations, letterhead, office sign (John Smith, speech-language pathologist—Alan Jones, speech-language pathologist), filing cabinets, form files, and so forth. Expense sharing is one precursor to a formal partnership. It is an arrangement undertaken for a limited time period, but the arrangement should be written and signed by both parties. The written agreement clarifies that both parties are adequately financed to cover costs for the duration of the arrangement, including monies that would cover any problems of split-up (phone bills, unpaid debts). Such agreement should also designate who moves and who stays, who gets the assets if any are shared, who pays the attorney if necessary for arbitration, and so forth.

3. *Partnership.*   Do not undertake a partnership or corporation with a colleague just because he/she is a friend (Foonberg, 1984). After a successful office or expense-sharing experience, if you want to establish a formal business structure, do it in the form of a partnership, not a corporation. It is easier to change the partnership and its operation than it is to change a corporation. If the partnership proves to be successful and the income to the practice creates the need for a tax shelter, then serious consideration of a corporation is in order. By now the practitioner/owner has had enough experience to determine whether the practice should be set up as sole owner or whether incorporation with one or two other colleagues sharing ownership is more desirable.

4. *Corporation.*   Incorporation is more expensive than any other type of organizational structure. The cost is high because of the professional assistance needed from consultants and others for predicting and analyzing the financial and tax situation of the practice and owners, for developing practice policies and by-laws, for designing fringe benefits for owners and employees, and for providing on-going consultation as needed.

The corporation represents the greatest complexity in terms of initial organization, expense, record keeping, and paper, and can provide the greatest advantages in terms of tax deductions and protection of personal assets.

Complexity can be advantageous because of the protection it provides (see Table 2–1). By contrast, simplicity offers the greatest risks but allows the greatest control and is easiest to change. The bases for deciding upon a practice structure depend upon one's professional and personal goals. It is not unusual to find that needs and goals change over time, requiring a change in the organizational structure of a practice. The purpose of making an informed decision about the structural framework is to use what works; if the owner/practitioner finds that he/she is working too hard just to maintain a particular structure, it is time to reconsider that structural choice.

JOINING AN EXISTING PRACTICE

If you have an opportunity to join a practice as a practitioner and co-owner, it will be important to know how to assess the practice, its quality of service delivery, goals of the practice, financial soundness and fiscal management, and personnel policies.

If you are offered an opportunity to buy-in, determine how long before your share of ownership will be realized, how the accounts receivable will be divided, and what your initial investment will be. If you do not already know how to read a financial statement, or if you find one too difficult to decipher, enlist the aid of an accountant or financial consultant to analyze the assets and liabilities of the practice (Marshall et al., 1982).

Investigate the operating policies of the practice; obtain copies of statements of policies given to clients and to staff. Find out what percentage of the accounts receivable are outstanding, whether outstanding bills are ever collected, and what percentage of clients are seen at reduced fees. Find out how employees are provided incentives, whether professionals are allowed a percentage of income over a salary base, and what are permissable expenditures for owners and employees (i.e., business expenses, fringe benefits). Find out what the distribution of profits to shareholders was at the end of the last fiscal year. Determine if fees are based on any systematic cost accounting and what cost containment measures are practiced (see Cost Analysis, Chapter 9, this book).

Before anyone in the professional community knows that you are considering joining a practice, ask colleagues and other professionals in the community about the general impression and reputation of that practice and its practitioners. There are always mixed reactions to any professional practice, but most reactions about ethics and professional services of a practice should be favorable before you begin

Table 2–1.   Organizational Structure Complexity*

	Structure	Sources of Revenue	Partner/Co-owner, Employees
I.	**Sole Proprietorship**		
a.	solo practice	fees only/direct pay	none
b.	solo practice	fees only/direct pay	independent consultant (salary on percentage of income generated)[†]
c.	solo practice	fees only/direct pay	salaried employee
d.	solo practice	fees and private 3rd party payment	consultants/employees
e.	solo practice	fees and private and public 3rd party payment	consultants/employees
II.	**Partnership**		
a.	partnership	fees only/direct pay	one partner
b.	partnership	fees only/direct pay	one partner independent consultant[†]
c.	partnership	fees only/direct pay	one partner salaried employee
d.	partnership	fees only/direct pay	two or more partners consultants/employees
e.	partnership	fees and private 3rd party payment	two or more partners consultants/employees
f.	partnership	fees and private and public 3rd party payment	two or more partners consultants/employees
III.	**Corporation**		
a.	corporation	fees only/direct pay	none
b.	corporation	fees only/direct pay	independent consultant[†] (salary based on percentage of income generated)
c.	corporation	fees only/direct pay	one co-owner
d.	corporation	fees only/direct pay	two or more co-owners
e.	corporation	fees only/direct pay	two or more co-owners consultants/employees
f.	corporation	fees and private 3rd party payment	co-owners consultants/employees
g.	corporation	fees and private and public 3rd party payment	co-owners consultants/employees

*Least complex at I.a; most complex at III.g.

†An independent consultant, as used in Table 2–1, is a licensed/certified speech-language pathologist and/or audiologist who is capable of working with no supervision in practice and is hired on an as-needed or regularly scheduled basis to practice in the office of the owner. Salary is based on percentage of income generated. An independent consultant is not employed in the traditional sense, and no withholding or social security is taken from the salary. The independent consultant is self-employed and works on the basis of an arrangement with the owner/practitioner.

serious negotiations with that practice. Determine the long-term goals of the current owners in order to draw some conclusions about what effect you might have on the practice and what their intent is in asking you to join. When a professional joins an operation as a new stockholder, either the practice must grow, or the other stockholders will have reduced income (Marshall et al., 1982).

Before initiating a new practice or joining an existing practice, remember that in group practice, there is the potential for compromising profit as well as professional philosophy. If the compromises are satisfactory to you and in line with your professional goals, then proceed. Your reward with a group practice will be more free time and less responsibility than you would have in solo practice.

Appendices

APPENDIX 2–1
STEPS FOR INCORPORATING A PRACTICE*

	Date Done	Attorney	Accountant	Owner(s)

1. Incorporation Meeting. Have a meeting of the future stockholders to decide:

    a. The corporate name

    b. Location of the principal office

    c. The purposes for which the corporation is to be formed

    d. The scope of the activities

    e. Classes and number of shares

2. Corporate Name. Check with the secretary of state to see if the corporate name is available. Reserve name if available.

3. Directors. Determine directors; list names and addresses.

4. Officers. Establish corporate officers.

5. Target Date. Schedule a sequence of steps for target date for completion.

6. Multiple Corporations. Determine if stockholders of this corporation are also stockholders of other corporations. If they are, determine if stock ownership qualifies this corporation as a member of a controlled group.

7. Assets and Liabilities. If the corporation is to take over a going business, determine what assets and liabilities are to be turned over to the corporation, and which shares or notes are to be issued in exchange. Consider assumption of liabilities; determine whether or not real estate is to be transferred.

8. Notices. Send notice of incorporation to all debtors, creditors of former business.

9. Employment I.D. and Social Security. File application for social security identification number (Federal Form SS-4) and for employer identification number (E.I.N.).

	Date Done	Attorney	Accountant	Owner(s)

10. Workmen's Compensation and Unemployment Insurance. File for coverage under Workmen's Compensation and Unemployment Insurance with the Bureau of Unemployment Compensation.

11. Credit Transfer from Unemployment Compensation. If the corporation qualifies for merit rating by transfer from a former business, file Employer's Report on Change in Status of Business.

12. Election under Sub-Chapter S. If the corporation is going to elect to be taxed as Sub-Chapter S, prepare and file Form 2553, Election by Small Business Corporation, within 30 days of the incorporation date.

13. Fiscal Year. Determine the date of the fiscal year and set up tax calendar.

14. Final Returns. If the new corporation is taking over an established business, file sales tax, FICA tax, and unemployment tax final returns for the old business within 30 days after the corporation takes over the operation of the new business.

15. County Tax Assessor Notification. If the corporation is taking over an established business which has already paid personal property tax, notify the county assessor.

16. Property Tax. File personal property tax within 90 days of commencing business.

17. Officers' Salaries. Establish officers' salaries and fill out Form W-4 authorizing the corporation to withhold wages.

18. Depository. Furnish selected bank with resolution authorizing who is to sign checks and negotiate loans.

19. Notify Utilities. Notify utilities so accounts can be changed over to the corporation on an effective date.

20. Insurance. Establish list of insurance needs and contact insurance agents.

    a. Group insurance

    b. Income protection insurance

	Date Done	Attorney	Accountant	Owner(s)

   c. Disability insurance (provided by corporation to relieve the business of responsibility for providing income to a disabled associate for an extended period)

   d. Other

21. Accounting Methods. Determine or elect the accounting methods desirable for this business.

22. Books and Records. Design chart of accounts, ledgers, and journals appropriate for particular business operations.

23. Death Benefit. Determine if the corporation will elect to provide $5,000 death benefit.

24. Medical Reimbursement Plan. Determine if the corporation will adopt a Medical Reimbursement Plan for employees.

25. Valuation. Determine how business is to be valuated.

26. Buy-out Plans. Determine buy-out plan in event of premature death. Determine buy-out (i.e., buy–sell agreement) in event one partner wishes to leave the practice, or a new partner wants to come in. (May not be funded through insurance.) Methods of sale terms, conditions, and time line.

27. Policies. Determine operating policies and liquidation procedures.

(Record these decisions in minutes of the directors' or shareholders' meetings.)

APPENDIX 2–2
ELECTION BY A SMALL BUSINESS CORPORATION (SUB-CHAPTER S) IRS FORM 2553 AND INSTRUCTIONS

Department of the Treasury
Internal Revenue Service

Instructions for Form 2553

(Revised May 1983)

Election by a Small Business Corporation

(Section references are to the Internal Revenue Code, unless otherwise specified.)

Paperwork Reduction Act Notice.—We ask for this information to carry out the Internal Revenue laws of the United States. We need it to ensure that you are complying with these laws and to allow us to figure and collect the right amount of tax. You are required to give us this information.

A. Purpose.—To elect to be treated as an "S Corporation," a corporation must file Form 2553. The election permits the income of the S corporation to be taxed to the shareholders of the corporation except as provided in Subchapter S and section 58(d). (See section 1363.)

B. Who May Elect.—Your corporation may make the election only if it meets the following tests:

1. It is a domestic corporation.
2. It has no more than 35 shareholders. A husband and wife (and their estates) are treated as one shareholder for this requirement. All other persons are treated as separate shareholders.
3. It has only individuals, estates, or certain trusts as shareholders.
4. It has no nonresident alien shareholders.
5. It has only one class of stock. See sections 1361(c)(4) and (5) for additional details.
6. It is not an ineligible corporation as defined in section 1361(b)(2). See section 6(c) of Public Law 97–354 for additional details.
7. It has a calendar tax year or other permitted tax year as explained in Instruction G.
8. Each shareholder consents as explained in the instructions for Column D.

See sections 1361, 1362 and 1378 for additional information on the above tests.

C. Where to File.—File this election with the Internal Revenue Service Center where the corporation will file Form 1120S, U.S. Income Tax Return For An S Corporation. You should keep a copy for the corporation's files.

If the corporation's principal business, office or agency is located in	Use the following Internal Revenue Service Center address
New Jersey, New York City and counties of Nassau, Rockland, Suffolk, and Westchester	Holtsville, NY 00501
New York (all other counties), Connecticut, Maine, Massachusetts, New Hampshire, Rhode Island, Vermont	Andover, MA 05501
Alabama, Florida, Georgia, Mississippi, South Carolina	Atlanta, GA 31101
Michigan, Ohio	Cincinnati, OH 45999
Arkansas, Kansas, Louisiana, New Mexico, Oklahoma, Texas	Austin, TX 73301
Alaska, Arizona, Colorado, Idaho, Minnesota, Montana, Nebraska, Nevada, North Dakota, Oregon, South Dakota, Utah, Washington, Wyoming	Ogden, UT 84201
Illinois, Iowa, Missouri, Wisconsin	Kansas City, MO 64999
California, Hawaii	Fresno, CA 93888
Indiana, Kentucky, North Carolina, Tennessee, Virginia, West Virginia	Memphis, TN 37501
Delaware, District of Columbia, Maryland, Pennsylvania	Philadelphia, PA 19255

D. When to Make the Election.—Complete Form 2553 and file it either: (1) at any time during that portion of the first tax year the election is to take effect which occurs before the 16th day of the third month of that tax year (or at any time during that year, if that year does not extend beyond the period described above) or (2) in the tax year before the first tax year it is to take effect. An election made by a small business corporation after the 15th day of the third month but before the end of the tax year is treated as made for the next year. For example, if a calendar tax year corporation makes the election in April 1983, it is effective for the corporation's 1984 calendar tax year.

For purposes of this election, a newly formed corporation's tax year starts when it has shareholders, acquires assets, or begins doing business, whichever happens first.

E. Acceptance or Non-acceptance of Election.—IRS will notify you if your election is accepted and when it will take effect. Until then, do not file Form 1120S. If you are now required to file Form 1120, U.S. Corporation Income Tax Return, continue filing it until your election takes effect.

You will also be notified if your election is not accepted.

F. End of Election.—Once the election is made, it stays in effect for all years until it is terminated. During the 5 years after the election has been terminated, the corporation can make another election on Form 2553 only if the Commissioner consents.

See section 1362(g). However, the 5-year waiting period does not apply to terminations made under Subchapter S rules in effect for tax years beginning before January 1, 1983. See sections 1362(d), (e), and (f) for rules regarding termination of election.

G. Permitted Tax Year.—Section 1378 provides that no corporation may make an election to be an S corporation for any tax year unless the tax year is a permitted tax year. A permitted tax year is a tax year ending December 31 or any other tax year for which the corporation establishes a business purpose to the satisfaction of IRS. The tax year requirement applies to any election made after October 19, 1982. See section 1378(c) for additional requirements when a 50 percent shift in ownership occurs in an existing S corporation.

H. Investment Credit Property.—Although the corporation has elected to be an S corporation under section 1362, the tax imposed by section 47 in the case of early disposition of investment credit property will be imposed on the corporation for credits allowed for tax years for which the corporation was not an S corporation. The election will not be treated as a disposition of the property by the corporation. See section 1371(d).

Specific Instructions

Part I.—Part I must be completed by all corporations.

Name and Address of Corporation.—If the corporation's mailing address is the same as someone else's, such as a shareholder's, please enter this person's name below the corporation's name.

Employer Identification Number.—If you have applied for an employer identification number (EIN) but have not received it, enter "applied for." If the corporation does not have an EIN, you should apply for one on Form SS–4, Application for Employer Identification Number, available from most IRS or Social Security Administration offices. Send Form SS–4 to the IRS Service Center where Form 1120S will be filed.

Principal Business Activity and Principal Product or Service.—Use the Codes for Principal Business Activity contained in the Instructions for Form 1120S. Your principal business activity is the one that accounts for the largest percentage of total receipts. Total receipts are gross sales and gross receipts, plus all other income.

Also state the principal product or service. For example, if the principal business activity is "Grain mill products," the principal product or service may be "cereal preparation."

Number of Shares Issued and Outstanding.—Enter only one figure. This figure will be the number of shares of stock that have been issued to shareholders and have not been reacquired by the corporation. This is the number of shares all shareholders own, as reported in column E, Part I.

Form **2553** (Rev. May 1983) Department of the Treasury Internal Revenue Service	**Election by a Small Business Corporation** (Under section 1362 of the Internal Revenue Code) ▶ For Paperwork Reduction Act Notice, see page 1 of instructions. ▶ See separate instructions.	OMB No. 1545–0146

Note: *This election to be treated as an "S corporation" can be approved only if all the tests in Instruction B are met.*

Part I

Name of corporation (see instructions)	Employer identification number (see instructions)	Principal business activity and principal product or service (see instructions)
Number and street		Election is to be effective for tax year beginning (month, day, year)
City or town, State and ZIP code		Number of shares issued and outstanding (see instructions)
Is the corporation the outgrowth or continuation of any form of predecessor? . . . . . ☐ Yes ☐ No If "Yes," state name of predecessor, type of organization, and period of its existence ▶		Date and place of incorporation

A If this election takes effect for the first tax year the corporation exists, enter the earliest of the following: (1) date the corporation first had shareholders, (2) date the corporation first had assets, or (3) date the corporation began doing business. ▶

B Selected tax year: Annual return will be filed for tax year ending (month and day) ▶
See Instructions before entering your tax year. If the tax year ends any date other than December 31, you must complete Part II or Part IV on back. You may want to complete Part III to make a back-up request.

C Name of each shareholder, person having a community property interest in the corporation's stock, and each tenant in common, joint tenant, and tenant by the entirety. (A husband and wife (and their estates) are counted as one shareholder in determining the number of shareholders without regard to the manner in which the stock is owned.)	D Shareholders' Consent Statement. We the undersigned shareholders, consent to the corporation's election to be treated as an "S corporation" under section 1362(a). *(Shareholders sign and date below.)	E Stock owned		F Social security number (employer identification number for estate or trust)	G Tax year ends (Month and day)
		Number of shares	Dates acquired		

For this election to be valid, the consent of each shareholder, person having a community property interest in the corporation's stock, and each tenant in common, joint tenant, and tenant by the entirety must either appear above or be attached to this form. (See instructions for column D, if continuation sheet or a separate consent statement is needed.)

Under penalties of perjury, I declare that I have examined this election, including accompanying schedules, and statements, and to the best of my knowledge and belief it is true, correct, and complete.

Signature and Title of Officer ▶   Date ▶

See Parts II, III, and IV on back.

Item B.—The tax year selected must be a permitted tax year as defined in instruction G.

A newly formed corporation may automatically adopt a tax year ending December 31.

Generally, a corporation may automatically change to a tax year ending December 31, if all of its principal shareholders have tax years ending December 31, or if all of its principal shareholders are concurrently changing to such tax year. If a corporation is automatically changing to a tax year ending December 31, it is not necessary for the corporation to file Form 1128, Application for Change in Accounting Period. A shareholder may not change his or her tax year without securing prior approval from IRS. For purposes of the automatic change, a principal shareholder is a shareholder who owns 5% or more of the issued and outstanding stock of the corporation. See temporary regulations section 18.1378–1 for additional details.

If a corporation wants to change to a tax year ending December 31, but does not qualify for an automatic change as explained above, it may want to complete Part IV and indicate in an attached statement that it wants to change to a tax year ending December 31. Also, the corporation can apply under section 442 to change its tax year to a tax year ending December 31, by filing Form 1128 before filing Form 2553.

If a corporation selects a tax year ending other than December 31, it must complete Part II or IV in addition to Part I.

Column D.—Shareholders' Consent Statement.—Each person who is a shareholder at the time the election is made must consent to the election. If the election is made during the corporation's first tax year for which it is effective, any person who held stock at any time during that portion of that year which occurs before the time the election is made must consent to the election although the person may have sold or transferred his or her stock before the election is made. Each shareholder consents by signing in column D or by signing a separate consent statement, described below.

The election by a small business corporation is considered made for the following tax year if one or more of the persons who held stock at any time during that portion of that year which occurs before the time the election is made did not consent to the election. See section 1362(b)(2).

If a husband and wife have a community interest in the stock or in the income from it, both must consent. Each tenant in common, joint tenant, and tenant by the entirety also must consent.

A minor's consent is made by the minor or the legal guardian. If no legal guardian has been appointed, the natural guardian makes the consent (even if a custodian holds the minor's stock under a law patterned after the Uniform Gifts to Minors Act).

Continuation Sheet or Separate Consent Statement.—If you need a continuation sheet or use a separate consent statement, attach it to Form 2553. The separate consent statement must contain the name, address, and employer identification number of the corporation and the shareholder information requested in columns C through G of Part I.

If you wish, you may combine all the shareholders' consents in one statement.

Column E.—Enter the number of shares of stock each shareholder owns and the dates the stock was acquired. If the election is made during the corporation's first tax year for which it is effective, do not list the shares of stock for those shareholders who sold or transferred all of their stock before the election was made but who still must consent to the election for it to be effective for the tax year.

Column G.—Enter the month and day that each shareholder's tax year ends. If a shareholder is changing his or her tax year, enter the tax year the shareholder is changing to. If the election is made during the corporation's first tax year for which it is effective, you do not have to enter the tax year of shareholders who sold or transferred all of their stock before the election was made but who still must consent to the election for it to be effective for the tax year.

Signature.—Form 2553 must be signed by the president, treasurer, assistant treasurer, chief accounting officer, or other corporate officer (such as tax officer) authorized to sign.

Part II.—Items I and J of Part II are completed by a corporation that selects a tax year ending other than December 31, and that qualifies under section 4.02, 4.03, or 4.04 of Revenue Procedure 83–25, 1983 Internal Revenue Bulletin No. 15, at page 13. Items I and J are completed in place of the additional statement asked for in section 7.01 of the procedure. Sections 4.02, 4.03, and 4.04 provide for expeditious approval of certain corporations' requests to adopt, retain, or change to a tax year ending other than December 31. The representation statements in Part II of Form 2553 highlight the three types of requests provided for in the revenue procedure. A corporation adopting, retaining, or changing its accounting period under the procedure must comply with or satisfy all conditions of the procedure.

The revenue procedure applies only to the tax years of corporations which are electing S corporation status by filing Form 2553. A corporation is permitted to adopt, retain, or change its tax year only once under the procedure. It is not necessary for the corporation to file Form 1128 when adopting or changing its tax year under the procedure.

Items I and K of Part II are completed by a corporation that is making a request as specified in section 8 of the procedure. Section 8 provides that if a corporation wants to adopt, retain, or change to a tax year not specified under section 4.02, 4.03, or 4.04 of the procedure or certain subsections of temporary regulations 18.1378–1, it should attach a statement to Form 2553 pursuant to the ruling request requirements of Revenue Procedure 83–1, 1983 Internal Revenue Bulletin No. 1, at page 16. The statement must show the business purpose for the desired tax year.

Approval of tax year selections made under section 4.02, 4.03, or 4.04 of Revenue Procedure 83–25 are generally automatic; however, a request under section 8 is not automatic. If a request is made under section 8, the corporation may want to make the back-up request under Part III. See section 8 of the procedure for details.

Part III.—Check the box in Part III to make the back-up request provided by temporary regulations section 18.1378–1(b)(2)(ii)(A). This section provides that corporations requesting to retain (or adopt) a tax year ending other than December 31, may make a back-up request to adopt or change to a tax year ending December 31, in case the initial request for a fiscal year is denied. In order to make the back-up request, a corporation requesting to retain its tax year ending other than December 31, must qualify for an automatic change of its tax year under temporary regulations section 18.1378–1(b)(1).

Part IV.—Check the box in Part IV to request the IRS to determine your permitted tax year under the provisions of temporary regulations section 18.1378–1(d). If you check the box in Part IV, enter "See Part IV" in the space in item B, Part I, for month and year.

You may attach a schedule to Form 2553 showing any additional information you want the IRS to consider in making the determination. IRS will notify you of the permitted tax year determination. The tax year determination by IRS is final.

Part II—Selection of Tax Year Under Revenue Procedure 83–25

I Check the applicable box below to indicate whether the corporation is:
- ☐ Adopting the tax year entered in item B, Part I.
- ☐ Retaining the tax year entered in item B, Part I.
- ☐ Changing to the tax year entered in item B, Part I.

J Check the applicable box below to indicate the representation statement the corporation is making as required under section 7.01 (item 4) of Revenue Procedure 83–25, 1983 Internal Revenue Bulletin No. 15, at page 13.

- ☐ Under penalties of perjury, I represent that shareholders holding more than half of the shares of the stock (as of the first day of the tax year to which the request relates) of the corporation have the same tax year or are concurrently changing to the tax year that the corporation adopts, retains or changes to per item B, Part I.

- ☐ Under penalties of perjury, I represent that shareholders holding more than half of the shares of the stock (as of the first day of the tax year to which the request relates) of the corporation have a tax year or are concurrently changing to a tax year that, although is different from the tax year the corporation is adopting, retaining, or changing to per item B, Part I, results in a deferment of income to each of these shareholders of three months or less.

- ☐ Under penalties of perjury, I represent that the corporation is adopting, retaining or changing to a tax year that coincides with its natural business year as verified by its satisfaction of the requirements of section 4.042(a), (b), (c), and (d) of Revenue Procedure 83–25.

K Check here ☐ if the tax year entered in item B, Part I, is requested under the provisions of section 8 of Revenue Procedure 83–25. Attach to Form 2553 a statement and other necessary information pursuant to the ruling request requirements of Revenue Procedure 83–1, 1983 Internal Revenue Bulletin No. 1, at page 16. The statement must include the business purpose for the desired tax year. See instructions.

Part III—Back-Up Request by Certain Corporations Initially Selecting a Fiscal Year (See Instructions.)

Check here ☐ if the corporation agrees to adopt or to change to a tax year ending December 31 if necessary for IRS to accept this election for S corporation status (temporary regulations section 18.1378–1(b)(2)(ii)(A)). This back-up request does not apply if the fiscal tax year request is approved by IRS or if the election to be an S corporation is not accepted.

Part IV—Request by Corporation for Tax Year Determination By IRS (See Instructions.)

Check here ☐ if the corporation requests the IRS to determine the permitted tax year for the corporation based on information submitted in Part I (and attached schedules). This request is made under provisions of temporary regulations section 18.1378–1(d).

☆U.S. Government Printing Office: 1983—381-108/141

APPENDIX 2-3
SAMPLE CERTIFICATE OF INCORPORATION

OFFICE OF THE SECRETARY OF STATE
CERTIFICATE OF INCORPORATION OF
____

Charter No. ____________________________

The undersigned, as Secretary of State of the State of Texas, hereby certifies that duplicate originals of Articles of Incorporation for the above corporation duly signed and verified pursuant to the provisions of the Texas Business Corporation Act have been received in this office and are found to conform to law.

ACCORDINGLY the undersigned, as such Secretary of State, and by virtue of the authority vested in him by law, hereby issues this Certificate of Incorporation and attaches hereto a duplicate original of the Articles of Incorporation.

Dated ______________________________

____
Secretary of State

APPENDIX 2–4
SAMPLE ARTICLES OF INCORPORATION

ARTICLES OF INCORPORATION
OF

____

We, the undersigned natural persons of the age of 21 years or more, at least two of whom are citizens of the State of Texas, acting as incorporators of a corporation under the Texas Business Corporation Act, do hereby adopt the following Articles of Incorporation for such corporation.

ARTICLE ONE

The name of the corporation is:

ARTICLE TWO

The period of its duration is perpetual.

ARTICLE THREE

The purpose or purposes for which the corporation is organized are:

To engage in the business of establishing, maintaining, and operating offices for speech, language, and hearing assessment and intervention and all related activities, and to engage in the wholesale and retail buying, selling, leasing, renting, maintaining, using, operating, installing and distributing of all materials, equipment and personal property appurtenant or incident to and useful in the business.

To purchase, own, convey, or otherwise use and enjoy real and personal property of all kinds required for the operation of said business, and in connection therewith to acquire, construct, maintain and operate buildings and equipment deemed necessary or convenient in connection therewith.

ARTICLE FOUR

The number of shares which the corporation shall have authority to issue is _________ THOUSAND (___ ,000) of the par value of ___________ DOLLARS ($___________) each.

ARTICLE FIVE

The corporation will not commence business until it has received for the issuance of its shares and consideration of the value of ___________ THOUSAND DOLLARS ($___________), consisting of money, labor due, or property actually received.

ARTICLE SIX

The post office address of its initial registered office is ___________________________ ___________________ , and the name of its initial registered agent at such address is ___________________________________ .

ARTICLE SEVEN

The number of directors constituting the initial Board of Directors is three (3), and the names and addresses of the persons who are to serve as directors until the first annual meeting of the shareholders or until their successors are elected and qualified are:

Name   *Address*

ARTICLE EIGHT

The names and addresses of the incorporators are:

Name   *Address*

IN WITNESS WHEREOF, we have hereunto set our hands this _________________
day of ____ .

THE STATE OF TEXAS
COUNTY OF ___________

I, ____ , a Notary Public, do hereby certify on
this _______ day of _______ , _______ , personally appeared _______ , who, being by me
first duly sworn, severally declared that he is one of the persons who signed the foregoing
document as incorporator, and that the statements therein contained are true.

____
Notary Public, ___________ County, Texas

APPENDIX 2–5
SAMPLE MINUTES AND BY-LAWS

MINUTES

AND

BY-LAWS

OF

(Clinic)
____

INCORPORATED UNDER THE LAWS OF THE
STATE OF __________

MINUTES AND BY-LAWS OF THE ORGANIZATIONAL MEETING OF THE
DIRECTORS OF

____

The organizational meeting of directors was held at ______________________________ on
______________________________, 19______ at ____________________ m.
The following were present:

being all the directors of the corporation.

____ was appointed chairman of the meeting
and ____ was appointed secretary.

The secretary then presented and read to the meeting the waiver of notice of the meeting, subscribed by all the directors named in the articles of incorporation, and it was ordered that it be appended to the minutes of the meeting.

The secretary then presented and read to the meeting a copy of the articles of incorporation and reported that on ________________________________ , 19______ the original thereof was filed in the office of the Secretary of State of the State of ____________ and that the Secretary of State issued a formal Certificate of Incorporation to the company on that date. The secretary presented the Certificate of Incorporation annexed to the approved duplicate of the articles of incorporation as filed and it was ordered appended to the minutes of the meeting.

The chairman then stated that nominations were in order for election of directors of the corporation to hold office until the first annual meeting of shareholders and until their successors shall be elected and shall qualify.

The following persons were nominated:

No further nominations being made, nominations were closed and a vote was taken.

After the vote had been counted, the chairman declared that the foregoing named nominees were elected directors of the corporation. The chairman then stated that the newly elected directors would assume their responsibilities immediately.

The secretary then presented a proposed form of by-laws prepared by ________________________ , counsel to the corporation. The proposed by-laws were read into the minutes, considered and upon motion duly made, seconded and carried, were adopted as and for the by-laws of the corporation and ordered appended to the minutes of the meeting.

The chairman of the meeting then called for the election of officers of the corporation. The following persons were nominated to the office preceding their name:

President   ____

Vice-President   ____

Secretary-Treasurer   ____

No further nominations being made the nominations were closed and the directors proceeded to vote on the nominees. The chairman announced that the foregoing nominees were elected to the offices set before their respective names.

The secretary submitted to the meeting a seal proposed for use as the corporate seal, a specimen share certificate proposed for use as the corporate certificate for shares, the corporate record book, and the share transfer ledger. Upon motion duly made, seconded and carried, it was

RESOLVED, that the seal now presented
at this meeting, an impression of which is
directed to be made in the minutes of this
meeting, be and the same hereby is
adopted as the seal of the corporation, and
further

RESOLVED, that the specimen share certificate presented to this meeting be and hereby is adopted as the form of certificate for shares to be issued to represent shares in the corporation, and further

RESOLVED, that the corporate record book, including the share transfer ledger, be and hereby is adopted as the record book and share transfer ledger of the corporation.

Upon motion duly made, seconded and carried, it was

RESOLVED, that the treasurer of the corporation be and hereby is authorized to pay all charges and expenses incident to or arising out of the organization of the corporation and to reimburse any person who has made any disbursement thereof.

Upon motion, duly made, seconded, and carried, it was

RESOLVED, that an office of the corporation be established and maintained at ________________________ in the City of ____________ , State of ____________ , and that meetings of the board of directors from time to time may be held either at the principal office or at such other place as the board of directors shall from time to time order.

Upon motion, duly made, seconded and carried, it was

RESOLVED, that for the purpose of authorizing the corporation to do business in any state, territory or dependency of the United States or any foreign country in which it is necessary or expedient for this corporation to transact business, the proper officers of this corporation are hereby authorized to appoint and substitute all necessary agents or attorneys for service of process, to designate and change the location of all necessary statutory offices and, under the corporate seal, to make and file all necessary certificates, reports, powers of attorney and other instruments as may be required by the laws of such state, territory, dependency or country to authorize the corporation to transact business therein.

The chairman then stated that it was desirable to designate a depository for the funds of the corporation. Thereupon, on motion duly made, seconded, and unanimously adopted, it was

RESOLVED, that the treasurer be and hereby is authorized to open a bank account in behalf of the corporation with the ______________ Bank located at ______________ , ______________ and a resolution for that purpose on the printed form of said bank was adopted and was ordered appended to the minutes of this meeting.

The Secretary then presented to the meeting a proposal from ____ , and addressed to this corporation. Upon motion duly made, seconded, and carried, the said proposal was ordered read into the minutes by the Secretary and was as follows:

"I, ____ , propose to purchase ______________ shares of stock in ______________________________ in exchange for $____________ in cash."

The Secretary then presented to the meeting a proposal from __________________ , and addressed to this corporation. Upon a motion duly made, seconded, and carried, the said proposal was ordered read into the minutes by the Secretary and was as follows:

"I, ____ , propose to purchase ______________ share of stock in ______________________________ in exchange for $____________ in cash."

The proposals were taken up for consideration and the following resolution was, on motion unanimously adopted.

"WHEREAS, proposals have been made to this corporation, which proposals have been read into these minutes, and

WHEREAS in the judgement of the Board of Directors the assets proposed to be transferred to the corporation are reasonable and worth the amount of the consideration demanded therefor, and that it is in the best interests of this corporation to accept the said offers as set forth in said proposals,

NOW THEREFORE, it is RESOLVED that said offers, as set forth in these minutes, be and the same is hereby approved and accepted, and that in accordance with the terms thereof, this corporation shall, as full payment for said property, issue to said officers ______________________ shares of common stock, in __________________ , and,

It is further RESOLVED, that, upon the delivery to this corporation of said assets and the execution and delivery of such proper instruments as may be necessary to transfer and convey the same to this corporation, the officers of this corporation are authorized and directed to execute and deliver the certificates for such shares to be issued and delivered on acceptance of said offers in accordance with the foregoing."

The chairman called attention to the provisions in paragraph 6, Article VII, of the by-laws, pertaining to reimbursement of employee expenses and provision of employee benefits. The Board reviewed a list of possible reimbursements and benefits proposed by the corporate accountant. Thereupon, upon motion duly made, seconded, and carried, it was

RESOLVED, that the policy of this corporation shall be to reimburse employees for expenses which they incur in performing corporate business and to provide employees with employee benefits, as described below:

(1) TRAVEL. Employees traveling on corporate business will be reimbursed for the cost of transportation, meals, lodging, and incidentals (telephone calls, tips, laundry, and so forth). Employees will be reimbursed for the actual cost of meals, lodging, and incidentals or receive a flat per diem of ____________ ($____________) Dollars per day for each full day of travel. Rates of reimbursement of transportation costs depend upon the mode of travel, as explained below:

(a) Travel by corporate automobile. Employees traveling in an automobile owned by this corporation will be reimbursed only for out-of-pocket costs paid for servicing the vehicle (gasoline, oil, repairs, tolls, parking, and so forth).

(b) Travel by commercial carrier. Employees traveling by commercial carrier will be reimbursed for the actual fare paid by them.

(c) Travel by privately owned vehicle. Employees traveling in their personal vehicles will be reimbursed at the rate of _______ ($.____) cents per mile for authorized business travel. When two or more employees travel in the same privately owned vehicle, only one employee will be reimbursed for the cost of transportation.

(2) AUTHORIZED MEALS. Employees will be furnished or reimbursed for the cost of certain meals, as follows:

(a) Meals on the premises. Employees who are required to reside on the corporate premises, as a condition of their employment, will be furnished all meals eaten on the premises. Such meals will be furnished in kind or by reimbursement of actual costs to the employees of food brought to the premises for their consumption thereon. Other employees required to eat on the premises for the convenience of the corporation also will be furnished meals in kind or will be reimbursed for the actual cost of such meals.

(b) Supper money. Employees who work 2 or more hours overtime on any regular work day, or 4 or more hours on a Saturday, Sunday, or holiday, and who are not furnished meals on the corporate premises, will be paid supper money at the rate of _____________ ($ _____________) dollars for each such overtime period.

(c) Business Meetings. Employees may be reimbursed for the actual cost paid by them for meals at which corporate business is discussed. Such reimbursement will cover the cost of the meals of the employees as well as those of authorized guests of the corporation attending such meetings.

(3) CASH PAYMENTS. Employees who use their personal funds to make minor purchases for the corporation, or pay such items as freight bills, will be reimbursed for the actual cost of such payments. The Treasurer is authorized to maintain a petty cash fund of not more than _____________ ($ _____________) Dollars for the payment of such items.

(4) MEDICAL BENEFITS. All officer-employees and other key employees designated by the Board of Directors will be reimbursed for up to the actual cost incurred by them for medical services, hospitalization, medicine and drugs for such employees and their families, including the premiums on insurance policies which provide these benefits according to the medical and health plan adopted by the Board of Directors and attached at the end of these minutes.

(5) SICK PAY. All full-time employees will be paid at their regular rates of salary or wages during periods of illness. Termination of such payment, in the event of extended illness, will be at the discretion of the Board of Directors in each individual case.

(6) SALARIES OF EMPLOYEES. The annual, weekly, or hourly rate of pay of the employees of the corporation shall be set by the President of the corporation. The President's salary will be set by the Board of Directors by contract with the President.

The Board noted, during the course of its discussion of the reimbursement and benefits enumerated above, that other benefits should be provided to employees, but that further investigation would be required to ascertain the most desirable plans for providing the benefits. Therefore, upon motion, duly made, seconded, and carried, it was

RESOLVED, that the President hereby is authorized to contract with _______________ for plans which will provide the following insurance coverage to all present employees and to all future employees upon completion of one year of service with the corporation:

(1) Group accident, health and major medical insurance plans.
(2) Group term life insurance plans, providing up to the maximum coverage deemed necessary for each employee.
(3) Professional liability insurance.

The Chairman next presented to the Board the following contract for consideration:

WHEREAS, there has been presented to and considered by this meeting a proposed employment contract between ____ and this corporation, to employ _____________________________________ as president of the corporation; and

WHEREAS, said proposed employment contract is for a 5-year term, at the annual salary of ____ ($_____________) Dollars per year plus any bonus the Board might award;

NOW THEREFORE, BE IT RESOLVED, that the terms and conditions of the proposed employment contract presented to and considered by this meeting be and the same is hereby approved.

WHEREAS, there has been presented to and considered by this meeting a proposed employment contract between ____ and this

corporation,   to   employ ______________________________ as
secretary-treasurer of the corporation; and

WHEREAS, said proposed employment contract is for a 5-year term, at an annual salary of ____ ($____________) Dollars per year plus any bonus the Board might award;

NOW THEREFORE, BE IT RESOLVED, that the terms and conditions of the proposed employment contract presented to and considered by this meeting be and the same is hereby approved.

Upon motion duly made, seconded, and carried, it was

RESOLVED, that the Board of Directors of the corporation be, and it hereby is, authorized to issue from time to time the authorized shares of capital stock of the corporation for money paid, labor done, or personal property or real estate leases thereof actually acquired by the corporation, upon such terms as the Board of Directors in its discretion may determine.

Upon motion duly made, seconded, and carried, it was

RESOLVED, that the corporation proceed to carry on the business for which it was incorporated, and further

RESOLVED, that the signing of these minutes shall constitute full ratification thereof and waiver of notice of the meeting by the signatories.

There being no further business before the meeting, on motion duly made, seconded, and carried, the meeting was adjourned.

Dated: ______________________________

____
Chairman

____
Secretary-Treasurer

A true copy of the following papers referred to in the foregoing minutes is appended hereto:

Waiver of notice of the meeting
Certificate of Incorporation and Articles of Incorporation
By-laws
Specimen share certificates*
Resolution designating depository of funds*
Health and Accident Plan*

____
*Not included in these Appendices.

WAIVER OF NOTICE OF THE ORGANIZATION MEETING OF THE DIRECTORS OF ____

We, the undersigned, being all the directors named in the articles of incorporation of the above corporation hereby agree and consent that the organization meeting thereof be held on the date and at the time and place stated below and hereby waive all notice of such meeting and of any adjournment therefore.

Place of meeting

Date of meeting

Time of meeting

____

____

Dated:

APPENDIX 2–6
SAMPLE MINUTES—BOARD OF DIRECTORS MEETING

MINUTES OF THE ANNUAL MEETING OF THE
BOARD OF DIRECTORS OF

____

____

Date

The annual meeting of the Board of Directors of the company was held at
_______________________ . Present at the meeting and constituting a quorum of the full
board were the following persons:

The President, ____ , called the meeting to
order and presided during the meeting. ____
served as Secretary.

The minutes of the previous meeting, held on _____________________ , were
approved as read.

The President presented the following items for discussion:

—

—

—

—

After due discussion, agreement was reached regarding the move of office location to
_______________________ within the next 2 months.

The final item of business was the election of officers of the Board of Directors. The
election resulted in the following:

_______________________________   — President
_______________________________   — Secretary
_______________________________   — Vice-President

There being no further business to come before the meeting, upon motion duly made,
seconded, and unanimously carried, the meeting was adjourned.

____

Secretary

APPENDIX 2–7
MINUTES—SHAREHOLDERS MEETING, SAMPLE 1

MINUTES OF THE ANNUAL MEETING OF THE SHAREHOLDERS OF

____

The annual meeting of the shareholders was held on _____________ at _____________.
The shareholders present in person at the meeting were

Shareholder   *Shares*

The total number of shares issued and outstanding and entitled to vote being
_____________ shares, it was announced that a quorum was present for the transaction of
business.

The Chairman, _______________________________________ , called the meeting to
order and presided during the course of the meeting; _______________________________
served as secretary of the meeting. The minutes of the previous meeting, held on
_______________________ , were approved as read.

The Chairman reviewed the financial report for the previous fiscal year ending
_______________________ . The report was discussed and accepted by the shareholders. It was decided that the Sub-Chapter S election would be continued for another fiscal
year.

Additional discussion resulted in the following resolution:

RESOLVED, that the actions taken during the previous year on behalf of the Corporation by its Directors be, and they are hereby ratified and approved.

The Chairman then stated that the election of a Board of Directors was in order. The
following persons were nominated and elected to serve for the ensuing year and until their
successors have been elected and qualified:

____
____
____

There being no further business to come before the meeting, upon motion made and
seconded, and unanimously carried, the same was adjourned.

____

                                                  Secretary

APPENDIX 2–8
MINUTES—SHAREHOLDERS MEETING, SAMPLE 2

MINUTES OF THE ANNUAL MEETING OF SHAREHOLDERS OF

____

The annual meeting of the shareholders of the corporation was held at _____________ on _______________________ 19___________ at ____________ m.

The meeting was called to order by ____ , the chairman of the corporation.

The secretary then reported that the meeting had been called pursuant to a notice of meeting and/or waiver of notice thereof in accordance with the by-laws. It was ordered that a copy of the notice and waiver of notice be appended to the minutes of the meeting.

The secretary then read the role of shareholders from the stock transfer ledger. The following shareholders were present in person or by proxy:

Shareholder	Shares	In Person	By Proxy

The chairman stated that a majority of the total number of shares issued and outstanding was represented and that the meeting was complete and ready to transact any business before it. It was ordered that proxies be appended to the minutes of the meeting.

The president then gave a general report of the business and finances of the corporation and the secretary reported the following changes of shareholders since the last such report:

The chairman then stated that the election of directors of the corporation was now in order. The following were nominated as directors:

Upon vote, all of the nominated persons were then duly elected directors of the corporation to serve until the next annual meeting of shareholders or until their successors are elected and shall qualify.

There being no further business, the meeting was, on motion, adjourned.

Dated ____________________________

____
Secretary

RATIFICATION

We, the undersigned shareholders, or assignees thereof, have read these minutes and do hereby approve, ratify, and confirm all business transacted as reported herein.

____

____

The following have been appended to the minutes:
Waiver of Notice

WAIVER OF NOTICE OF THE ANNUAL MEETING OF SHAREHOLDERS

We, the undersigned shareholders, hereby agree and consent that the annual meeting of shareholders of the corporation be held on the date and at the time and place stated below for the purpose of electing directors of the corporation and the transaction thereat of all such other business as may lawfully come before said meeting and hereby waive all notice of the meeting and any adjournment thereof.

Date of meeting

Time of meeting

Place of meeting

Dated ____________________

____

APPENDIX 2–9
REGISTERED OFFICE OR AGENT CHANGE

**STATEMENT OF CHANGE OF REGISTERED OFFICE OR REGISTERED AGENT
OR BOTH BY A ___________ DOMESTIC CORPORATION**
(State)

The name of the corporation is ____
____

The address, including street and number, of its present registered office as shown in the records of the Secretary of State of the State of ___________ prior to filing this statement is ____
____
____

The address, including street and number, to which its registered office is to be changed is
____
____
____

(Give new address or state "no change")

The name of its present registered agent, as shown in the records of the Secretary of State of the State of _____________ , prior to filing this statement is ________________________
____
____

The name of its new registered agent is ______________________________________
(Give new name or state "no change")

The address of its registered office and the address of the business office of its registered agent, as changed, will be identical.

Such change was authorized by its Board of Directors.

____
President or Vice-President

Sworn to ___________
   (date)

____
Notary Public

______________________ County, _______ .

Submit two (2) copies with genuine signatures and notary seals on each. Filing fee for a business (for profit) corporation is $____________ .

APPENDIX 2–10
SALE OF STOCK

OFFER OF SALE OF STOCK
FOR

____

I, _______________________________________ , Offer to the ___________________________ ,
the total of my share of stock in the _______________________________ , with the following
terms:

1. cash purchase of $_______________ , payable at closing;

2. payment of earnest money of $______________ (______________ dollars) within five (5) calendar days of the signing of this offer (to be applied to the balance of purchase payment);

3. seller (_______) will relinquish the name of _______________________________ , and its use;

4. seller retains possession of all furniture in personal office as well as few items of private possession in use in general office (e.g., rug on waiting room wall);

5. seller and purchaser (the Corporation) divide equally all equipment, furniture, and consumables within the total office (except for letterhead, stationery, and other items bearing the name of _______________________________ which the purchaser retains);

6. seller receives all due salary through date of closing;

7. seller receives prorated share of profit from Corporation due the owners (e.g., distributions as determined by accountant's audit) for the portion of the fiscal year completed at time of closing;

8. seller and purchaser retain respective vehicles;

9. seller is released from responsibility for any expenses encumbered by the Corporation and its representatives after the closing date;

10. seller is released from lease agreement for current office space (at _______________) at the time of closing;

11. expenses encumbered by Corporation between this signing and closing date will be only those immediate and necessary for ongoing office operation and will be mutually agreed upon by seller and purchaser;

12. seller and purchaser will forfeit credit cards owned by the Corporation between this signing and closing, at which time seller permanently relinquishes such credit cards;

13. seller may privately pay seller's portion of Corporation group insurance until other insurance arrangements are made, but not to exceed three months after closing date;

14. any legal and accounting fees encumbered as a result of this transaction are the individual responsibilities of seller and of buyer;

15. closing of this transaction will occur within thirty (30) calendar days of the signing of this offer and not later than the last day of _______________________________________ .

The signing of this offer by seller and buyer represents a legally and professionally binding agreement.

___________________________   ___________________________
           seller   buyer

___________________________   ___________________________
           date   date

Projected date of closing: _______________________

APPENDIX 2-11
SAMPLES OF FORMS AND DOCUMENTS RELATING TO DISSOLUTION OF CORPORATION

_______________________________ Date

NOTICE OF EMERGENCY MEETING OF THE BOARD OF DIRECTORS OF
____

Date:
Time:
Place:

The meeting is called at the request of _______________________________________ for the purpose of discussing the immediate and equitable dissolution of the Corporation known as the _______________________________ .

LETTER TO DIRECTORS TO CALL MEETING

(LETTERHEAD)

TO: Board of Directors
RE: Notice of meeting

Please be notified that a meeting of the Board of Directors is called for _______________ , at _____________ at _________________________ . The meeting is called at the request of ____ for the purpose of discussing and voting on the operating policies of the _______________________ for the duration of the office lease at the _______________ Building.

**INSTRUCTIONS AND FORM FOR FILING ARTICLES OF DISSOLUTION
WHEN NO SHARES HAVE BEEN ISSUED
AND THE CORPORATION HAS NOT COMMENCED BUSINESS**

**ARTICLES OF DISSOLUTION
BY INCORPORATORS OR DIRECTORS
(Article 6.01)**

1. The name of the Corporation is _______________________________________
____

2. The date of issurance of its Certificate of Incorporation was _______________ .

3. None of its shares has been issued.

4. The Corporation has not commenced business.

5. The amount, if any, actually paid in on subscriptions for its shares less any part thereof disbursed for necessary expenses, has been returned to those entitled thereto.

6. No debts of the Corporation remain unpaid.

7. (Check either Statement A or Statement B below)

_______________ A majority of the Directors elect that the Corporation be dissolved.

_______________ A majority of the Incorporators elect that the Corporation be dissolved.

____
____
____
____

(Must be signed by a majority of Directors if 7A is checked, or by a majority of Incorporators if 7B is checked)

Sworn to _______________________
          (date)

____
                    Notary Public

_______________________________ County, Texas

(Notary Seal)

INSTRUCTIONS

1. Submit an executed original and a copy of the Articles of Dissolution. The documents must be signed by:

   a. A majority of the incorporators

                      or

   b. A majority of the directors

2. Attach a certificate from the Comptroller of Public Accounts indicating that all franchise taxes have been paid. The corporation should specifically request a tax certificate for purposes of Dissolution.

3. Attach the remittance for the filing fee for the Articles of Dissolution. The check should be made payable to the Secretary of State.

   Filing fee for For-Profit Corporations—$25.00

4. Return the documents to:

   Secretary of State
   Statutory Filings Division
   Corporations Section
   P.O. Box 13697
   Austin, Texas 78711-3697

NOTICE OF SPECIAL SHAREHOLDERS' MEETING TO DISSOLVE

TO ALL SHAREHOLDERS:

You are hereby notified of a special shareholders' meeting to be held at the principal office of the Corporation at _____________________ , _____________________ , on _____________ , _____________ , at _____________ .m., for the following purposes:

1. To consider and act upon the advisability of dissolving the Corporation.
2. To consider and act upon any other business that may come before the meeting.

Dated: _____________ , _____________ .

____

By: _________________________________

SHAREHOLDERS MEETING

PROPOSED ITEMS FOR SHAREHOLDER VOTE
(REGARDING DISSOLUTION)

ITEM   VOTE
                                                              (Mark "YES" or "NO")

1. The dissolution will be effective ________________________ .

2. For the duration of the lease with ____________________ ,
   the lease itself will be divided into two documents
   separating responsibility for equal rent payments and
   for separate and equal portions of space.

3. Each party shall be responsible for own expenses in the
   modification of each office space, where common walls
   are established, the cost shall be shared equally by the
   two parties.

4. Reconstruction may begin ____________________________ .

5. Notification of employees will be done by a letter
   signed by both parties on ____________________________ .

6. Employment offers may be tendered to any employee
   by either shareholder at any time following the
   notification.

7. Letter informing patients and families of the dissolution of
   the Corporation and the separation of the practices and
   the future whereabouts of each employee shall be
   prepared and dispersed to patients and families on
   ____________________________ . The letter shall be
   signed by both parties.

8. After ____________________________ :

   a. Credit cards bearing name ____________________
      will be relinquished, as will any other charge
      accounts in the name of the Corporation.

   b. The name ____________________________ will not be
      used by either party in any way, nor modified in
      any way to produce a close fascimile thereof.

   c. Checks written on Corporate account will be signed
      by both parties.

   d. All creditors will be notified of the dissolution by
      letter, signed by both parties, and will be asked for
      a final statement of the account, as of __________ .

   e. Furniture and fixtures ordinarily in the office of each
      party and considered the property of each may be
      kept by same;

   f. Income from previous patient billing (including
      ____________ through ____________) and other
      accounts receivable shall be deposited into the
      Corporate account.

   g. Letter to inform referral sources may be sent as
      signed by both parties.

h. Professional books and professional journals will be divided by the two parties at the same time and place as mutually agreed—such procedure shall continue until such previously paid subscriptions lapse.

i. Corporate records will be held by a mutually agreed-upon party for a minimum of 5 years for federal and state record retention requirements.

Name _______________________   Name _______________________

Date _______________________

SHAREHOLDERS MEETING
ITEMS FOR DISCUSSION AND DECISION

Date ________________________________

1. Method of determining relative value of furniture, fixtures, and vehicles.

2. Review of corporate records for the past 2 years to determine:
   a. Source and amount of income to Corporation by employees
   b. Source and amount of expenses to Corporation by employees
   c. Means of compensating employees for back salary which has not been paid by Corporation to employees
   d. Means of compensating employees for inequitable ratio between income production and expenditures of Corporate money
   e. Means of paying debts incurred by Corporation and its employees before and after ______________ (date on which shareholders voted to dissolve the Corporation) (e.g., outstanding expenses will be paid equally by each party and and not from Corporate banking account)
   f. Drawing of consultation money from Corporation without deducting FICA and withholding, and so forth (e.g., consultation money)

3. Means of protecting name of ________________________________ from use by anyone after the time of Corporate dissolution.

4. Amount of time for maintaining current group insurance policy and the eventual disposition of such policy.

5. Disposition of any money remaining in Corporate account at time of its closing.

6. On ________________________ , the # ____________________ will be disconnected and no longer be a working number.

7. On ________________________ , the # ____________________ will be used only for the recorded message for incoming calls.

UNANIMOUS WRITTEN CONSENT OF SHAREHOLDERS TO VOLUNTARY DISSOLUTION OF ____________________ , INC.

The undersigned shareholders of record of ____________________ , a Texas Corporation, whose shares constitute all of the issued and outstanding shares of the Corporation, hereby consent to the voluntary dissolution of the Corporation according to the following plan of dissolution:

That the Corporation is being liquidated pursuant to section 333 of the Internal Revenue Code and will distribute all of its property and assets during the calendar month of ____ ;

That all liabilities and obligations of the Corporation will be paid or discharged, or that adequate provision will be made therefore;

That, after the provision for, or the payment of, the known debts and liabilities of the Corporation, the officers of the Corporation are authorized and directed to distribute the remaining assets of the Corporation to the shareholders of record in the following manner: (1) with respect to any cash by distributing to each such shareholder of record a proportion of such cash equal to the proportion that the shares owned by such shareholder bears to the total issued and outstanding shares of this Corporation; and (2) with respect to assets other than cash, by distributing to each shareholder of record an undivided interest in each of such assets equal to the proportion that the shares of this Corporation owned by such shareholder bears to the total issued and outstanding shares of this Corporation;

That the distribution of the assets shall be made to the shareholders of this Corporation on the following conditions: (1) that on demand made by the Board of Directors, each shareholder surrender, for cancellation, the certificate or certificates evidencing her ownership of capital stock of this Corporation; and (2) that such distribution shall be in complete satisfaction of the rights of each shareholder as a shareholder of this Corporation;

That the officers of this Corporation be, and they hereby are, authorized to do such acts and to take such steps as may be necessary or convenient to carry this plan into effect, including, but not limited to, the execution of such instruments as may be required to vest title to the assets of this Corporation in the shareholders.

IN WITNESS WHEREOF, each of the undersigned shareholders of record has signed his/her name and the date of signing and the number of shares of the Corporation held by her of record on said date.

Name   *Date*   *Number of Shares*

ARTICLES OF DISSOLUTION OF
______________________________ , INC.

Pursuant to the provisions of Article ______ of the ______*(state)*______ Business Corporation Act, the undersigned corporation adopts the following Articles of Dissolution for the purpose of dissolving:

1. The name of the Corporation is ____

2. The names and addresses of its officers are:

   Name   *Office*   *Address*

3. The names and addresses of the Directors are:

   Name   *Address*

4. A written consent to dissolve, a copy of which is attached, has been signed by all shareholders of the corporation, or in their behalf by their duly authorized attorneys.

5. All debts, obligations, and liabilities of the Corporation have been paid, discharged, or adequate provision has been made therefor.

6. All remaining property and assets of the Corporation have been distributed among its shareholders in accordance with their respective rights and interests.

7. There are not suits pending against the Corporation in any court.

Dated this _____________ day of _____________ , _____________ .

By: _________________________________

By: _________________________________

STATE OF _______________
COUNTY OF _____________

Before me, the undersigned authority, on this _____________ day of _____________, 19 _____________ , personally appeared ____ , who, being by me first duly sworn, declared that he/she is the President of the above Corporation, that he/she signed the foregoing document as such officer of said Corporation, and that the statements therein are true and correct.

Notary Public in and for the state of _______
My Commission Expires: _______________

STATE OF _______________
COUNTY OF _____________

Before me, the undersigned authority, on this _____________ day of _____________, 19 _____________ , personally appeared ____ , who, being by me first duly sworn, declared that he/she is the Secretary of the above Corporation, that he/she signed the foregoing document as such officer of said Corporation, and that the statements therein are true and correct.

Notary Public in and for the state of _______
My Commission Expires: _______________

NOTICE TO CREDITORS AND CLAIMANTS
OF INTENT TO DISSOLVE

____

TO ALL CREDITORS OF AND CLAIMANTS AGAINST _______________________________ :

NOTICE IS HEREBY GIVEN that _____________________ , whose principal office is located at _____________ , _______________ , _____________ , intends to dissolve.

Dated _____________ , _______________ .

By: ____

CERTIFICATE OF MAILING OF NOTICE
OF INTENT TO DISSOLVE

____

The undersigned hereby certifies that he/she is the duly elected, qualified, and acting Secretary of _______________________ and that on _____________ , _______________ , he/she sent by registered mail, to all known creditors of and claimants against the Corporation, a notice of the intent to dissolve the Corporation, a copy of which notice is attached hereto as Exhibit A.

Dated: _____________ , _______________ .

____

ASSUMPTION OF LIABILITIES
OF

____

CORPORATION TO BE DISSOLVED

Each of the undersigned shareholders of _______________________ , a ___________
(state)
Corporation, hereby assumes and agrees to discharge the known liabilities and obligations

of the Corporation not in fact discharged or otherwise adequately provided for in the

dissolution of the Corporation, but only to the extent of the property and assets distributed

to (her/him) by the Corporation pursuant to the dissolution of the Corporation.

Name   _Date_   _Number of Shares_

RECEIPT OF DISTRIBUTION
BY SHAREHOLDERS REGARDING THEIR HOLDINGS
IN CORPORATION TO BE DISSOLVED

In complete satisfaction of the rights of each of the undersigned as shareholders in
_______________________ , a ____(state)____ Corporation, and in consideration of
their assumption of the Corporation's liabilities (to the extent of the property received by
each of them pursuant to the dissolution of the Corporation), the undersigned, constituting
all of the shareholders of the Corporation, hereby acknowledge receipt of all of the right,
title, and interest of the Corporation in and to all of its property, both real and personal,
tangible and intangible, whether known or unknown, in dissolution of the Corporation.

Dated: _____________________ , _________ .

____

____

Executed on _____________________ , _____________ , at _____________ ,

_____________ County, _____________ .

By: _________________________________
                     Shareholder

By: _________________________________
                     Shareholder

Chapter 3

Financial Considerations

Before planning for financial needs at the office, plan for them at home. You will need enough money to support yourself and your family for at least 18 months without expecting any profit from your practice. Opening a new practice or modifying an old one costs a lot of money without any immediate financial return; the demise is slow but certain if you cannot sustain the practice until it begins to pay for itself. Foonberg (1984), a successful attorney in private practice, states that a beginning practitioner should have some combination of the following sources of income:

1. A year's* living expenses in a savings account;
2. A working spouse with enough income to support the family for one year;
3. A bank loan for the funds to live on for a year (very difficult to get without cosigner or other kind of guarantor);
4. Wealthy parents, in-law, or other to
   a. lend the money
   b. give the money
   c. guarantee the bank loan

It is easier to anticipate living expenses than to plan capitalization for opening and operating a new practice. Nevertheless, you must try. Disregarding the obvious fact that you do not *know* the answers, begin to develop an operating plan for the practice by asking yourself the following questions. It is from a consideration of the issues listed below that the goals and plans for your practice will evolve.

1. What population of clients will you serve? Age? Type of disorder? Socio-economic level?

---

*Attorneys and some other professionals advise initial financial budgeting for a 1-year period. It has been my observation from my own practices and those of my colleagues that 8 to 18 months is a more realistic time frame.

2. Do you intend to work alone?
3. If you intend to eventually bring a colleague into the practice with you, do you want partners? Employees? Independent consultants?
4. Will you see groups and individuals? How large is the largest size group? How old is the largest size group?
5. Will you be spending most of your working day in the office? Will you be doing out-of-the office contracting?
6. Will you work at night? Weekends?
7. What percentage of time per week are you willing to spend in direct client contact?
8. What kind of payment will you accept from clients? Direct pay? Public insurance? Private insurance?
9. Will you bill monthly or require pay per session?
10. How will you notify the public and professionals and other referral sources of your practice?
11. What kind of insurance do you need personally and professionally for the practice?
12. Is office location crucial?
13. What kind of space and how much will you need for the office, including secretarial space, office/therapy rooms, waiting rooms?
14. What kind of files and record-keeping system will you use?
15. What special consultants will you need? Accountant? Attorney? Insurance? Computer?
16. What furniture will you need for the first 3 years?
17. What equipment will you need for the first 3 years?
18. What supplies will you need for the first year? Therapy materials? Consumables? Stationery?
19. What amount of money are you prepared to borrow? For what duration? How will you pay it back?
20. Do you want or need a secretary or clerk? An answering service or machine?

As you begin to conceptualize your practice and your professional objectives, you may spend more time than you prefer with the issues of money and management.

The biggest money/management mistake made by professionals is to expect that revenue from the practice in the first year (or two) will finance the operations. Do not forget how far in debt you may be, how many clients forget to pay their bills, and how many unexpected expenses will be encountered. Experienced private practitioners who move or expand their businesses do not necessarily encounter these same monetary problems. Most of their clientele are established and waiting for a change to occur so that services may resume.

As you visualize your practice, begin to project operating costs on a monthly basis (see Table 3–1).

As monthly item costs are specified, you will develop a better understanding of the amount of money you need to borrow to capitalize your operations for the first year. One item to include in the monthly item and expense lists is the cost of the borrowed money (i.e., interest). Other easily forgotten items are property and sales taxes, withholding deposits, workers compensation, and payroll taxes. Mon-

Table 3–1. Estimates of Operating Costs for Private Practices

Item	Cost per month
Equipment/maintenance	$ _______
ordinary	_______
special	_______
Supplies/materials	_______
ordinary	_______
special	_______
Files/records	_______
Furniture	_______
Space/rent	_______
Janitor/maintenance	_______
Utilities	_______
Remodeling	_______
repairs/improvements	_______
Telephone	_______
Announcements	_______
advertisements	_______
other	_______
Stationery/business cards	_______
Postage	_______
Dues/subscriptions	_______
Automobile	_______
transportation	_______
maintenance	_______
Personnel	_______
Insurance	_______
office	_______
personnel	_______
automobile	_______
other	_______
Answering service/recorder	_______
Legal and accounting fees	_______
other consultation fees	_______
Working capital	_______

ies should be set aside as part of the payroll for quarterly payroll taxes. Failure to make withholding deposits is a criminal act.

You now have one half of the data necessary for the development of a profit and loss projection for your practice. A profit and loss projection shows operating expenses, item by item, that are subtracted from a reasonable estimate of the month's gross revenue. A reasonable estimate of revenue can be drawn from predictions of client services. However, such an estimate is difficult-to-impossible to make prior to establishing your practice. So many variables affect one's practice—from political climate to time of year—that an educated guess must be made by the new practitioner. My suggestion is to find colleagues in practices similar to the one you are planning. Ask them for a monthly average of clients per clinician. To make a ballpark estimate of revenue, take one-third of that number for the first 3 months of your practice and one half of that number for the second 3 months.

You are almost ready to begin talking with an accountant and legal advisor. First, however, you may want to avoid embarrassment and save time by being familiar with the terminology used in discussing financial operations. I guarantee that if your accountant suspects your unfamiliarity with the vernacular of the business world, he/she will become your devoted tutor on the subject (at a nominal fee per hour, of course).

What follows is a very basic introduction to the terminology used to discuss money and its management:

accounting: a system of maintaining a record of monetary events.

accounts receivable: money owed you for work done. Until you send a bill, you do not have an account receivable (Foonberg, 1984).

accrual concept of accounting: net income is measured as difference between revenues and expenses rather than between cash receipts and expenditures.

asset: property owned by a business that is valuable because it can or will be converted into cash. Possibly it could benefit future operations, and it was acquired at a measurable cost.

audit: review of accounting records by independent (outside) accountants.

balance sheet: lists what the practice owns, less its debts, which equals its net worth. Sometimes it is called a financial statement. When used with cash flow projections, it can chart progress of the practice and its financial status.

bill: the document sent to first inform clients that the work is done and payment is now due.

billing: the process of preparing and sending a bill.

capital expenditures budget: listing of planned purchases and items for operation.

cash flow projection: a forecast of actual cash surplus or deficit for each period. The cash flow statement subtracts bills paid by the office from cash actually collected. (Profit and loss statement shows payments due, but not necessarily received.) Projected cash flow usually includes:
- cash on hand
- money collected from patients
- money from loans and payable to notes (principal, interest)
- cash disbursements (money needed to live on)
- payroll and withholding taxes (11.7% social security; state and federal income taxes; unemployment tax, disability tax withheld from employee)
- amount due purchase of business (if applicable)
- operating expenses (rent, utilities, etc.)
- cash flow monthly—difference between total cash available and total disbursements for each month represents a positive flow.

cost concept of accounting: accounting values the resources of a business at cost rather than market value.

credit entry: (in a journal or ledger sheet) the record of a decrease in any asset account; the record of an increase in an equity account.

debit entry: (left hand entry) record of an increase in any asset account; the record of a decrease in an equity account.

depreciation: portions of the cost of an asset (i.e., an audiometer) charged off to expenses according to a predetermined plan. The entire cost can be written off (deducted from taxes) as a one-time expense at the time of purchase, or the life of the asset is determined and the expense is charged off over the expected life of that asset. In other words, each year, only that portion of the asset by which value is expected to decline for that year is deducted from taxes as an expense. A replacement fund can also be established that runs parallel to the depreciation period so that a new asset (another audiometer) can be funded when the life of the old one expires.

depreciation rate: the percentage of original cost charged off in a year.

dividend: portion of profits distributed to stockholders.

equities: claims against assets by owners or creditors.

expenditure: payment for an asset.

expense: a decrease in owners' equity resulting from the operation of the business.

income statement: a record of profit and loss in a given period. Net income is the difference between revenues and expenses (not between cash receipts and expenditures). This term is used in conjunction with the accrual concept of accounting.

journal: chronological recording of transactions (an accounting log).

ledger: transactions are transferred (posted) from the journal to the ledger(s) for categorizing and totaling transactions.

liability, current: usually a monetary obligation which becomes due within a certain time period (one year, 90 days, etc.).

liquidity: the formula for determining liquidity of a business (basically what you are worth if you have to sell-and-run) is:

$$\frac{\textbf{cash + marketable securities + accounts receivable}}{\textbf{current liabilities}}$$

mortgage: a pledge of real estate as security for a loan.

note receivable: debts that are evidenced by a note or other written acknowledgment.

overhead rate: method of allocating overhead to various products manufactured or services rendered (what you pay to keep operating).

posting: transfer of an entry from the journal to a ledger account.

profit and loss projection: shows operating expenses as well as inventory purchases for a period of time (i.e., month, quarter) and subtracts that from an estimate of the time period's gross revenue. This is used for determining whether the management and financing are appropriate. In other words, if the profit and loss sheet shows a loss, it is a signal for increased revenue, tighter management, and so forth. If the profit and loss projection shows a profit, it is an indicator of adequate financing and profitable operations.

proprietor: the owner of an unincorporated business.

realization: the time at which a service is rendered or a product is delivered.

statement: the document sent after the first bill, informing the client that all or part of the money asked for on the first bill is still due (Foonberg, 1984).

stockholder: an owner of an incorporated business, the ownership being evidenced by stock certificates.

The accountant will help you understand tax implications of various forms of organizational structure. You may also want to discuss this matter with a small business tax specialist or attorney. When you have made the decision about the structure your practice will take, the accountant will set up an appropriate accounting system for you. The most commonly chosen fiscal year is July 1 to June 30. You may pay one of the accountant's bookkeepers to help your secretary learn the accounting and bookkeeping system. You will probably want the accountant to keep close watch on your books during the initial period of your practice. This will allow early modifications to be made and errors to be corrected.

Your accountant will be able to advise your bookkeeper or secretary about methods useful for maintaining an accurate record of accounting and payment periods as well as procedures for recording expenditures in proper categories (see Appendix 3–3).

Do not become immobilized by your financial records. You *do not* have to learn how to keep books. You *do* have to know enough to use the information given by your accountant and bookkeeper. You will make financial decisions; they will help you keep track of those transactions that are based on your decisions.

Now you are ready to go to the bank.

BORROWING

If you have never borrowed money before and have no credit history,
If you have only a few credit cards—all of which are charged beyond their limit,
If you have always used cash for purchases and have no credit record,
If you are a single female,
If you do not have a rich relative or friend who would like a tax write-off by loaning you start-up money,
Then, don't quit your job yet.

I know someone who did that, on her way to the bank, to get an unsecured loan for operating expenses to open a private practice. The good news is that I got the loan, and 20 years later I am still in private practice. The bad news is that my loan officer was fired the week after he approved my loan.

How to Apply for a Loan

Obviously, 20 years ago it was possible to blunder into a bank with no collateral and walk away with a small loan. It may still be possible, but there are ways to prepare for requesting a loan that will increase one's chances of having that request approved. A loan officer will want to know the following things as the initial step in considering your loan request:

1. Personal financial information (a financial statement completed on a form that will be provided by the bank);
2. Evidence of security or collateral for the loan, such as certificates of deposit, mortgage, stocks, savings, and so forth. (This is particularly important for first-time borrowers who have no positive credit or loan history);
3. Evidence of experience in the profession (take a copy of your resume);
4. History and some level of opinion and marketing needs statement regarding the initiation of such a professional service in the community (they will want to know how the practice will survive, and what makes you think you can make a go of it);
5. Your willingness to transfer all of your personal and business banking to their bank;
6. How you will charge fees, how you will manage your cash flow and creditors, what time-line you are projecting for the break-even point;
7. The size and duration of the loan;
8. What plans you have for paying back the loan if the practice fails.

Be prepared for questions about your prospective practice and about your own professional and management acumen by having the following available (see ''Loan Package'' in Appendix 3–7, this chapter):

1. A business plan with a cover letter (see Appendix 3–6, this chapter);
2. Information on your business structure (sole proprietorship, etc.);
3. Fee schedule, projected cash flow for one year, and projected profit and loss statement;
4. Formal or informal market analysis (competition, need, etc.);
5. Plan for public relations and referral sources;
6. Sources of fee payments (private pay, Medicare, insurance, etc.);
7. Office plan with space, furnishings, equipment;
8. Names of accountant and attorney;
9. Outline of accounting plan;
10. Personal tax returns for past 2 years;
11. Copy of any previous loans made to you (especially ones you have paid off).

Loan approval will depend on the loan committee's decision about *you*. Therefore, your *self-presentation* is as important as your presentation of information. After your presentation to the loan officer, he/she should be able to discuss your profession and your proposed practice knowledgeably with the loan committee. He/she should also be able to vouch for your personal integrity. Your presentation to the loan officer should establish: your professional knowledge, the community's need for your services, sources of money available to pay your fees, your ability to manage money in your practice, and your ability to repay the loan regardless of the success of your practice. It is usually advisable to take out term life insurance to guarantee loan repayment in the event of your death. Some banks may even require it.

The term of the loan and the amount of unsecured money requested will affect your chances for approval. Banks have to spend less time and labor in arranging short-term commercial loans than in arranging formal long-term loans. Banks also consider the risk involved in making the loan. The longer the loan term requested and the higher the amount of the loan request, the greater the bank's risk.

Cost of the Loan

Cost of the loan—the interest charged for the privilege of using someone else's money—will depend upon the prime interest rate (the rate charged borrowers in good standing who borrow $1,000,000 or more) and upon the number of points (interest rate points) above the prime rate that the bank decides to charge you. The bank may give you a choice of the following ways to determine the cost of your loan:

1. *Floating Rate.* This rate is based on the prime rate. The borrower is charged prime plus X percentage points. As prime changes according to various national economic indices, so does the borrower's rate.
2. *Fixed Rate.* The borrower's loan rate is fixed at a certain rate above prime and does not vary, regardless of the fluxuations of the prime rate.

For example, at the time of this writing, prime rate is 9.5 percent. Many banks are charging 14 to 14.5 percent for short-term (6-month loans) of a small amount (under $20,000). This is a fixed interest rate. Regardless of whether prime rises to 12 percent or drops to 6 percent, the interest rate for that particular loan will remain the same throughout the life of the loan. If you feel psychic and have confidence that the prime rate will drop, when or if you are given the choice, you might elect to take a floating rate (e.g., prime plus 2 points). Should the prime rate drop to 8 percent, the interest rate on your loan would fall to 10 percent. However, should the prime rate jump to 20 percent, your interest rate would be increased to 22 percent. (This did happen in the early 1980s, if you recall.)

When obtaining a loan tied to the prime rate, it is important, where possible, to establish floors and ceilings for the loan. A *floor* guarantees the bank that your interest rate will never fall *below* a certain rate, regardless of how low the prime rate falls. Similarly, a *ceiling* protects the borrower from having to pay interest *above* a certain rate, no matter how high prime may become.

Cash or Credit

An important consideration in obtaining a loan is the form in which you take the loan. Although it may be very difficult to estimate how much money you will need for the next year or two, you may decide that you should apply for more credit approval than your current projection indicates in case you need more. You may request all in cash at the outset; or, you may try to secure approval for a specified line of credit. With the latter, you withdraw only that portion in cash that is necessary to meet current expenses (and only pay interest on the cash taken), leaving the remaining approved credit untapped until you need it. In that way, you do not have to pay interest on money you may not need. Do not ask for cash; ask for a credit line. This gives you the flexibility to decide how and when to draw upon that credit.

Early Payback

Request a loan that carries no penalties (additional charges) for early pay-off of the principle. Many notes (documents describing the terms of a loan) do not allow early pay-off; that is, the note must be paid as originally agreed upon with the interest rate on a predetermined payment schedule (e.g., $500/month for 36 months). Through this type of note, the bank will continue to receive your payment, which includes a sizeable interest portion, for a predictable period of time. The longer you pay interest, however, the more money the loan costs. By securing a loan that allows early pay-off, you can save money in case you do not need the money as long as you originally projected. The interest payable on loans is tax deductible, but the tax savings are usually not as great as the interest savings obtained from early pay-off. There are exceptions to this early payback rule, of course. If you happened to have 7.5 percent fixed mortgage rate against your office purchase over 25 years, it would not pay you to spend money to pay-off that note.

Payback Schedule

Ask the loan agent for an amortization schedule, which is a payoff schedule reflecting each month's payments throughout the term of the loan. This schedule describes exactly how much money will go toward paying off the principal and how much goes toward the interest. Taxes are shown when appropriate, such as with office or land purchases. At the end of the tax year, you will have the information necessary for your accountant to use to prepare your income tax. An amortization schedule also illustrates graphically exactly how much the loan is costing you. This can be a great motivation for collecting fees from your clients.

Bank Hopping

It is possible that, when a fixed rate loan is obtained, interest rates will drop rapidly. If the bank will not let you refinance the loan unless you pay off a portion of the principal, consider obtaining a short-term loan for a small amount from another loan agent ($2,000 for 90 days). Pay off some of the principal on the original note, and refinance it at a lower rate of interest. If necessary, use some of the money from refinanced loan No. 1 to pay off loan No. 2 within the same time period. You have now established credit at two banks and have two banking relationships for future needs. Of course, the illogical possibilities of this sort of caper are endless and can be dangerous. If it seems advisable, do it with integrity and keep track of what you are doing.

Your Banker

Good credit derives from paying notes in a timely manner *and* from maintaining good contact with your loan officer. Even when you do not need money at the moment, give your loan officer a call to mention that things are going well. There is no substitute for honest, direct, and personal contact, especially in the business world.

The trend in many banks now is to promote women bankers as the banking agents for businesswomen. If, as a female practitioner, you are invited to change affiliation from a male to a female loan representative of the bank, be careful. Do not impulsively give up a contact with a loan officer who knows you and who has obtained loan approval for you. Be sure that the unknown loan officer has as much seniority and influence with the loan committee as your current loan officer. Do not leave a position of advantage for a political reason that may be irrelevant to your banking needs.

Other Loan Agencies

Because of the competition between banks and savings-and-loan agencies that was created by changing federal regulations, it is possible to negotiate with banks and savings-and-loan companies to find the best possible deal for your financial position. Some things to look for include the following:

1. Find a banker or savings-and-loan representative who will cover some of your inadvertent overdrafts (from time to time), without sending then back to the depositor marked ''insufficient funds'';
2. Investigate the possibility of free check printing or reduced charges for check printing;
3. Seek preferential treatment from various departments of the bank or savings-and-loan regarding consideration of personal and professional loans;
4. Select a banker who will provide relative ease for obtaining short-term notes on signature only for operating expenses during moves or other times of temporary low income when your collateral is otherwise obligated;
5. Select a bank that makes no service charge on various accounts.

Government agencies also are involved in loaning money to small businesses or business people. Two agencies that provide such possibilities include the following:

1. The Small Business Administration (SBA) is a federally funded program that sets modest loan ceilings and provides its clients with some management assistance. Small Business Administration loan procedures are complex and requirements are stringent, taking several months to qualify.
2. The Farmers Home Administration (FHA) makes term loans to small businesses in rural areas (where cows outnumber people), when the applicant is unable to get funds from another source. The FHA application is even more extensive than the SBA procedures and requires extensive impact study of the proposed business, description of the jobs to be created, and other information.

Foonberg (1984) suggests getting a rich friend or relative to finance the start-up costs by offering them tax advantages in the following manner:

1. You select furniture and equipment; list prices for which the equipment can be obtained.
2. Give the list to friends and relatives.
3. Have the friend or relative buy the equipment in his/her name and deliver it to you.
4. Have the friend or relative lease the equipment to you (*with a lawyer drafting the lease*).
5. The friend or relative can receive the following advantages:
   a. investment credit tax benefits
   b. depreciation expense benefits (technically, cost recovery)
   c. interest deduction if he/she borrows the money
   d. the ability to claim he/she is in the equipment leasing business or to deduct appropriate expenses

FEES

One of the most difficult tasks of entering private practice for the first time is fee setting. Even more difficult is discussing fees with clients and asking for payment when that becomes necessary. Setting appropriate fees and collecting past due accounts is a technique that can take several years to develop. The new practitioner should remember that people believe that they get the value they pay for; if services are free, then their value is zero.

It is important to remember you own bankers' and creditors' expectations regarding your obligations to them, when you are considering clients who owe you money, or who ask you for reduced or deferred fees. Some clients will expect professionals to act as a form of friendly home bank, extending interest-free credit when requested. Unless you have been able to secure interest-free loans yourself, it will be difficult for you to extend such terms to your clients.

When discussing overdue payments with clients, it is important to be direct and honest in stating that you do not have the cash to extend credit to them and that, in fact, you frequently must borrow in order to continue your own professional/personal pursuits. If the practitioner does not feel that his/her services are sufficiently significant to a client for that client to borrow money or defer purchases in order to secure services, then the practitioner should consider the ethics of serving that person at all. If the services are not considered by the professional, as well as by the client and family, to be one of the most important investments for that person, then the services should not be offered.

A clinician in any setting should not be afraid of making money; money is the vehicle through which service delivery can be maintained. If the practice fails after the first year, or as soon as the loan runs out, clients will be without services. Those clients would have been the foundation of the practice and a source for its growth. If a practice closes and reopens later, the clients may be wary of making a commitment for the second time. The practitioner who does not succeed on his/her first attempt probably will not succeed on a second attempt (Foonberg, 1984).

Fee-for-service is not only necessary for maintaining a bank balance, but it also serves as one component of the professional interaction with the client. Payment of fees is a representation of clients' recognition and acceptance of their own responsibilities in the intervention process. Without enforcement of that tangible responsibility, clients' other responsibilities in the interaction are lessened by implication as well as by action.

Society has the obligation to provide health and certain allied health services to those who need them but are unable to afford them. Professionals who provide those services, share those obligations. There are some people—among them speech-language pathologists and audiologists—who believe that professionals should bear this responsibility alone. The professional who feels the obligation to single-handedly provide free services to society should not go into private practice unless he/she is independently wealthy and looking for a worthy charity or is subsidized totally by some organization or group. Reasonable fees must be charged to clients and collected in all appropriate situations for services rendered in private practice. By definition and by function, if one works for him/herself, the venture is private and the support is private—hence the terms *self-supporting* and *private enterprise*. If one works for the public, for society, that person is supported by public funds. Many publicly supported programs employ professionals as service providers for persons who cannot or choose not to pay for private care. If a person is able and wants to choose private care, then that person must not expect help from society or the provider in paying for the services. Those who are unable to pay for services should have services available to them through publicly and privately endowed programs; it is toward these ends that professional associations should advocate.

Professionals in (re)habilitation services must apply different criteria for fee setting than many other professionals whose work is done ''by the job.'' Surgeons, for example, do not charge by the hour but rather by the service (one cataract operation: $__,000). The same principle is true for most physicians, architects, and engineers whose services usually are one-time assignments and are relatively short term. By contrast, many specialists in communication disorders do not find it at all unusual to begin working with a 2 or 3 year old and continue working with that child for 10 or 15 years. In one sense, we take the child ''to raise''; in some instances, we also take the family to raise. A few other professionals, such as psychologists and psychiatrists, face analogous situations for long-term care.

As D'Asaro (1971) pointed out, some of the conflict regarding fees in our profession has come from the large numbers of clinicians who supplement their income by moonlighting. By working in their homes or client's homes, their overhead is negligible; cost accounting, marketing, and bank loans are usually unnecessary. Fees often are a fraction of those charged by full-time, private practitioners who must derive total income and fringe benefits from fees alone. However, the reliability of the moonlighters' services, as well as their availability over the long term, is unpredictable.

With few exceptions, the fee for direct delivery of services is the only source of income for the private practitioner. Attorneys demand and receive retainers for a future time when their services may be needed. No one retains a communication specialist because no one really knows why they might need one until they do. Everyone has been sick or injured to one degree or another and has an idea of how devastating a major illness or accident could be; thus, the success of health and life insurance companies. Attorneys receive substantial bonuses, or bill their clients over-and-above the agreed-upon fee when they accomplish unusually good results. When someone talks better or hears better, however, it usually is assumed to be part of the natural order of things. The communication specialist is merely one of the influences and rarely is credited for being the central figure who might deserve hard-earned fees. This nightmarish fact fits in rather nicely with the professional preparation many of us received. We learned that *good*, well-intentioned communication specialists did not take advantage of clients by taking money from those who had already suffered so much. Enough reward was to be found in exhausting all personal and professional resources to help the communicatively impaired. This same self-righteous, but unrealistic attitude has been responsible for many of the injustices our profession has suffered—not the least of which have been poor self-image, poor public image, and low-reimbursement rates from funding sources. Little wonder more of our profession have not sought the harsh realities of private practice.

Initial Agreement

The practitioner must establish an agreement with the client and/or family about fees and payment schedule. The owner/practitioner should handle all issues regarding direct payment from the client; other office personnel can deal with insurance companies. Money that insurance companies owe the client is an arrangement between the client and the insurance company; it is *not* the concern of the practitioner, except in whatever way the practitioner can facilitate reimbursement from the insurance company to the client.

Agreement regarding charges for services and payment schedule should occur before any services are rendered. The practitioner should be specific, receive verbal confirmation from the client (parent, or spouse, when appropriate), and have the written agreement signed by clients before they leave the office. Misunderstandings regarding fees are common with new clinicians because of their negligence in putting the fee agreement in writing. At the same time as fees are arranged, the client and family should be informed of other policies regarding the practice.

Setting Fees

One of the most important considerations for the new practitioner is to set fees high enough at the beginning. It is much more difficult to raise fees than it is to set an initial fee that may be adequate for at least two years. It is usually better to establish a standard fee with no preannounced exceptions. If you think you may want to make exceptions in certain instances, you should clearly define in advance the types of exceptions you will make, the percentage of low-pay or partial-pay clients you expect to carry at one time, without jeopardizing your practice, and the lowest amount you will accept from any client. Exceptions to the full-and-timely payment policy may relate to the following:

1. **Client Finances:**
   a. Be certain you know how many low-paying clients you can carry at once;
   b. Extract other kinds of obligations from the low-paying client, such as homework assignments, independent work, timely payment of the special fee (i.e., $1.00 cash before any session) in order to maintain a bond of commitment.
2. **Third-Party Payment:**
   Be careful about promising your clients that you will wait for payment until they receive notice from their insurance companies. You may end up offering several months of services for which you will never collect, creating a client who has become dependent on you for services.
3. **Mid-Therapy Increases:**
   a. Whenever you increase your fees, you will find that you have quite a few reliable clients who have been with you since your fees were lower and will continue to see you in the future.
   b. You may decide to increase fees with new clients only and maintain the old fee schedule with long-term clients.

Numerous factors influence the development of a fee schedule, including the following:

1. What services cost, including direct and indirect costs (see Chapter 9)
2. Factors not usually built into cost analysis, such as
   - the 5- or 10-minute conferences in the waiting room after the session
   - the necessary phone calls and reports to parents, insurance companies, physicians, teachers, tutors
   - consultation with colleagues about a particular aspect of intervention or assessment
   - continuing education, formal or informal, to remain current with regard to various clients and their communication disorders
   - clients who do not pay at all, who pay partial fee, or who defer payment (all with your permission, of course)
   - clients who leave without paying their bills or leave bad checks
   - clients who do not show up for appointments
   - a margin of profit above the direct and indirect cost factors
     The practitioner must remember that much time is spent in indirect patient services; unless this is built into the fee schedule, either as part of the hourly rate or as additional charges, the hourly fee that one receives per patient is greatly reduced.
3. What the market will bear (i.e., the economic area served, the sources of funding)
4. What other professionals charge within the same region
5. What skilled workers and tradesmen charge in the community
6. What other communication disorder specialists within the same community charge (ask them directly, have someone call)
7. Cost of living increases and other economic factors
8. What third party payers pay as maximum payment

As one performs a cost analysis every year, it is important to reflect future costs. Analyzing the past fiscal year and adding a correction factor for the coming year is one way of predicting future costs. A source of information is the *Cost of Living Index* of the Bureau of Labor Statistics. Regional information can be obtained relative to geographic and socioeconomic populations.

It does not take many years of cost analysis and prediction of future costs to show most practitioners that initial costs are widely underestimated and fees are too low. After an initial adjustment in fees, which most new practitioners have to make, changes in the fee structure do not have to be made more than every 2 or 3 years. Fee schedules usually follow the economy, with adjustments for inflation as well as recession.

Some practitioners find that they are eligible for certain private grants, or that they are recipients of private endowments, gifts, or contributions. Some philanthropic organizations donate or contribute money, or use a practice as the site of their philanthropic projects for a year or two. In these circumstances, it may be possible to establish a sliding fee schedule or a scholarship program for certain clients who qualify on the basis of financial need. The resulting fee adjustment should be based on a detailed cost analysis of services that are provided on a low-fee basis. Only through such an analysis can a practice determine the amount of fee reduction and the number of clients to which contributions can be applied (ASHA, 1985).

Even though costs may be predictable, income from fees varies with the seasons, vacation time and holidays, the economy, political situation, and the health of clinicians who are earning the fees. For all of the reasons cited here, and many others not elaborated at this time, it is usually a good rule of thumb to charge 30 or 35 percent more for services than would be indicated by cost analysis.

Flower (1984) describes four different approaches to establishing fee schedules: unit of service approach, functional approach, relative value approach, and pragmatic approach.

1. **Unit of Service.** This approach assumes that the time expended in providing a service is the primary determinant of the fee. Each block of time in direct client contact is assigned a unit value; 30 minutes of intervention = 1 unit; 1 hour = 2 units, and so forth. Fees are assigned on the basis of units per client.
2. **Functional Approach.** This approach bases fees on estimates of actual costs of providing each particular service. It requires more elaborate cost-analysis procedures than the unit of service approach.
3. **Relative Value Approach.** In this approach units are established that are converted into fees. One service is selected as the basis for computation. That service is usually chosen as the basis because of the frequency of its use by clients and because of its small demand for special equipment, materials, and staff. Annual schedules are analyzed for each procedure's frequency; frequencies are then converted according to assigned values and a total is computed. Relative value scales often state or imply ordinary or average length of time for a procedure or service; for example, 2 years, 200 sessions for X disorder. It should be noted that several professional associations, among them the American Speech-Language-Hearing Association, have attempted to design relative value scales.

The Federal Trade Commission (FTC) has ruled that such scales are illegal, when imposed on any practitioner by any group, because the scales suggest price fixing and imply restraint of trade. Flower (1984, p. 225) points out that there are growing pressures to exclude professional practices from the purview of FTC regulations.

4. **Pragmatic Approach.** This is an approach that apparently concedes to environmental and operational factors other than rigid adherence to systematic application of cost accounting principles. Some factors included are what other professionals charge, how long the service continues (duration), and third-party coverage.

Who Sets the Fees?

The practitioner should guard against conveying to clients the impression that fees are related to third-party coverage of services. Because most practitioners offer to help clients with insurance claims, clients tend to assume that the originally quoted fee schedule is dependent upon insurance coverage. When some clients find that insurance will not cover fees charged, they refuse to pay the total fee or pay only that portion that is not covered by insurance. The statement of operating policies that is given to clients should clearly indicate that fee arrangements are between the practitioner and client, that they are not related to insurance coverage, and that they are the total responsibility of the client.

If the practitioner is not protective of his/her right to set fees, it will take little time for fee schedules to be determined by third-party payers and clients. Fee schedules are set by the practitioner, not by a third party. Third-party payers usually set a maximum amount of coverage for any service included in its policy; sometimes the policy owner does not understand that charges for services may not approximate insurance coverage.

It is more difficult than it appears to retain complete fee-setting control. Sometimes the practitioner feels honor-bound to continue services, regardless of pay received or promises made that are not followed by actual payments. This situation is different from that in which the practitioner has decided to make an exception to the fee schedule for a particular client.

Foonberg (1984) notes that attorneys usually find that clients who fuss about paying a retainer will be the same clients who fuss about paying the bill after the work is done. It may be appropriate to harbor suspicions about the client who complains about fees for the initial interview or screening. In all likelihood, that client will be the same one who will not pay until insurance coverage is established, will not pay any charges not covered by the insurance policy, or will refuse to pay when charged for missing an uncancelled session. When warning signs appear, take special care that the client is clear about charges, billing schedule, and any late payment charges incurred. If the warning signs seem particularly strong with any individual client, establish a pay-each-visit policy with him/her. This policy is cumbersome if used with all clients, but it serves to protect the practitioner from a no-pay encounter.

Policies Involving Payment

In many practices, clients are charged for failing to attend a scheduled session without cancelling the session in advance. Typically, 24-hours advance notice is required for cancellations. Exceptions are made for sudden illness and other emergencies, but such a policy tends to reduce the frequency with which some clients leave a practitioner with an unexpected empty hour in the middle of a long day. Another reason for an advance cancellation policy is to strengthen the client's commitment to the intervention process. Attendance and payment of fees are part of the client's responsibility for the therapeutic interaction and are not to be taken lightly nor honored only when convenient.

Another aspect of the client's payment responsibility is the *timely* payment of charges for services rendered. If a client does not pay charges within a certain time period after receiving a statement and bill for charges, the client can be charged an additional amount. For example, a late charge of 5 percent can be added to the total bill when payment is 1-month overdue; when a bill becomes 2-months overdue, a 10 percent charge can be added; at the end of the third month without payment, a notice can be sent to the client or family (via registered mail) indicating that legal action will be pursued unless full payment is made within 10 to 20 days. After the time period has elapsed with no payment forthcoming, a letter may be sent stating that legal action will be pursued. At that point, the account can be automatically filed through civil court and legal action begun (see Appendix 3–8). Frequently, the final letter from the practitioner, or the letter from the court indicating that such processes have been undertaken, is enough to bring about payment. It has been my experience that this format is more effective and provides the professional a better alternative for collecting fees than a collection agency. Rarely is the delinquent payment, less charges from the collection agency, worth the hostility and subsequent bad public relations that can result from aggressive bill collectors' attempts to collect from a former client.

Cash Payments

It has been the temptation of more than one practitioner who was paid in cash to pretend that charges were never made and payment never received. This temptation can be unbearable when the client says, ''I never keep records anyway, I don't want to bother with a check.''

In this day of professional liability suits, blackmail, accusations, and frequent audits by IRS, this temptation to pocket cash payments should be considered carefully. The best advice is to count the cash in front of another person (i.e., a secretary); give the client a receipt, keeping a carbon copy; and put the cash entry into deposit records, accounts-paid column, and/or any other appropriate record. Economic honesty at this basic level is just as important to a sound practice as professional integrity.

When You Must Decide Between the Money and the Client

When you feel that you must choose between doing the work and not getting paid and not doing work and not getting paid, what do you choose (Foonberg, 1984)?

A client who withholds payment deliberately is also a client or family who will not participate completely in the mutual responsibility of the therapeutic process. It is not an unusual occurrence for a client who has complained about fees and never paid for services to disappear without notice after months of free professional help. It is not unusual for that same client to turn up in a colleague's office at some later point, shouting the evils of your practice and your integrity (usually related to your obvious greed).

A serious and responsible client and family will pay their bills, negotiate payment deferrals when necessary, and adhere to professional advice. These are the clients and families who deserve your efforts—not just because of their fiscal responsibility, but because that level of responsibility is usually a sign of commitment to the professional interaction and a willingness to persist in good faith with the clinician.

Barter

There is a possible alternative in situations of financial hardship where the clinician cannot refuse services. Rappoport (1983) advocates barter as a viable means for a client to participate in the therapeutic relationship while contributing services or goods of value to the therapist. Barter may take many forms, limited only by the abilities of the clients and needs of the therapists. Rappoport stresses that the value placed on barter must be a realistic value and genuinely needed or desired by the clinician.

Application of barter to a practice will not fit every situation, but its possibility offers clients and practitioners increased options for service delivery and payment. The approach, when used appropriately, appears to be in line with good ethical practice.

Group Rates Versus Individual Rates

Some practitioners establish fee schedules that differentiate between group and individual fees. Sometimes group rates are 15 to 20 percent lower than individual fees. The argument for lower fees for persons in groups is that less revenue is needed from each person in a group-hour than from each person in an individual-hour session. Reduction of fees for groups seems to have several effects upon clients, as well as upon bookkeeping processes. For example:

1. Having two fees rates is more complex and can cause problems when a client is seen occasionally for individual therapy concurrent with regular group therapy.
2. When other group members are absent, does the lone group member get charged individual rate or group rate?
3. Clients often feel that since group rates are lower, group therapy must be of less value and a dilution of individual therapy. This, of course, is not the case in most work done with many clients, particularly in preschool and school-age

language impaired people. Group work is more intensive, more concentrated, and generally more effective in teaching spoken and written communication skills. This is especially true for teaching clients how to maintain a topic, repair conversation breakdowns, listen, and follow group instructions. These things cannot be done individually, but are absolutely essential to an intervention program.

If a uniform fee schedule is charged in all situations, clients rarely, if ever, express concern.

Settling Bills for a Child After a Divorce

When working with children of divorced parents, meet with both parents and get a written statement regarding who is responsible for which portion of the child's bills. If a meeting is not possible, obtain each parent's written agreement to a contract mailed to them, spelling out their responsibility for the child's treatment.

Fees and Consulting

Setting fees for consulting work can be done on a slightly different basis than direct client contact. The basis of most fee structures for consultation is a consultant's billing rate. Billing rate is the dollar amount a client pays for a certain time period, such as a working day or hour (i.e., $50/hour; $400/day).

Kelley (1978) suggests that the billing rate for a consultant include the following considerations:
1. Salary
2. Employee benefits
3. Overhead expenses
4. Profit
5. Competition
6. Economic conditions
7. Fairness to both professional and client

Salary considerations would include:

a. value of service to client;
b. client responsibilities to consultants;
c. provider skills required;
d. provider education and experience.

Employee benefits are those benefits that may or may not be tax free. They include insurance, sick leave, job training, and other fringe benefits.

Overhead expenses are

a. directly related to business operations (rent, fire insurance, typing costs, etc.);
b. expenses incurred while serving clients (long distance calls on behalf of the client, etc.).
c. indirect expenses of operating a professional practice such as:
   - Typing

- Telephone
- Automobile
- Travel
- Postage
- Duplicating
- Professional liability insurance
- Collision and personal insurance coverage
- Time used in travel

Profit must be figured on the basis of time lost from one's practice and costs incurred as a result of the consultation as well as on the basis of income from the consultation.

Considerations of *competition* relate to the fees charged by other consultants in the same field and in the same geographic area.

Economic conditions demand that one consider how inflation or recession affects one's own practice as well as the business of one's potential clients.

Fairness to both professional and client is a prime consideration in setting the fee. What minimum and maximum levels will you accept? If, in your perception, you have undercharged, you may feel that you can cut corners; if, in your client's perception, you have overcharged, they may feel they can ask for additional services that were not part of the original agreement. The best financial agreement is one that is satisfactory to both parties. It is important to recognize that consultation includes time spent in activities related to the consulting work, but for which you cannot charge; for example, updating yourself in certain areas specific to the consultation.

Other Fee Arrangements

Other fee arrangements possible in consultation work include a *fixed fee* and a *fee by stages*. A *fixed fee* is often used for work such as a government project where one might be writing a grant or doing grant review. The risk involved with fixed fees is that the fee is set by estimating the amount of time the actual work will require. The actual work may take much less or much more time, causing one party to lose in the arrangement. Attorneys sometimes use *fee by stages* (Foonberg, 1984), in which work is broken into stages with an estimate for each stage, progressively setting the fee for each stage. For example, research and preparation: X dollars; drafting of proposal: X dollars; implementing of proposal: X dollars; evaluation and extension of proposal into action: X dollars; and, other services not covered: X dollars.

Some consultants in service-related fields can make use of a *retainer fee*, which is taken as a sign of trust and an intention to use services on a prepayment basis. The consultant can specify services for a fixed *retainer fee* for a fixed period of time. Services beyond the agreement are billed separately. If a *retainer fee* is used in some way by a consultant, it is important that its use be defined early in the arrangement.

Collecting Fees

One of the most difficult areas of fee management is that of slow and delinquent accounts. After an account becomes delinquent, chances of obtaining payment decreases in proportion to the length of time it is delinquent. Fee collection time is another good time to remember your banker; if money owed to you gets too far behind money you have collected, you have entered the banking business, and service delivery has become a sideline.

Keeping accounts receivable (money owed to you) low, and cash flow high, is essential to any practice. If there is no cash flow, there is no practice. With that thought in mind, try to incorporate some or all of the following principles for collecting accounts receivable:

1. Use a formal payment agreement. Put it in writing and have it signed by the client.
2. Require full, or large payments in advance for purchases, such as hearing aids.
3. Send bills on a routine basis, if you do not require cash at each visit.
4. Contact slow payers, as soon as they are identified, with a form letter or handwritten note on the bill.
5. Apply a penalty charge (processing fee) on unpaid and overdue accounts.
6. Notify nonpayers of the time remaining before you take legal action.
7. Do not let clients wait for their insurance reimbursement before they begin payment.
8. Itemize bills and charges by dates and services—not by time.
9. Make some notation about every account with the client or family (telephone, hall visit, physician contact, etc.); if necessary, note all such contacts on the statement.
10. If the bookkeeper is prepared properly to represent the office, have him/her make telephone calls to clients with overdue accounts.

Some professionals use credit cards or cash-by-visit payment. Credit cards may produce more frequent payments, but the cost of using a credit card can erase the gain. Cash-by-visit payment method is fairly cumbersome and requires extra bookkeeping; however, it may produce a 99 percent collection rate, justifying the extra trouble.

You, as owner of the practice, should review your accounts receivable at least every 2 weeks. You may be surprised at the *number* of clients who owe you money. You also may be surprised about *who* owes you large amounts of money. Begin action—form letters, notes, calls, and so forth—on the largest and longest overdue bills; do not work them alphabetically. You may need to tell some clients that you cannot continue to work with them until they pay their overdue bills.

Be sure you have a systematic way of handling overdue accounts. One such system might include the following steps:

1. One month overdue: a notice on the statement with 5 percent charge;
2. No payment in two or more weeks: a letter from the bookkeeper;

3. Two months overdue: a notice on the statement with 10 percent charge;
4. No payment in two more weeks: a phone call from you or the bookkeeper;
5. Three months overdue: a notice on the statement indicating 10 percent charge and impending legal action;
6. No payment in two more weeks: a formal notice that legal action has been started and intervention will no longer be scheduled until action has been taken to clear up the account;
7. Any person who gets to item No. 6 and wants to reenter an intervention program must pay each visit.

Before discussing overdue payment with a client, have the following information before you:

1. The client's chart with dates and items of services provided;
2. The amount the client owes and services included in this total;
3. Amounts owed by this client for previous services or for other family members;
4. A history of previous payments made, including amounts and dates of most recent payments;
5. Time and content of initial fee discussion with client, including what each of you said;
6. Obligations of client under the fee agreement.

In the discussion, obtain a commitment from the client regarding amount and exact date the next payment can be expected. Record that information on the payment sheet. Follow up this conversation with a letter summarizing and noting the agreed upon payment amounts and dates of payment.

A common mistake in billing and collection practices of many professionals is that services are not itemized and dated. Many of us, as consumers, insist that we receive itemized bills, yet we do not always practice that when we bill for our services. Foonberg (1984) emphasizes the necessity for recounting in writing everything that has been done on the client's behalf. Such documentation would include telephone conversations, consultation with colleagues, report writing, and any other pertinent or related activities. He recommends sending brief notes on letterhead stationery to the client or family concerning progress. Foonberg suggests that people do not like to pay for time, but are happy to pay for ''stationery''— reports and other paperwork that provide evidence of professional attention and care for the client.

Billing and collection for consultation should be as systematic as billing and collection for direct delivery of client services. Bills should be sent regularly with itemized activities and brief periodic updating reports.

Small Claims Court

Unfortunately, there are some people who have no intention of honoring their payment arrangements with the practitioner. Often such offenders are people who can afford to pay but choose to ignore their responsibilities. In such circumstances, small claims court* is a final collection option. Claims vary from $150 to $5,000, depending on the state; however, several claims can be made by one party against another. Usually all that is involved is a small filing fee and presentation of the complaint with evidence. A secretary or bookkeeper can handle the matter quite easily. An attorney is not necessary, and the owner/practitioner need not take time from practice to pursue the claim. Frequently, once a client has received a notice from the court that a suit has been filed, payment is forthcoming. If that does not happen, the owner must decide whether to take the final step, turning the court's decision into cash. This is an important decision and must be weighed carefully, for it may entail rather harsh action, such as attaching part of a paycheck.

Some people have difficulty understanding that the only commodity a professional has is his/her time and service. Professional advice is intangible and can be viewed as fairly insignificant, particularly when obvious and immediate progress is not apparent to the client or family. Even the most successful practitioners find that, on occasion, problems arise with cash flow that can be directly attributed to overdue accounts. Some ways to avoid serious problems with collections can be summarized as follows:

1. Do your best work. Clients are more likely to be satisfied with services and pay for them if your best interests and efforts are apparent.
2. Maintain periodic contact with the family for informal progress reports and interchanges.
3. Include the client or family at each step of service. If the client and family know what is being done on their behalf, such as teacher conferences, changing of goals, and retesting, they will be more committed to services than if they are uninformed.
4. Monitor payment trends so delinquent and slow accounts can be identified for early action.
5. Itemize and date all action taken on the client's behalf.

Remember, the larger the amount owed by a client, the less impressed that client will be with your services.

VALUATION AND SALE OF THE PRACTICE

The monetary value of a practice in speech-language pathology/audiology is difficult, if not impossible, to determine. For one thing, if an owner/practitioner intends to leave a busy practice with long-term clients and a steady supply of referrals, it is conceivable that the long-term clients and supply of referrals will disappear with the owner. In a profession as closely tied to reputation and success as speech-language pathology/audiology, an old practice without the ''old'' practitioner or practitioners may be of no more value than a newly established practice. Even with the passing of the Laurel Crown of Approval from the exiting practitioner to the entering practitioner, the new practice will not be the same. To look at the value of a practice and try to predict what it will be worth to a new owner/practitioner is to compare apples and oranges. The comparison is particularly apt in

---

*In some states, certain forms of practice—for example, non–Sub-Chapter S corporations, professional corporations, and others—may not use small claims court, but rather must employ an attorney to file in the state district court. Check the requirements of your state before instituting court action.

small practices, in which the reputation and personality of the owner/practitioner are central to the delivery of services.

Formulas for determining the purchase value of professional practices stem primarily from law and accounting, in which long-term relationships and sizable retainers can be passed to another professional (e.g., a junior partner who has been groomed to know and receive clients when the time comes).

The question is, of course, *if* someone indicates a serious interest in buying part or all of a practice, how can the value be measured by buyer and by seller? Some formulas suggested by colleagues in our profession and related professions are:

1. Fifty percent of the past year's gross revenues, with a pay-off schedule acceptable to both parties and assuming certain considerations about the practice;
2. One year's gross income, using a 3-year averaging period with acceptable pay-off schedule, interest free;
3. Book value of fixtures and equipment, plus 1 year's receipts.

Some issues regarding transfer of ownership include the following:

1. How long should the transition period take? It seems clear that anyone buying a practice should be a part of the administration and service delivery before the sale occurs. The transition period of at least 2 years should include sharing client schedules, referral contacts, and financial and administrative responsibilities. The existing practitioner can use the final year of the turn-over period to reduce the number of new clients and cut back the number of office hours.
2. From where will referrals come? The ideal buy-in situation is one in which referrals are built in, such as for the sole practitioner (of speech-language pathology/audiology) in a multidisciplinary professional center. Other good situations involve being the recipient of referrals from an institution that would more readily accept change of owner/practitioner than take the effort to look for other sources of service. Offering specialized services, with a reputation built around that specialty, helps one acquire predictable sources of referrals.
3. How many other clinicians in the same area will draw from the same referral sources? Obviously, a broad supply of clinicians with the same specialty, experience, and reputation within a 5-mile radius reduces the appeal of a practice to a prospective buyer.
4. How different is the philosophy of service delivery between buyer and seller? No matter how eager the selling practitioner is to leave, sale of a practice will not be satisfying unless the seller feels that some part of the years of work devoted to the practice will not evaporate with its sale.

Some specific considerations in negotiating and consummating a professional practice are as follows:

1. Draw up a formal contract for sale specifying all contingencies and conditions before beginning the transition period;
2. Use an attorney or other advisors for the contract of sale *and for the formal transition contract;*
3. Draw up a formal transition contract to cover the time period during which both practitioners will be part of the practice; specify roles, financial obligations,

authority, and allocation of expenses and revenue for each (including any fringe benefits paid by the practice);

4. Inform clients, referral sources and colleagues of the transition;
5. Obtain written permission from each client (or responsible person) to transfer records to the new owner;
6. Agree upon the use of the *name* of the practice, both before and after the transition period;
7. Agree upon changes that may occur in letterhead and other stationery during the transition period;
8. Meet jointly with all referral sources and follow-up with notes or letters;
9. Meet with consultants pertinent to the practice, including the accountant and attorney; determine if they will or will not be used by the new owner and obtain the consultants' help in making the transfer; tax advantages can be missed if a sale is not made properly; other errors may be difficult to correct if financial advice and direction are not obtained early in the negotiations (*Guide to Private Practice*, ''Practice Issues,'' 1984).

If you think that you might consider sale of your practice, begin now to look for potential practitioners/owners. Consider having a partner or younger practitioner join your practice who might eventually want sole control of the practice. Be sure that a buy–sell agreement is in force from the beginning. Such agreement can always be modified, but it may be impossible at the time of sale negotiations to undo early carelessness.

Appendices

SHAREHOLDERS MEETING
ITEMS FOR DISCUSSION AND DECISION

Date _______________

1. Method of determining relative value of furniture, fixtures, and vehicles.
2. Review of corporate records for the past 2 years to determine:
   a. Source and amount of income to Corporation by employees
   b. Source and amount of expenses to Corporation by employees
   c. Means of compensating employees for back salary which has not been paid by Corporation to employees
   d. Means of compensating employees for inequitable ratio between income production and expenditures of Corporate money
   e. Means of paying debts incurred by Corporation and its employees before and after _______________ [date on which shareholders voted to dissolve the Corporation] (e.g., outstanding expenses will be paid equally by each party, and/and not from Corporate banking account)
   f. Drawing of consultation money from Corporation without deducting FICA and withholding, and so forth (e.g., consultation money)
3. Means of protecting name of _______________ from use by anyone other the time of Corporate dissolution.
4. Amount of time for maintaining current group insurance policy and the eventual dissolution of such policy.
5. Disposition of any money remaining in Corporate account at time of its closing.
6. On _______________ the # _______________ will be disconnected and no longer be a working number.
7. On _______________ the # _______________ will be used only for the recorded message for incoming calls.

UNANIMOUS WRITTEN CONSENT OF SHAREHOLDERS TO
DISSOLUTION OF _______________, INC.

The undersigned shareholders of record of _______________, a Texas Corporation, whose shares constitute all of the issued and outstanding shares of the Corporation, hereby consent to the voluntary dissolution of the Corporation according to the following plan of dissolution:

That the Corporation is being liquidated pursuant to section 333 of the Internal Revenue Code and will distribute all of its property and assets during the calendar month of _______________

That all liabilities and obligations of the Corporation will be paid or discharged, or that adequate provision will be made therefore.

That, after the provision for the payment of the known debts and liabilities of the Corporation, the officers of the Corporation are authorized and directed to distribute the remaining assets of the Corporation to the shareholders of record in the following manner: (1) with respect to any cash, by distributing to each such shareholder of record a proportion of such cash equal to the proportion that the shares owned by such shareholder bears to the total issued and outstanding shares of this Corporation, and (2) with respect to assets other than cash, by distributing to each shareholder of record an undivided interest in each of such assets equal to the proportion that the shares of this Corporation owned by such shareholder bears to the total issued and outstanding shares of this Corporation.

APPENDIX 3–1
ESTIMATED START-UP COSTS, PROFESSIONAL PRACTICE

Item	Estimated Amount

Office rental ($1,000.00/month)
  First and last months $2,000.00
  Two additional months $2,000.00
	$ 4,000.00

Secretary/Receptionist 12 months $800.00/month	9,600.00
Furniture/equipment (Office)*	10,000.00
Printing	2,500.00
Professional equipment and supplies*	4,000.00
Leasehold improvements	4,500.00
Miscellaneous Ongoing $1,000.00/month	12,000.00

Accountant/Legal Fees
  Telephone Installation
  City, etc., licenses   start-up
  Insurance   first four months
  Utility deposits, etc.
	6,000.00

Speech pathologist salary draw $1,800.00/month	21,000.00
TOTAL	73,600.00

*Audiological test suite and equipment not included.

APPENDIX 3–2
PROFESSIONAL OFFICE CHART OF ACCOUNTS—SAMPLE 1

Account
No.   *ASSETS*

_________ Cash in Bank—Office
_________ Cash in Bank—Payroll
_________ Client Costs Receivable
_________ Clinical Equipment
_________ Deposits–Lease, Utilities, etc.
_________ Desks and Chairs (accumulated
               depreciation)
_________ Typewriters (accumulated
               depreciation)
_________ Dictating Equipment
               (accumulated depreciation)
_________ Other Office Equipment
               (accumulated depreciation)
_________ Library (accumulated
               depreciation)
_________ Leasehold Improvements
               (accumulated depreciation)
_________ Returned Checks on Hand
_________ Transportation Equipment

LIABILITIES

_________ Bank Loans Payable
_________ Credit Cards Payable
_________ Equipment Contracts Payable
_________ Withheld Payroll Taxes
               Payable
_________ Other liabilities

CAPITAL

_________ (name) Capital
_________ (name) Draw (nondeductible)
_________ (name) Draw (deductible)

Account
No.   *INCOME*

_________ Fees Received
_________ Evaluation
_________   speech
_________   language
_________   hearing
_________ Screening
_________   speech
_________   language
_________   hearing
_________ Intervention
_________   speech
_________   language
_________   hearing
_________ Parent/Family Conferences
_________ Consultation
_________ Refunds
_________ Late Charges
_________ Gain (Loss) on Sale
               of Assets
_________ Other

EXPENSES

_________ Accountant
_________ Attorney
_________ Automobile
_________ Bank Charges
_________ Business Entertainment
               and Promotion
_________ Consulting Fees
_________ Contract Services
_________ Contributions
_________ Depreciation
_________ Dues, Professional
_________ Employee Meals and
               Incentives
_________ Equipment Rental
_________ Insurance:
_________   Auto
_________   Contents of Office
_________   Medical and Disability
_________   Malpractice
_________   Miscellaneous (Groceries,
               Petty Cash)
_________ Office Supplies
_________ Payroll

APPENDIX 3–3
PROFESSIONAL OFFICE CHART OF ACCOUNTS—SAMPLE 2

ASSETS

Current Assets

102 Cash in ______________ Bank
112 Accounts Receivable—Employees
116 Returned Checks on Hand

Property and Equipment

151 Furniture and Fixtures
152 Transportation and Equipment
153 Machinery and Equipment
154 Office Equipment
158 Leasehold Improvements

Accumulated Depreciation

161 A/D—Furniture and Fixtures
162 A/D—Transportation Equipment
163 A/D—Machinery and Equipment
164 A/D—Office Equipment
168 A/D—Leasehold Improvements

Other Assets

199 Suspense

LIABILITIES

Current Liabilities

201 Accounts Payable—Equipment
210 FICA Withholdings Payable
211 Income Tax Withholdings Payable
240 Notes Payable (Director) or
         (Shareholder)
241 Notes Payable (Director) or
         (Shareholder)
250 Notes Payable—Auto (co.)

CAPITAL

300 Common Stock
320 Retained Earnings
350 Shareholder's Undistributed
         Taxable Income
360 Basis for Stock (Shareholder)
361 Basis for Stock (Shareholder)

REVENUE

400 Speech and Language
         Therapy Fees
401 Speech and Language
         Evaluation Fees
402 Consultation Fees
403 Parent Conferences
404 Hearing Screening
405 Hearing Evaluation
490 Gain or Loss on Sale
         of Assets
499 Miscellaneous Revenue

COSTS AND EXPENSES

510 Professional Salaries
513 Consulting Fees
514 Payroll Taxes
521 Repairs and Maintenance
523 Operating Supplies
542 Business Promotion
543 Contributions
546 Travel (Out-of-Town)
547 Vehicle Servicing
550 Office Salaries
552 Office Contract Services
559 Accounting and Legal Services
560 Employee Benefits
568 Dues and Subscriptions
570 Office Rent
571 Insurance
574 Postage and Freight
575 Printing and Office Supplies
576 Telephone and Utilities
583 Interest Expense
588 Depreciation
589 Depreciation—Transportation
         Equipment
590 Depreciation—Machinery
         and Equipment
591 Depreciation—Office
         Equipment
592 Depreciation—Leasehold
         Improvements
594 Taxes and Licenses
595 Miscellaneous Expenses
597 Nondeductible Expenses

APPENDIX 3–4
FINANCIAL STATEMENT—SAMPLE 1

ASSETS   AMOUNT

Cash on Hand
Accounts, Notes & Contracts Receivable
    Due from
    Collateral
    How Payable
    Maturity Date
    Balance Due
Stocks & Bonds
    Name of Company
    Exchange List
    Number of Shares
    Market Price
    Total Market Value
Real Estate Owned
    Location
    Use, Description
    Cost
    Tax Assessment
    Monthly Income
    Monthly Payments
    Balance of Mortgage
    Lien Holder
    Current Value
Property and Equipment
    Office Equipment
    Furniture
    Automobile
    Boats
    Leasehold Improvements
    Current Value
Cash Value Life Insurance
    When Issued
    Beneficiary
    Name of Company
    Base Amount
    Cash Value
    Loan Outstanding Amount
Profit Sharing or Pension Benefits
    Amount

TOTAL ASSETS

LIABILITIES

Notes Payable
    Due to Whom
    Collateral
    Maturity
    How Payable
    Balance Due
    Annual Interest Rate

LIABILITIES (Cont.)   *AMOUNT*

Other Installment Loans
    Payable to Whom
    Collateral
    Payments per Month
    Balance
Bank Issued Credit Cards
    Issuing Bank
    Card Numbers
    Expiration Date
    Credit Limit
    Current Balance Owed
Mortgages and Liens on Real Estate
    From Real Estate Data Under ASSETS
    Balance of Mortgage
    Mortgage or Lien Holder
Income Tax Payable
    Accruals Including Real Estate Taxes, etc.
Loans Against Life Insurance
    See Cash Value of Life Insurance under ASSETS
    Loan Amount
Accounts and Bills Payable
    Payable to
    How Payable
    Balance
    Other (i.e., co-signer of note)

TOTAL LIABILITIES

CASH FLOW STATEMENT

Annual Income for the Year of _______________
    Salary
    Securities
    Dividends
    Business Income
    Other Income

TOTAL INCOME

Annual Expenditures for the Year of _______________
    Taxes and Assessments
    Mortgage Payments
    Rental Payments
    Contract Payments
       Department Store Accounts
       Automobile Payments/Lease
       Payments on Other Personal Property
    Payment on Notes
    Living Expenses
    Utilities
    Social Expenses
    Insurance Premiums
       Home Owners
       Automobile
       Life

Annual Expenditures (Cont.)   AMOUNT

    Health
    Professional Liability
    Disability

TOTAL EXPENDITURES

APPENDIX 3–5
FINANCIAL STATEMENT—SAMPLE 2

CURRENT ASSETS   AMOUNT

    Cash in Banks __________

    Accounts Receivable — Trade __________

    Refunds Due — Payroll Tax Deposits (Net) __________

    Refundable Telephone Deposits __________

    Prepaid Insurance __________

    Suspense __________

    TOTAL CURRENT ASSETS __________

PROPERTY AND EQUIPMENT, AT COST

    Furniture and Fixtures __________

    Transportation Equipment __________

    Machinery and Other Equipment (Clinic Equipment) __________

    Office Equipment __________

    Leasehold Improvements __________

    Less Accumulated Depreciation __________

    TOTAL ASSETS __________

LIABILITIES AND SHAREHOLDERS' EQUITY

Current Liabilities

    Current Portion of Long-Term Debt __________

    Accounts Payable—Trade __________

    Accounts Payable Credit Cards __________

    F.I.C.A. Payable __________

    F.W.T. Payable __________

    Accrued Payroll Taxes __________

    Accounts Payable—(Professional's) __________

Long-Term Debt

    Note Payable to Bank __________

    Less Installments Due Within One Year Included Above __________

    Loans Payable to Shareholders __________

TOTAL LIABILITIES __________

SHAREHOLDERS' EQUITY

    Common Stock, par \$_______ per share;
        _______ Shares Authorized;
        _________ Shares Issued and Outstanding __________

    Retained Earnings (Deficit)

    Shareholders' Undistributed Taxable Income (Loss) __________

    TOTAL LIABILITIES AND SHAREHOLDERS' EQUITY __________

REVENUE	AMOUNT

Screening Fees
Therapy Fees
Evaluation Fees
Consultation Fees
Other Revenue

TOTAL REVENUE

COSTS AND EXPENSES

Clinic Operating Costs (Schedule 1) (Appended)
Business Promotion Expenses (Schedule 2) (Appended)
General and Administrative Expenses (Schedule 3) (Appended)

TOTAL COSTS AND EXPENSES

NET INCOME (LOSS)

RETAINED EARNINGS (DEFICIT)

Retained Earnings — (Date)
Shareholders' Undistributed Taxable (Income) Loss
Nondividend Distribution to Shareholders
Retained Earnings (Deficit) — (Date)

SCHEDULE 1—CLINIC OPERATING COSTS

Professional Salaries
Consulting Fees
Payroll Taxes — Professional Salaries
Equipment Maintenance
Operating Supplies
Depreciation—Machinery and Other Equipment
Miscellaneous Operating Costs

TOTAL CLINIC OPERATING COSTS

SCHEDULE 2—BUSINESS PROMOTION EXPENSES

Business Promotion
Contributions
Travel (Out of Town)
Vehicle Servicing
Depreciation — Transportation

TOTAL BUSINESS PROMOTION EXPENSES

SCHEDULE 3—GENERAL ADMINISTRATION EXPENSES   AMOUNT

Office Salaries
Payroll Taxes — Office
Accounting and Legal Services
Employee Benefits
Professional Dues and Subscriptions
Rent — Clinic and Office
Insurance
Postage and Freight
Printing and Office Supplies
Telephone and Utilities
Interest Expense
Charge Card Fee
Depreciation — Furniture and Fixtures
Depreciation — Office Equipment
Taxes and Licenses
Miscellaneous General Expense

TOTAL GENERAL AND ADMINISTRATIVE EXPENSE

SOURCES OF CASH

Cash Receipts from Operations
Less Cash Disbursements for Operations:

TOTAL EXPENSES
LESS NONCASH CHARGES TO DEPRECIATION

NET CASH FROM OPERATIONS

Drawing Against Line of Credit at Bank
Less Repayments
Loans From Shareholders
Less Repayments
Sale of Common Stock

TOTAL CASH PROVIDED

APPLICATIONS OF CASH

Purchases of Property and Equipment
Placement of Refundable Deposits
Distribution to Shareholders

TOTAL CASH APPLIED

CASH BALANCE AT END OF PERIOD

APPENDIX 3–6
THE BUSINESS PLAN

The business plan describes a company's past and current operations, then demonstrates how desired investments or loans will further the company's goals and reward investors.

SAMPLE BUSINESS PLAN OUTLINE

I. *Cover Letter*
   A. Dollar amount requested
   B. Terms and timing
   C. Type and price of securities (collateral)

II. *Summary*
   A. Business description
      1. Name
      2. Location and plan description
      3. Product
      4. Market and competition
      5. Management expertise
   B. Business goals
   C. Summary of financial needs and application of funds
   D. Earnings projections and potential return to investors

III. *Market Analysis*
   A. Description of total market
   B. Industry trends
   C. Target market
   D. Competition

IV. *Products or Services*
   A. Description of services rendered
   B. Proprietary position: patents, copyrights, and legal and technical considerations, if applicable.

V. *Management Plan*
   A. Form of business organization
   B. Board of directors composition
   C. Officers: organization chart and description of responsibilities
   D. Resumes of key personnel
   E. Staffing plan/number of employees
   F. Facilities plan and any planned capital improvements
   G. Operating plan/schedule of upcoming work for next 1 to 2 years

VI. *Financial Data*
   A. Financial history (5 years to present)
   B. Five-year financial projections (first year by quarters; remaining years annually)
      1. Profit and loss statements
      2. Balance sheets
      3. Cash flow chart
      4. Capital expenditure estimates
   C. Explanation of projections

APPENDIX 3-7
THE LOAN PACKAGE

The outline of a complete loan package below illustrates the type of detailed presentations sometimes required by lenders, such as banks, and the Small Business Administration. However, this degree of detail is often unnecessary for stable businesses already known to the lender.

SAMPLE LOAN PACKAGE OUTLINE

I. *Summary*
   A. Nature of business
   B. Amount and purpose of loan
   C. Repayment terms
   D. Security or collateral (listed with market value estimates and quotes on cost of equipment to be purchased with loan proceeds)

II. *Personal Information* (on persons owning more than 20 percent of the business)
   A. Educational and work history
   B. Credit references
   C. Income tax statements (last 3 years)
   D. Financial statement (no older than 60 days)

III. *Firm Information* (whichever is applicable below—A, B, or C)
   A. New business
      1. Business plan
      2. Life and casualty insurance coverage
      3. Lease agreement
   B. Business acquisition (buyout)
      1. Information on acquisition
      a. Business history (include seller's name, reason for sale)
      b. Current balance sheet (less than 60 days old)
      c. Current profit and loss statements (less than 60 days old)
      d. Business's federal income tax statements (past 3 to 5 years)
      e. Cash flow statements for last year
      f. Copy of sales agreement with breakdown of inventory, fixtures, equipment, licenses, goodwill, and other costs.
      g. Description and dates of permits already acquired
   C. Existing business expansion
      1. Information on existing business
      a. Business history
      b. Current balance sheet (not more than 60 days old)
      c. Current profit and loss statements (not more than 60 days old)
      d. Cash flow statements for last year
      e. Federal income tax returns for past 3 to 5 years
      f. Lease agreement and permit data

IV. *Projections*
   A. Profit and loss projection (monthly, for one year) and explanation of projection
   B. Cash flow projection (monthly, for one year) and explanation of projection
   C. Projected balance sheet (1 year after loan) and explanation of projection

APPENDIX 3-8
JUSTICE OF THE PEACE AND SMALL CLAIMS COURT

Within the limitation of certain legislative rules, the plaintiff (the person or entity filing suit) has the option to file suit against the defendant (the person or entity being sued) in either the small claims court or the justice of the peace court.

Effective September 1, 1983, in Texas, the basic filing fee (filing fee and service of citation fee) is the same for a regular civil proceeding in the small claims court or the justice of the peace court ($27.00 total). Consult your state for relevant courts and costs.

Below is a list of differences in the two types of courts in Texas. Read them over and think about them. Weigh the pluses and minuses for both the plaintiff and the defendant. Then decide which court is appropriate for your situation.

JUSTICE OF THE PEACE COURT	SMALL CLAIMS COURT
Monetary Jurisdiction $0–$1,000.00	Monetary Jurisdiction $0–$1,000.00
The (state) Rules of Procedures and the (state) Rules of Evidence apply.	The (state) Rules of Procedure and the (state) Rules of Evidence do *not* apply.
A party that charges any type of interest (includes late fees) must file in J.P. court. These charges cannot be waived in order to file in small claims court. Failure to comply with this rule will result in the case being dismissed and the plaintiff forfeiting all costs.	A party that does not charge any type of interest (includes late fees) can file in small claims or J.P. court. These charges cannot be waived in order to file in small claims court. Failure to comply with this rule will result in the case being dismissed and the plaintiff forfeiting all costs.
An individual or individual doing business may represent himself/herself in court. ANY OTHER PARTY (I.E., A CORPORATION OR ASSOCIATION) MUST BE REPRESENTED BY AN ATTORNEY. Failure to comply with this rule will result in the case being dismissed and the plaintiff forfeiting all costs.	No attorney is required to represent either party; however, an attorney may represent a party in the case.
Only the plaintiff or the plaintiff's attorney may appear in the court or file pleadings. Only the defendant or the defendant's attorney may appear in court or file pleadings.	The plaintiff, plaintiff's attorney, or any other authorized agent may appear in court or file pleadings. The defendant, defendant's attorney, or any other authorized agent may appear in court or file pleadings.

FILING SUIT IN JUSTICE OF THE PEACE AND SMALL CLAIMS COURT

To File or Not to File

1. If someone wants to sue another person in justice of the peace court or in small claims court, he or she must file a *petition* (complaint) with the justice of the peace (J.P.) or the judge of the small claims court. The person who sues is the *plaintiff;* the person being sued is the *defendant.*
2. If someone is considering filing a complaint, he or she should try to learn something about the defendant *before* filing suit. If the defendant does not have anything (money or property) that could be seized legally by the constable, it is not likely he or she could recover the amount sought. It is always a disappointment to find out that the defendant is penniless *after* having (1) spent money to file the suit; (2) taken time off from work or school to appear for the trial; and (3) spent more money trying to collect on the judgment by using "post-judgment remedies," (see section entitled "Filing Suit"). "You cannot get blood from a turnip."
3. Consider whether the proposed defendant has any legal claims against the practitioner or practice that he or she might file if put to the trouble of defending against a lawsuit. For example, it may not be smart to sue someone for $100.00 if he or she could show that the practice or practitioner owes him or her $200.00.

Filing Suit

1. The civil clerk of the court will provide the plaintiff with a petition in which to state his or her claim.
2. Most cases are heard by the judge.
3. The plaintiff must provide the court with the correct name and address of the person to be sued. The court cannot do any detective work for the plaintiff.
4. Do not make allegations (statements) in the petition that are untrue.
5. Remember, the plaintiff is only making an allegation that he or she should recover money from the defendant. Assume that the defendant will contest the case, so be prepared to prove allegations. The "burden of proof" is on the plaintiff to convince the judge or jury of allegations made.
6. Once a plaintiff has filed the petition, a constable delivers a *citation* (notice that a lawsuit has been filed) to the defendant. If the defendant does not enter a *general denial* (answer) within the time stated in the citation, the judge will rule in favor of the plaintiff without hearing the defendant's side.

Counterclaims

1. If a defendant has a claim of damage or liability (responsibility) against the plaintiff, the defendant can file a *counterclaim* against the plaintiff in the court in the same suit the plaintiff filed.
2. If the defendant files a counterclaim, the defendant has the "burden of proof," that is, to convince the judge or jury that the defendant should win.

Witnesses

Bring witnesses and records to court for the trial. If an interpreter is needed, either for the deaf or a foreign language speaker, tell the clerk several days before the trial.

APPENDIX 3-9
SAMPLE LETTER TO CLIENT WITH SERIOUSLY OVERDUE BILL

Dear _______________________

Enclosed is a copy of your current bill with its overdue balance. As you remember, our fee agreement requires complete and timely payment of charges for services. This is the fourth statement you have been sent, but we have received no payment from you.

You must make arrangements to clear your balance immediately. Please call the bookkeeper and indicate the amount of payment you intend to make and the date we can expect to receive that payment.

If we have not heard from you within 5 days of receipt of this letter, we will be forced to pursue appropriate legal action. You will not receive another notice from this office regarding payment.

Sincerely,

Send by Registered (or Certified) Mail

APPENDIX 3–10
SAMPLE NOTES ON STATEMENT FOR OVERDUE PAYMENT

1. *Sample Note No. 1*
   a. Your payment is 1 month overdue. Please clear the balance. Thank you.

   (signed: Bookkeeper)

   b. Thank you for your immediate attention to your overdue balance.

   (signed: Bookkeeper)

2. *Sample Note No. 2*
   a. Your account is seriously overdue and a processing charge has been added. Please attend to this matter within 5 days.

   (signed: Owner)

   b. Your payments are delinquent, and a processing charge has been added to your balance. Please recall that the fee agreement you signed requires immediate and timely payment. You must clear the balance within 5 days.

   (signed: Owner)

3. *Sample Note No. 3*
   a. Your account is seriously overdue. See attached letter regarding action to be taken. (Enclose copy of signed fee agreement with letter outlining action.)

   (signed: Owner)

   b. Because your account is seriously delinquent we must pursue legal action if we do not receive full payment within 5 days. (Enclose copy of fee agreement)

   (signed: Owner)

Fee-for-service is not only necessary for maintaining a bank balance; it also serves as one component of the professional interaction with the client. Payment of fees is a representation of clients' recognition and acceptance of their own responsibilities in the intervention process. Without enforcement of that tangible responsibility, clients' other responsibilities in the interaction are lessened by implication as well as by action.

Society has the obligation to provide health and certain allied health services to those who need them but are unable to afford them. Professionals who provide those services share those obligations. There are some people—among them speech-language pathologists and audiologists—who believe that professionals should bear this responsibility alone. The professional who feels the obligation to single-handedly provide free services to society should not go into private practice unless he/she is independently wealthy and looking for a worthy charity, or is subsidized totally by some organization or group. Reasonable fees must be charged to clients and collected in all appropriate situations for services rendered in private practice. By definition and by function, if one works for him/herself, the venture is private and the support is private—hence the term *self-supporting* and *private enterprise*. If one works for "the public" or "society," that person is supported by public funds. Many publicly supported programs employ professionals as service providers for persons who cannot or choose not to pay for private care. If a person is able and wants to choose private care, then that person must not expect help from society or the provider in paying for the service; those who are unable to pay for services should have services available to them through publicly and privately endowed programs; it is toward these ends that professional associations should advocate.

Professionals in (re)habilitation services must apply different criteria for fee setting than many other professionals whose work is done "by the job." Surgeons, for example, do not charge by the hour but rather for the appendectomy, cataract operation [illegible]. The same principle is true for many others: lawyers, architects, and engineers whose services usually are defined assignments and are relatively short-term. By contrast, many specialists in communication disorders do, and it is not at all unusual to begin working with a 2- or 3-year old and continue working with that child for 10 or 15 years. In one sense, we take the child "to raise"; in some instances, we also take the family to raise. A few other professionals, such as psychologists and psychiatrists, face analogous situations for long-term care.

As D'Asaro (1971) pointed out, some of the conflict regarding fees in our profession has come from the large numbers of clinicians who supplement their income by moonlighting. By working in their homes or client's homes, their overhead is negligible; cost accounting, marketing, and bank loans are usually unnecessary. Fees often are a fraction of those charged by full-time, private practitioners who must derive total income and fringe benefits from fees alone. However, the reliability of the moonlighters' services, as well as their availability over the long term, is unpredictable.

With few exceptions, the fee for direct delivery of services is the only source of income for the private practitioner. Attorneys demand and receive retainers for a future time when their services may be needed. No one retains a communication

Chapter 4

The Office, Part I
Location, Structure, and Furnishings

Once the decision is made to pursue private practice, the next step is to determine how the private practice is to be established. Certain considerations about size and nature of the practice must precede specific decisions about location and design of the office. For example, decisions must be made for the first 3 years of practice regarding the following:

1. What population of clients will be served? Age? Type of disorder?
2. Do you intend to work alone, at least for a while?
3. If you intend to bring a colleague into the practice with you, will you want partners? Employees? Independent consultants? Full time? Part time?
4. If you do intend to bring a colleague into the practice with you, do you want a colleague of a different profession? Occupational therapist? Physical therapist? Social worker? Full time? Part time?
5. Will you see groups or individuals? How large is the largest size group? What age is the largest size group?
6. Will you be spending most of your workday in the office? And/or will you be doing out-of-office contracting?
7. Will you work at night? Weekends?
8. How much time per week do you intend to spend in direct client contact?
9. Where in the community do you want to work?
10. Is office location crucial to the type of clients you will see? Is location crucial to referrals?
11. What kind of space will be needed for the office, including office and therapy space, waiting room, parking or drive-through space?

12. What kind of files or records will be needed? What kind of system will you use for record-keeping?
13. Do you want a secretary/clerk? Full time?
14. What furniture will you need or want for the first 3 years?
15. What equipment will you need for the first 3 years?
16. What supplies will you need for the first year? Assessment tools? Therapy materials? Consumables? Stationery?

These considerations are crucial to office space planning for obvious reasons. The type and size of a practice, the number of employees, and the philosophy of service delivery are intrinsic to planning the kind of office that is necessary to accommodate the practice.

Geographic Location

Many new practitioners find that the geographic location of their practice is predetermined by personal factors. If, however, you happen to be unrestricted and unbiased in terms of choosing a location for your practice, consider the following criteria:

1. Go where you have family and friends. Many practices begin with friends, relatives, and professional acquaintances. Start your practice where they are. If no one knows you, it is going to be difficult to begin a practice. If you cannot start your practice where people know you, then find a place and make yourself known there. Being unknown lengthens the time you need to become established.
2. Choose a growing section of the country. Consider possible changes in economic patterns and new development of the community you consider. Decide before you choose a place whether you'll be happier in a rural or small town atmosphere, or if you need to locate in a city.
3. In choosing the area within a community, consider the following:
   a. What is the educational status, atmosphere, social life, professional life, economic life, recreational life, and quality of home life in the office area? The area in which you work should match your preferences for the type of client you want, proximity desired to certain parts of the community, safety of the area in terms of your spouse and children, and your own safety when leaving work at night or working alone late at night.
   b. What is the proximity of the office to major anticipated referral sources and clients, to public transportation for your staff and clients, to eating places, and to other professionals? It is not necessarily bad to locate an office in an area where there are other professionals, such as in a building that has other speech-language pathologists/audiologists. Other professionals can be a source of referrals, advice, and professional contact, as well as potential office sharers. Locate where the clients are (or will be) and find out what you can afford in the area where you *want* to practice. If you're embarrassed to give your office address to colleagues, or if you're uncomfortable working at night because of the location, it would be a mistake to select that site.

If you do not know the community or region in which you must open a practice or branch office, you can utilize several sources of information regarding the population and its demographics, including county, city, state, and U.S. census reports, which are easily attainable from various Bureaus of Census and from public libraries. Other sources include maps and local information available from the Chambers of Commerce, zoning commissions, and realtors. These can indicate access to various parts of the community, zoning ordinances, and range of office prices. Sometimes office space is priced more reasonably in a fringe professional/residential area than in the midst of a professional area, yet still offer the advantages of a professional area. It is important for a professional to observe zoning restrictions in any community, even though some areas are far more lenient about enforcing these restrictions than others. It is embarrassing, inconvenient, and bad business to be forced out of an office within a few weeks of opening because of a zoning violation.

In addition to physical location, the type of office can vary from a large professional complex to a small converted house. The physical location should be able to accommodate the number of clients who will be seeing you on a concurrent basis and provide adequate parking and good lighting. Sometimes it is a good idea to consider inexpensive space in an expensive building. Do not be afraid to make contacts and be assertive in finding space. If there is a particular building in which you want space for your office, send letters to the building manager and to existing tenants. When shopping for prices, determine true rental costs. Many commercial buildings are leased on the basis of ''total rentable space.'' This figure is based on measurement of the exterior dimensions of the space. The actual interior area with which you have to work is termed ''total useable space.'' There can be as much as 10 percent difference in these two figures. For example, you may find that the cost of your office space is $1.00/sq. ft. for 1,000 square feet of ''total rentable space,'' resulting in monthly rent of $1,000. However, your ''total useable space'' will be only 900 square feet. Much commercial space also carries an add-on factor of as much as 15 to 20 percent for ''common area'' costs. These include, among other items, halls, lobbies, restrooms, and janitorial closets shared by all tenants.

Office Size

Requirements for office size will vary depending upon arrangements of office space, number of employees, and number of clients to be seen concurrently. One way to estimate office space is as follows:

> Full time practitioners—150 to 200 sq. ft. for personal office, (smaller is adequate if there is a conference room).
> Full time therapy—120 to 150 sq. ft. (depending on the size of the groups and the ages of the people seen). Count on 1.5 therapy rooms per full time practitioner. Some of the therapy and testing can be done in the practitioner's office. Adults can be seen in the practitioner's office; group therapy requires a separate room.
> Secretarial area—150 to 200 sq. ft.
> Reception area, storage, filing cabinet—300 sq. ft.

A speech-language pathologist will need an office/consultation/adult therapy room, as well as an evaluation and therapy room for children. In many instances, a therapy room can also serve as a storage room. An audiologist will need at least an office/consultation room, a testing area, and additional space for fitting hearing aids and for conducting various sophisticated audiometric assessment procedures.

Negotiating an Office Lease

In addition to having an attorney review an office lease and evaluate it in light of comparable lease agreements in the area, the following are some items to negotiate and *get in writing:*

1. Be sure your rent is competitive for that location and office.
2. Specify that utilities be included in the fixed rental price.
3. Fix automatic rental increases at a designated percent and frequency. Do not allow the owner to put in an undetermined ''cost of living'' automatic rent increase. A cost of living clause should be specified and kept as small as possible (no more than 10 percent a year). Where such a ''cost of living'' increase clause exists, try to negotiate a decreased ''cost of living'' clause where the rental price would drop should taxes or other costs drop.
4. Specify parking for staff and clients. Be sure that you have enough parking per hour to accommodate some of the large groups who are seen concurrently.
5. Arrange a safe and convenient drop-off or drive-through area so that clients can be let off at the door without parking if they choose.
6. Assure access to the office nights and weekends, with no extra charge for air conditioning, heating, and electricity.
7. Specify the provision of building security on nights and weekends.
8. Specify that you have the first right of refusal for additional space in the same building or on the same floor when your lease renewal comes due.
9. Retain controls for air and heat thermostats in your office.
10. Arrange for adequate number of electrical outlets where needed.
11. Arrange to retain or purchase furniture from previous tenants (where available) at a reduced rate.
12. Specify the provision of janitorial service and the cleaning schedule. Define complete services, including cleaning supplies.
13. Arrange for owner to paint and clean space, and replace or clean carpets and drapes.
14. Specify length of lease with renewal options. The longer lease you negotiate, the more concessions you should expect from the owner.
15. Specify any special build-out modifications, or repairs. Get owner to pay for as much as possible.
16. Obtain permission to sublet.
17. Include a death and disability clause which provides for termination of your lease under specified conditions.
18. Specify that any intrusions for repairs affecting your office be in writing with advance notice.

Remember, if it's not in writing, it does not exist!

Delay the effective date of the lease as long as possible after signing because of the lag time in opening an office—printing announcements and stationery, purchasing furniture, and so forth. See if furniture or equipment can be stored prior to move-in and kept in a locked area. Many professionals prefer to have their own keys to certain areas, such as rooms with confidential files and delicate equipment. Sometimes it is necessary to put in the contract that this is required and, in the event of fire or other emergency, management will not be held responsible for destroying the door to get into locked office space.

Office Sharing

Some professional practices are engaging in the mutual use of a central reception area with other services shared as needed. Sometimes a monthly fee is charged for specific services such as telephone, answering service, receptionist, typing, billing, and so forth. Some practitioners opt for office sharing arrangements that include receptionists, waiting room, appointment and typing services, and for all other services hired independently. For example, bookkeeping, accounting, and legal services would be arranged independently by the various practitioners. If any lease sharing, space sharing, or any other arrangements are worked out, whether with a central office management area or with other professionals, it is imperative that all arrangements be put into writing and all facets of the agreement be written and signed by all parties.

Subletting

Whether one rents or buys, subletting can become an advantage in meeting office overhead costs and using spare office space. If handled appropriately, this arrangement can be advantageous to both the leaseholder and the sublet tenant. One way to consider office sharing or subletting, is to share the same office, using different hours. If you are not using office space, then perhaps someone else could be using it, paying you needed income for office costs. Specific and written arrangements should be made about hours, fees, and services. Scheduling hours when two professionals share the same office space can be a very difficult problem. Subletting minimizes freedom in the office use. The best arrangement is to rent by the hour for a fixed fee, specifying hours when the sublet tenant may use the space. If the sublet tenant wishes to use any of the other advantages besides the specified room, such as the answering services or clerical help, then a flat monthly fee should be charged in addition to the rental fee for space. It is important to maintain separation between the two professionals so that clinical liability does not become a problem. However, if you, as the primary tenant, carry accident liability for the office, that insurance would be applicable to the office, regardless of the individuals who were using the space at the time of the accident. An arrangement to sublet office space should not be allowed to evolve into a fee-splitting arrangement. That is, if the primary practitioner has too many clients and agrees to give the sublet tenant some of the overflow, no charge may be made for the referral. This holds whether it is called a referral charge or an additional charge for ''rent.'' Accepting a fee for client referral is unethical.

In some instances, professionals have set up a separate nonprofessional management/leasing company for subletting office space. The primary practitioner becomes the manager/lessor, providing certain physical facilities and nonprofessional services for a fee. The length of time that the office space is sublet should be written into the contract, as well as the manner for terminating the agreement. Charges for furnishings and utility services should also be specified. The professional should seriously consider the consequences of sharing office space. This arrangement can be disruptive, and some people have problems with invasion of personal space. Variations of subletting are possible, but should be arranged with extreme caution. One such variation includes subletting the office space during summer or holiday periods or for the duration of the primary tenant's vacation. This can have implications for the image of the office and the impact of the location upon the practice itself. Many clients and referral sources do not remember names of a practice (i.e., where an alleged abuse occurred) but merely refer to the "one in the brown building on X street."

Sometimes professionals choose to trade space for services. Foonberg (1984) discusses the use of extra space by a new practitioner in exchange for the contribution of a certain number of hours of services per month. Foonberg feels that assessing the cost of furniture use, equipment, and utilities, in order to equate this cost with the number of hours of services to be provided, is very difficult. This difficulty, he feels, outweighs the advantages for both parties. A better alternative is for the new practitioner to pay a rental fee, accepting or rejecting referrals and work assignments from the established practitioner as desired. In that way, the space, furnishings, and other office amenities are paid for on a rental or lease sharing basis, and any referral work or substitute work done by the new practitioner is remunerated at an agreed-upon rate for work performed.

Obviously there are advantages and disadvantages to sharing an office with other professionals. Success of this structure depends upon the arrangements that are made and that are set out in writing by all involved parties. Some of the advantages of office sharing include the following:

1. The sharing of common expenses such as waiting room and receptionists greatly reduces monthly occupancy expenses for both.
2. There is a known, fixed monthly income to the lessor from the office sharing contract.
3. There is flexibility to expand within the suite, or move out when a better arrangement occurs for the sublet tenant.
4. There is access to secretaries and equipment on an as-needed basis for the sublet tenant and the lessor obtains some reduction in his/her costs for such services.
5. Both have access to other professionals for advice and consultation.
6. The sublet tenant has the possibility of obtaining the lessor's overflow work, and the lessor can secure substitute work from the sublet professional.
7. The sublet tenant may avoid certain administrative problems, such as hiring a receptionist, negotiating lease clauses about the building, and so forth.
8. Both may profit from sharing a library of professional journals, books, and media materials.
9. Both may reduce overhead costs by sharing office costs.

Certainly, all of these advantages could become disadvantages if the office sharing arrangement is not properly negotiated. Even in the best of circumstances there can be disadvantages to office sharing such as the following:

1. Frequently a receptionist or a front office secretary who is shared by many different professionals will not necessarily know each client and may become rather impersonal with all clients. Some clients resent this kind of impersonal or automated behavior.
2. Sublet tenants may have difficulty assessing the office during off-hours. Sometimes getting in an office at night or on weekends and holidays may be a problem because of the original contract signed by the leaseholder.
3. If a library is shared, it may be that needed journals, books, and references are missing at the time when they are needed.
4. There may be different kinds of clients in the waiting room. This sometimes causes discomfort to adults or adolescents who are sensitive to being seen in the same office with children.
5. The decorations and interior design may be distasteful to the sublet tenant. Little flexibility is possible because the office has usually been designed and decorated before the sublet tenant moved in.

The design of office size, structure, and content is determined in large part by what services will be offered. An additional consideration is what the practitioner can afford. There are several design considerations specific to the practice of speech-language pathology/audiology. These include the following:

1. Sound treatment of rooms such as sound insulation material, acoustic tile, and so forth must be included;
2. Care should be given to the strength and design of the office floor in order to support any special equipment;
3. Electrical service, outlets, and fixtures must meet all requirements specified by guidelines of standards agencies such as American National Standards Institute (ANSI) requirements, standards of Professional Services Board (PSB) of the American Speech-Language-Hearing Association, Vocational Rehabilitation Standards, and so forth.

Leasing/Purchasing Office Space

Most professionals still practice in rented office space, although there is an increasing awareness by professionals of certain advantages and conveniences in building and owning their office space. Along with this interest in owning office space is an increasing trend on the part of architects and developers to construct office facilities especially designed for professionals. The argument is that office space that is designed for professionals, specifically therapists, will increase efficiency and prove to be a profitable investment in terms of tax advantages and opportunities for subletting. The problems, however, counterbalance the advantages. The potential owner must consider the expense and energy involved in any construction project, the time needed to build and manage an office, and the real financial differences between renting and buying.

In calculating financial differences between owning and renting, the practitioner should (1) consider all annual costs to himself/herself as owner and as renter; (2) figure tax and depreciation deductions for both owning and renting; and (3) perform cost comparisons with that information.

In deciding whether or not to build, it would be helpful to pick a few desirable locations; estimate the amount of square footage that one would need for the next 5 to 8 years; find out the per-square-foot construction costs in each area; determine the length of the best mortgage arrangement (75% mortgage at 12% interest rate); and add the necessary cash outlay at the initiation of the building and loan arrangements (remaining 25% of the mortgage plus construction loan). It would also be helpful to calculate annual costs in terms of mortgage payments versus rental payments, costs of utilities and insurance, and any maintenance and repair costs. By doing calculations on paper it is easier to predict necessary cash outlay and cost of the loan. Then one can compare the figures with the advantages and disadvantages of owning an office *before* any money is spent.

At this time, in many desirable office areas, owning costs more in outright expense than renting because of mortgage loan costs, maintenance, and other operating costs. However, if tax factors are taken into account, the cost differential between buying and renting is much less. The cost of ownership may have a slight advantage over the cost of renting. Continuing inflation will result in ever-increasing rental costs, whereas a well-designed professional office may mean significant savings in the long run in spite of increased property taxation.

Some basic considerations of the buyer-versus-rent proposition include land cost variations, financing, estimates of future annual costs, tax consequences, and management and design of the building (Ridgewood Financial Institute, 1984). Land costs vary from residential to commercial. Zoning problems are a greater factor in commercial building than in residential building. In some land areas, certain site improvements, such as water run-off and access to major thoroughfares, can become a problem. The value of any property in the future will not be in the office, itself, but in the location and the potential use for it by prospective buyers.

Securing financing for residential purchases is usually a simple process. However, securing financing for commercial purchases is more complex. Construction loan costs must be added to long-term mortgage costs. Building costs, as well as costs of interior furnishing and fixtures, can increase rapidly during construction. One should estimate at least a 10 percent increase in annual costs of labor materials, improvements, and taxes.

If a building purchase still seems desirable, one viable option is to buy an existing building in a good location. Buying and remodeling an existing building takes less time and energy than building a new building. Financing is less difficult, zoning for office use may already have been accomplished, and a long-term mortgage can sometimes be worked out to include assumption of the previous loan at its previous interest rate. The tax advantage of owning a building lies primarily in the depreciation that can be deducted on personal tax returns. Current and projected personal and professional financial circumstances should be worked out carefully with an accountant or other consultants before embarking on the design of office plans. Certainly after the decision has been made to build or to buy a building, professional help will be necessary for the design or remodeling of the building, financing, zoning, insurance, and other legal matters. Talking with a contractor early in the project is also a good idea.

Deciding whether to buy new space, remodel an old building, or rent depends upon personal and professional goals and finances and the type of practice that is anticipated.

Office Design and Furnishings

A diagram of the entire office arrangement should be done before any build-out plans are begun. Clients' access to the office; ease and efficiency of client flow within the office; and number and size of consultation/treatment rooms, waiting areas, business areas, and storage space should be carefully planned before any action is taken.

As Fox (1971) indicated, design and function of an office are best when the client is not aware of business workings of the office.

Equipment, Instruments, and Furnishings

Office design and planning should be accomplished before actual purchases are made. Necessary furniture and equipment should be listed and diagrammed into office design space. In this way, consideration can be given to future office needs, as well as to space planning for reduced or increased use of office space. Major considerations in equipping and furnishing the office are parallel to previous decisions about office location and purchase. One must consider both what is affordable and what is necessary. A crucial consideration in equipment planning is to avoid duplicating equipment that can be easily accessed in out-of-the-office locations. It may be unnecessary to buy a copy machine at the outset when one is easily available within one's own office building.

Speech-language pathology practices usually require relatively few and relatively inexpensive instruments and materials. On the other hand, audiologists require fairly complex and expensive equipment. The importance of space planning is accentuated for them due to the necessity of placing equipment in spaces which meet certain standards.

Some professionals believe there are advantages to leasing major pieces of equipment rather than buying. Leasing allows immediate deduction of payments as a business expense; does not demand immediate large scale cash flow; and minimizes bookkeeping and tax reporting. However, in many instances, the leasing adds significantly to the long-term cost of equipment or furniture. Time payments almost always include an interest charge or a carrying fee that represents the amount of money the selling company is ''loaning'' you until you pay the total cost of the purchase. It is best to consult a tax specialist about the most advantageous way to treat items for tax purposes, especially where cash flow is not a major consideration. Initial short-term rental of equipment may be preferable to purchase. Even if new items are purchased, small loans from a bank can cost less than the cost escalation built into lease/purchase agreements.

Office furnishings represent a philosophy and convey the personality of the practice and its owner. Just as the practice is very personal, so are its furnishings. Even if office furnishings have to be bought one piece at a time, it is essential that the quality convey what the practitioner intends. In addition to obvious factors of economic considerations, major considerations in furnishing an office are (1) comfort, (2) utility, (3) safety, and (4) aesthetics.

Office furnishings must be comfortable for the clients, but especially for employees, who spend most of their waking hours there. Furnishings and equipment should be efficient and highly usable. Wall furnishings and decorations must be safe, and the entire office concept should be personally pleasing. Expensive decoration and furnishings at the outset of a new practice are neither necessary nor practical. Office changes can be anticipated in the first few years, and moves may not accommodate furniture already bought.

Minimum requirements for office space and design include

1. Office and consultation rooms (for children and adults)
2. Treatment rooms (for children and adults)
3. Storage area and files
4. Reception and waiting areas
5. Business and secretarial area
6. Some sound control from room to room
7. Nearby water for drinking
8. Accessible toilets
9. Wheelchair accessibility (barrier free entrance to building, doors in the office, space in the waiting room)
10. Electrical outlets
11. Heating and cooling controls
12. Adequate lighting

Minimal equipment, necessary for almost any office, includes

1. Secretarial chair and desk
2. Dictaphone, recorder and receiver (or cassette recorder, with a dictaphone receiver and headset for the secretary)
3. Typewriter

Some people believe that a postage scale, meter, and copy machine are essential at the outset. The practitioner needs to make sure that these purchases are necessary and not just desirable, particularly if early cash flow is a problem.

Minimal furniture requirements include (1) Desks; (2) Chairs (for staff, for clients, and for the waiting room); (3) Lamps; (4) Clocks; (5) Plants; (6) Bookshelves; (7) Filing cabinets; (8) Typing table(s); and (9) Therapy tables (adult and children).

When furnishing the waiting room, remember that children stand in chairs; both children and adults spill things on chairs, sofas, and floors; and everyone has dirty hands and feet. Attention to these basic facts should steer a practitioner away from carpeting the waiting room, selecting light colored furniture, and buying overstuffed chairs and sofas. Usually it is not a good idea to have a children's play area in the waiting room for siblings of clients. Parents will think of this as a babysitting area and leave their children beyond the required amount of time, often unattended, for free child care services.

The only way to furnish and equip a professional office is to design the best possible office arrangement for the services to be provided and the number of people to be served. On the basis of this design, determine which furnishings and equipment are absolutely necessary for the first 3 years. The practitioner can be as creative as money and energy allow. Furniture and equipment bought at the initiation of a new practice should be bought with at least a 3 year goal in mind. The 3 year term frequently coincides with a loan from the bank, the lease for office space, and the predictable direction of a new practice. When this first 3 year period is half over, the practitioner can begin planning for a second period, ranging from 5 to 10 years. At this point, the practitioner may feel free to develop new designs for the practice, new furniture and equipment, new personnel, and new office space.

As initial preparation for purchasing furniture and equipment, it is helpful to define the function or functions that will be required of each area—the subdivisions, if appropriate (child area, adult area); reception area; typing and telephone area; bookkeeping area; office/consultation room; testing and therapy rooms for adults and for children; and areas for audiological assessment and services. The specification of functional areas can help avoid unnecessary furniture duplication and the need to rearrange a room or an area for every different group of clients or parents. A checklist for each functional area should be at least in two parts—the desirable, and the necessary and affordable. As one makes this list, it becomes easier to budget for future items that are considered high priority as soon as they become affordable. Goals may be set for the purchase of high-priority items by the second or third year of practice.

Equipment and furniture for use by staff can be classified in terms of *individual* equipment/furniture and shared equipment/furniture. Certain items can be shared, but other items yield inefficiency if shared. A primary purpose in equipping a professional office is to maximize productivity of the professional staff. If staff functioning is inhibited by insufficient or inadequate equipment and furnishings, then productivity will be decreased and the savings projected from not buying additional pieces of equipment or furniture will quickly be negated. As the staff grows and the number of clients increase, the design, as well as equipment and furnishings, changes. The office space may have to be modified for greater efficiency, but not at the expense of reducing quality of services or productivity of the professional staff. Some equipment and materials will be in demand at all times by each professional staff member. These include items such as file cabinets, clocks, consultation and therapy tables, tape recorders, flashlights, stop watches, and other items specific to the service delivery itself. Other items such as a typewriter, copy machine, or telephone answering device, will serve more than one staff member.

The practitioner will quickly learn how to predict whether a new piece of business or office equipment, or professional supply, will pay for itself in time saved and in productivity. Office and business equipment should expand the efficiency of both office and clinical staff. Professional equipment and supplies should increase productivity of the professionals and reduce time and energy required when such supplies and equipment are not available. The weighing of equipment cost against gains in productivity and efficiency is basic to a cost effective practice. The successful practitioner soon learns how to predict cost effectiveness within a certain margin before expenditures are actually made.

Selecting Equipment Dealers and Consultants

Equipment dealers and consultants must be chosen on the basis of their accessibility and their service; references from colleagues can be helpful in choosing dealers and consultants. Business equipment, as well as professional equipment, requires prompt and accurate assistance at the time of purchase and whenever repairs and reordering become necessary. A reputable dealer will also make clear the payment schedule and the difference between purchases and a lease/purchase plan. Some companies allow payment on a deferred schedule, which means that no payment is required until x period after delivery. It is important, when obtaining any new equipment, to inspect it and check out its functioning before the dealer or company representative leaves the premises. If equipment is shipped to your office, be sure to inspect the statement and the piece of equipment itself before signing a release of damages with the freight company.

Essential items for audiology practice differ in type and in cost from a speech-language pathology practice. In addition to items necessary for basic office supplies, the audiologist will need an examination table and a sound room. The audiology test suite can double as a consultation area. Although some professionals build their own sound rooms, a commercial sound room with exact specifications is qualitatively better. Construction costs of a sound room are not much less than a commercially built and installed sound room. If the practitioner is not an audiologist, he/she will need diligent help from an audiologist in designing a list of essential items for basic equipment and accessories for an audiology suite. Such items will include basic equipment and tools for hearing aid dispensary and specialized audiometric procedures. If certain medically-related tests are added to a practice, a physician should be within the immediate office building area. An audiological suite, even more than other functional areas of a practice, must have adequate lighting, electrical outlets, ventilation, and usually a water source.

More and more members of the profession are dispensing products as a part of their practice. Prosthetic appliances and computer adaptations for the communicatively impaired are drawing the speech-language pathologist into dispensing of products along with the audiologists, who have been involved in hearing aid dispensing for some time. Standard procedures for buying and repairing equipment should include these products as well. An inventory is necessary for reporting property and assets in journals and bookkeeping ledgers.

Telephones

As with any other piece of equipment, the telephone must serve the practice. The practitioner must estimate number and kind of telephones and determine whether it is more desirable to rent or to buy. An important fact to note is that telephones need to be ordered at least 4 weeks before they are needed. The old estimate of 2- or 3-day waiting period is obsolete. In rapidly developing communities, sometimes the wait is as long as 3 weeks, 4 if problems arise. Reserve the telephone number far in advance to use in printing the stationery.

LETTERHEAD STATIONERY AND BUSINESS CARDS, PROFESSIONAL RECORDS, AND OTHER FORMS

The first things many people see about a practice are the stationery and business cards. These printed representatives of a practice are one of the most important public relations features of a practice. Reputation of a practitioner, appearance of practitioner and his/her office, telephone and front office reception, and letterhead stationery and business cards are crucial to the presentation of a practice to the general public and clientele. It is vital that the practitioner not skimp on quality or design of the letterhead stationery and business cards, nor on any other forms that will be seen by the public. The quality of paper used for stationery, as well as the name and logo used on the stationery, should convey the quality of the practice. Designers at print shops, other professionals, and artist consultants can be of service to the practitioner in making these decisions.

When buying more mundane office consumables, consider the following:

1. For billing clients, buy stationery with window envelopes that do not have to be addressed.
2. Match the letterhead typeface on statements and return envelopes with that of the stationery and business cards.
3. Buy cheap envelopes for paying bills from your own office, rather than using expensive letterhead stationery.
4. Some professionals feel that providing self-addressed stamped envelopes with the billing statements results in greater return of payments. Try your own market research. Do not provide self-addressed, stamped envelopes with statements for 6 months; then enclose self-addressed stamped envelopes for the next 6 months. Compare the difference between income received from the two methods, with the expense of including stamped envelopes.
5. Order all printing needs at once, if possible, including announcements, stationery, and forms. Reproduction will be only sightly more expensive than the paper itself, because the original artist's rendering of the letterhead and logo account for most of the expense. Have the printer keep the original and the dye cut for future reprints, so that additional orders will be less costly.
6. When ordering announcements to be mailed, be sure to order business cards to include with each announcement.
7. While waiting for the printing to be done, prepare the mailing list and start addressing envelopes for the announcements.

Office Forms

Collect from cooperative colleagues and business associates various kinds of forms already in use in other offices. From these determine which forms you will need for your specific practice. The only important rule of thumb in using forms is that a form must expedite the necessary paperwork, not encumber it. All forms disseminated to the public should bear your letterhead and be on quality paper. Usually it is not necessary that the public see routine forms. These mainly provide guidelines for work to be done at the clerical level. Some forms critical for administration of clinical aspects of a practice may include the following:

1. New Client Information
2. Client Case History (adult history, child history)
3. Screening Forms
4. Schedule of Appointments
5. Reappointment Cards
6. Client Ledgers
7. Payroll Record Forms
8. Billing Statements
9. Insurance Claim Forms

In-office administrative and clerical forms may include the following:

1. Thank-you Forms for Referral Sources (from which a formal letter on letter-head stationery is typed)
2. Client Status Report
3. Discharge Summaries
4. Telephone Messages
5. Plan of Treatment
6. Evaluation Forms
7. Employee Application Forms
8. Employee Attendance Forms
9. Employee Insurance Forms

Forms used only to expedite office work, which will not be stored, can be done on inexpensive scratch paper. Forms that will be stored in client folders but are not for public consumption—such as telephone messages, conversations on the telephone with teachers, and so forth—can be on plain note pad or inexpensive typing paper. Forms that are used as a shortcut for producing perfunctory letters, such as thank-you notes, can also be done on inexpensive scratch paper or dittoed on mimeograph paper and merely filled in by the professional for the secretary to type on letterhead stationery and mail. Forms that will be seen by the public, including billing statements, notice of overdue accounts, letters to clients' teachers, letters to referral sources, and formal reports, should be produced on letterhead stationery or other formal printed stationery. Carbons can be stored in client records. The copy for storage need not be on expensive paper. Any forms and ledgers used for bookkeeping and accounting or for possible legal use should be kept on a predetermined form as worked out with the accountant or other consultant.

Forms should be considered periodically for revision before being sent to the printer for duplication. In the course of a practice, opinions change, situations vary, and consequently information given or requested on various forms may change. As the supply of any particular form dwindles and time comes for reprint or recopy, the opportunity presents itself for revision of the form.

Records: Things-That-Go-Bump-in-the-Night

Almost in mockery of the freedom from bureaucracy that one seeks in a private practice is the annoying realization that records still must be maintained. The option for the practitioner is not *whether* records will be kept, but *how* records will be kept. Whether the practitioner chooses a computer or a ''Big Chief'' tablet, the protective value of records is not to be taken lightly. If you, as a practitioner and as a person, have succeeded in discovering how to avoid death, taxes, lawsuits, balancing a checkbook, borrowing money, buying insurance; *and* if you never need to communicate any aspect of client care to anyone else; *and* if you never intend to plan, project, expand, change, or liquidate your practice—*then* you may not have to keep records. However, for most of us who are not yet that clever, keeping records is necessary.

The protective value of records can apply to most aspects of any professional practice, including the following:

1. The protection and long-term care of clients
2. The legal protection of the practice and its owner
3. The fiscal protection of the practice and its owner
4. The operational protection of the personnel who create, manage, and service the practice

With these considerations in mind, one may choose to return to the relative freedom of an agency where someone else worries about how to keep records. Otherwise, one can proceed to determine which records are necessary for the practice and how conveniently and efficiently they may be maintained. Whether the most conventional record storage system is used for fairly simple files, or whether the most complex computerized system is used for a massive program, certain principles of record keeping must be served. These include the following:

1. Client Protection
   a. Privacy of records.
   b. Correct charge for services.
   c. Ease of retrieval of information for professional reports or insurance claims.
   d. Ease of retrieval of information from inactive or old records.
2. Clarity and Accuracy
   Can be read and understood 3 months later by a person who is not familiar with the original information.
3. Accessibility
   Anyone who needs information should be able to get it immediately.
4. Usability
   Any professional or office personnel should be able to use and understand the system.
5. Personnel Protection
   a. Contracts for wages.
   b. Operating agreement in a corporation.
6. Legal Requirements
   a. Tax reporting.
   b. Filing deadlines, claiming deductions.
7. Reducing Paperwork
   Minimizing the need for narrative input by coding and charting.
8. Expanding
   a. Records should be able to be expanded within themselves.

     b. Different types of records should be accommodated by the system.
9. Reasonable Economy
   The practitioner should find that the record-keeping system enhances and eases the workload rather than adding to the time, energy, and cost of the program.
10. Ease of Change to Another System as Desired
    From a Big Chief Tablet to a ledger book to a computer to microfiche files.
11. Communication with Another Party as Desired
    Information for internal revenue, client's physician, client, employees, owner, and so forth.
12. Minimizing Space Requirements
    The records system and storage of the system should not claim an inordinate amount of office space. When this occurs, then the cost of the record-keeping system increases because of cost of office space.
13. Permanence
    Client files may be needed for as long as 30 years. Sometimes clients reenter a therapy program after several years of absenteeism, or legal or educational questions arise that necessitate tracing original records.
14. Coordination and Compatibility
    The record keeping system should allow for the insertion and/or coordination of records from other professionals or agencies serving a client.

A record-keeping system should facilitate administrative and financial process of a practice, as well as facilitate and improve the quality of service delivery. Administrative and financial records to be included in a record-keeping system include the following:

1. Chart of accounts (coding system for use of money and receipt of revenue)
2. Financial statement (profit and loss statement with current balance)
3. Contracts with other agencies (hospitals, kindergartens, and so forth)
4. Personnel contracts (wages, benefits)
5. Consultation contracts
6. Payment records for fees for services
7. Disbursement of money among staff (wages and profits)
8. Deductible and nondeductible expenditures
9. Client billing forms and payment history
10. Collection letters
11. Loan agreements
12. Office contract (lease or purchase agreement)
13. Partnership or director's agreements (operating, buy-sell)

Clinical services files may need to include the following:

1. Client Information
   a. Intake Sheet
   b. Insurance Information
   c. Case History
   d. Intervention Plans
   e. Progress Notes
2. Charges
   a. Agreement for Billing and Payment

b. Summary of Test Files
c. Summary of Reports
d. Significant Occurrences Regarding Intervention
e. Summary of Therapy (dates, length, objectives)

Certainly information stored in each section depends upon preferences and needs of the practice itself. Some practices rely on computer use, either through buying computer time and services from record-keeping consultants, or by buying their own computers and gradually transferring information from traditional records. Some ongoing practices have found it easier to begin computer use with administrative and financial data, particularly client and billing information. Gradually administrative and clinical data are entered and used as desired. Frequently, the last information to go into a computer system is the client's clinical record. Flower (1984) discusses several systems designed for clinical records, including the *unit record*, the *problem oriented record*, the *practice oriented record* and the *CASE information system*.

1. The *unit record*, not necessarily computerized, is a system whereby all information regarding services provided to a single client is collected and compiled according to some format, and may include identifying information, pertinent case history information, initial test results, special tests and treatment, progress, correspondence, and termination. This system most closely parallels the traditional file folder method.

2. The *problem oriented record* system categorizes client information into sections of data base, problem lists, initial plan, and progress notes. Fashioned after the medical model of intake and treatment, this system does not require a computer. The data base incorporates identifying information about the client complaint, history, exam results, and laboratory tests. The problem list is categorized into any of several topics such as medical problems, social problems, psychiatric problems, and so forth. Initial plan and progress notes are related to the problem list, the attempts made to rectify those problems, and ultimate outcome. Kent (1980) and Flower (1984) discuss the application of *problem oriented record* systems to speech-language-hearing services.

3. The *practice oriented record* system developed from the principle that recording systems are not just for storage but also for communication. Therefore, such systems must record and provide retrieval of comprehensive pieces of information. This system, more than the other two, almost requires computerization. Storage of operational data is accomplished through client profiles, organized into components of client identifier, highlight section, problem-listing section, client services section, physician orders summary, and notes section. Client information can be retrieved by section, if desired, without calling up the complete file.

4. The *CASE information system* is one of the few fully developed record systems designed for speech-language-hearing services (American Speech-Language-Hearing Association, 1976). *CASE* is an acronym for *Comprehensive Assessment and Service Evaluation* and was originally formulated for the support of public school speech-language-hearing programs. Many aspects of the system, however, allow for application in any program and can be adapted to adult services (Flower, 1984). The system was designed to be evaluation oriented,

providing comprehensive client information that can be used for planning, documenting change, describing staff practices, and analyzing appropriateness and effectiveness of services that were rendered. The *CASE system* provides two levels of information—one, concerning individual clients, and the other documenting information about all services.

Naming the Thing

We professionals in speech-language-hearing services have finally decided what to call ourselves—almost. Even more difficult than knowing what to call ourselves as professionals has been knowing how to name communication disorders and knowing what to call the services we extend to people with those disorders. The terminology, taxonomy, and/or diagnoses used to describe speech-language-hearing disorders and services have presented a major obstacle for many years in terms of public image and more recently in terms of insurance. Another recent resurrection of the word problem has centered around the nomenclature necessary for universally accepted record-keeping systems (i.e., computers). At this point, there are several major classifications employed by medical care institutions. These are the *Standard Nomenclature of Diseases and Operations* (1961) and the *International Classification of Diseases (ICD) 1978*. Mental health programs have relied on revisions of the *Diagnostic and Statistical Manual of Mental Disorders*. (Currently, the third revision is in use—*DSM III*, 1980). Important contributions to the development of a taxonomy regarding speech-language-hearing services have been the *CASE information system* and the *Iowa Quality Assurance Program System* (1977). The *Rehabilitation Codes* (1967) have also offered some useful applications for speech-language-hearing services. The *Physicians' Current Procedural Terminology (CPT,* 1981), which is intended for physician use, can be adapted in some ways for use by speech-language-hearing professionals. Some insurance forms require the use of *CPT* codes on claim forms.

Speech-language-hearing services cover many areas of human behavior and physical state. Because of overlapping physical and mental disorders that manifest themselves in speech, language, and/or hearing impairment, a classification system based solely on physiological disorders or solely on psychological dysfunction has been both limiting and confusing. Just as confusing is the situation in which there is no evidence of physical or mental pathology that can account for the communication disorder. A reasonable solution to date has been to adapt either standard classification codes of other professions to speech-language pathology/audiology or merely to make up something on the spur of the moment. The *International Classification of Diseases* (ICD) now provides a supplementary classification known as the *V Code*. The supplementary *V Code* may be particularly applicable to our profession because it permits the clinician to describe the client complaint, rather than requiring the clinician to provide a diagnosis, as do the other codes.

In determining a coding system for speech-language-hearing problems, it has been difficult to know what is the *primary disorder* and what is the *secondary disorder*, or to know what is the *primary cause* or *contributing factor* of the disorder itself. For example, hearing disorders frequently result in problems of both spoken and written language, articulation, voice, and academic achievement. If the choice in a coding system is to put the causative or contributing factors as the primary code listing, many disorders of speech, language, hearing, and their resulting symptoms have no primary listing because no apparent causative factor can be proven. The coding system used by the mental health profession, *DSM III*, lends itself slightly more to applications than the coding of diseases or neurological disorders; however, the use of any other profession's health code, even when applicable, subordinates the profession of speech-language pathology/audiology to another profession's theories and perceptions regarding the etiology and the treatment of disorders. The *DSM III*, as well as other classification systems, does not include several categories necessary for documenting speech, language, or hearing disorders. Complicating the issue of developing a coding system specific to our profession are the many areas of professional and philosophical disagreement among speech-language-hearing professionals. To touch the tip of the iceberg, there is, for example, disagreement regarding such terms as *delay/disorder, speech/language, language/learning,* and so forth. The turmoil within the profession, which resulted from trying to arrive at a standardized taxonomy, has indeed been a longstanding one. The American Speech-Language-Hearing Association has attempted on several occasions to develop a detailed procedural coding system. Currently it is engaged in wrestling with the various problems of developing such a system.

A taxonomic system must allow for a type of categorization that can clearly describe the client regarding his/her disorder or disorders, and permit recommendations for intervention. The problems in achieving such a system include the following:

1. Professional disagreement within the profession regarding use of terminology describing the profession and its services;
2. The desire to avoid the appearance of subservience.

The sense of urgency that has been generated by the need for a coding or taxonomic system for current technology hopefully will bring the profession a little closer to a nomenclature appropriate for speech, language, and hearing that meets all the special needs of such a profession.

Clinical Reports

Clinical reports of varying types are inherent to all professional practices. In many agencies, including hospitals and public schools, legal or institutional regulations require that reports be kept of impressions and interactions formed in the delivery of services to the communicatively impaired clients. The degree of attention paid to formal report writing and record maintenance is related to the following:

1. Requirements of the employment institution;
2. The law;
3. The need to transmit information from one professional to another;
4. The necessity to supplement a clinician's memory about client interactions and dates over time;
5. Numerous other personal, professional, and clinical reasons.

The reluctance with which many professionals approach report writing is usually directly related to the amount of time required to accurately convey critical information. The danger in avoiding reporting—and the attraction to a computerized system of reporting—lies in the shortcuts and shorthand systems that may be employed but that may distort the clinical impressions that could be more accurately conveyed in a narrative report. Whatever the record-keeping system preferred by a practitioner, it is imperative that clinical reporting be done in such a way that it be of maximum help to the delivery of clinical services.

Organization of Traditional Filing Systems

When organizing client records in file folders, space-saving and ease of access become immediate concerns. One way of organizing files is to separate current clients from previous clients and to break down the current client files by type of intervention. *In-process* files are those that contain the records of a current client undergoing intake and evaluation, reevaluation, or other treatment planning procedures. *Current* files are those files that contain folders of clients currently seen in an intervention or long-term evaluation program. *Permanent*, *old*, or *inactive* files are those files that contain folders of clients seen in the past who have now terminated, moved, or been furloughed from intervention. These files should be fairly accessible but not as conveniently located as *current* files. Any files older than 5 years can be stored in an even less convenient spot. A separate filing category may also be necessary for clients who have been seen for only a single session or who have been seen only through a screening program. Screening files can be kept according to school, with year noted on the file label, and with children's screening forms filed alphabetically inside the folder.

However client records are stored, they should not be destroyed. At least once a year, a request is made for reports, records, or information on clients who were seen 15 to 20 years earlier. If nothing else, it is a humbling experience to look back over files that are many years old and note the naivete and professional simplicity with which we have dealt with clients in the past. A secretary or clerk should routinely review all current files to make sure that original documents provided by clients or their families have been copied and originals returned, that all release forms are signed, and that all clients currently seen have a copy of current clinic policies and have signed the fee agreement.

ADMINISTRATIVE AND FINANCIAL RECORDS

Once an accounting method, tax year, and bookkeeping system have been chosen, it is necessary to set about keeping records suitable for business purposes. Records may be kept correctly to report taxable income and to figure taxes. The law does not require any special kind of records. It is up to the practitioner to choose the system best suited to his/her business—one that will clearly show gross income, deductions, and credits. Methods of bookkeeping and accounting are discussed in Chapter 3, this book. Records of a business must be kept as long as they may be required by the Internal Revenue Service.

Whether administrative and financial records are kept in single ledger, double ledger, books and journals, or a computer program, such records must do the following:

1. Identify source of receipt. The money one receives can come from many sources. Records must identify the source of receipts in order to prove whether they are from business or nonbusiness sources.
2. Keep track of deductible expenses. Some expenses are quickly forgotten or lost by the time a tax return is prepared.
3. Figure depreciation allowance. Record the assets to be depreciated in the permanent record. A record of cost and other information on assets is necessary in order to figure depreciation deductions. If assets are sold or become fully depreciated, or if capital improvements are made to those assets, only a permanent record can show how much of their cost was not recovered by the owner.
4. Take advantage of capital gains laws. Good records indicate the date an asset was acquired, what it was used for, and whether it was sold, traded, destroyed, or otherwise disposed of.
5. Determine earnings for self-employment tax purposes. Records will show how much of the earnings require payment of self-employment taxes.
6. Support items reported on tax returns. Any examination of tax returns by the IRS may result in requests for explanation of items reported. Records can speed up this examination with support from sales slips, invoices, receipts, and other documents.
7. Retain copies. Any records used to support an item of income or deduction on a tax return must be kept until the statute of limitations runs out. Employers must keep all employment tax records for a specified period of time, as well. Records should be kept that verify owner's basis of property for as long as they are needed to figure the basis of the original or replacement property.
8. Copies of filed tax returns should be kept. These are useful in preparing future tax returns and may be helpful in later claims for refunds. Such returns are also helpful for settling an estate.

Almost without exception, a business checkbook must be maintained in an orderly manner, regardless of the financial record-keeping system. This is the basic source for record keeping as well as the basic source of documented expenditures in many businesses.

Some small businesses use an automatic data processing (ADP) system. If this system is used, it must include a method of producing from punched cards, or other machine-sensitive data media, legible records that will provide proof of tax liability. (Machine-sensitive data media include magnetic tapes, discs, punched tapes, and punched cards.) According to the IRS (IRS, Pub. No. 334, 1983), an ADP system is acceptable if it complies with the following guidelines:

1. Prints out a general ledger and its source references for the same period as the tax year.
2. Provides an audit trail so that details, such as invoices and vouchers of the summary accounting data, may be identified and made available upon request.
3. Provides a way to trace any transaction back to the original source, or forward to a final total. If printouts or transactions are not made when they are processed, the system must be able to make a record of those transactions.
4. Has adequate storage facilities for machine-sensitive data media, printouts, and any other supporting documents. Records must be kept in the same way as records under a manual accounting system.

5. Full descriptions of the ADP part of the accounting system and the controls used to insure accurate and reliable processing should be available.

In general, sketchy financial records, regardless of the system used, which only approximate income deductions or other items affecting tax liability, will not be considered adequate by the IRS. Entries must be supported by cancelled checks, paid bills, duplicate deposit slips, or any other items. The support items should be filed in an orderly manner and stored in a safe place.

Decisions and problems involved in filing, storage, retrieving, and preserving the records of a practice deserve the attention of the practitioner/owner. In many ways, a private practice that coordinates human services with business requirements complicates the record-keeping process. Clearly, good records significantly influence the quality of professional services and can help the practitioner remain financially solvent and administratively efficient. Various management agencies provide advice, as well as products, for both traditional and computerized storage and retrieval systems. These range from color-coded filing systems to floppy discs for computers to microfiche storage.

Appendices

APPENDIX 4–1
STARTER LIST: OFFICE SUPPLIES AND FURNISHINGS

Accounting forms
Advertisement copy
Announcement cards
Appointment calendar and cards
Audiometric equipment
Billing statements
Billing and posting forms
Business cards
Calculators and related supplies
Calibration equipment
Chalk board and accessories
Client Public Information materials
Clocks
Copier and related supplies
Desk lamps
Dictation equipment
Door signs
Envelopes
File folders and indexing supplies
Filing cabinets
Framed diplomas and certificates
Hearing aid dispensary supplies
  and equipment
Insurance payment forms
Letterhead stationery
Magazine rack and magazines
Mailing labels
Memo paper and pads

Office chairs and tables
Office decorations
Office desks
Office lamps
Office signs
Paper clip holder and clips
Pencil holders, sharpener, pencils
Pens
Petty cash box
Rubber stamps and pads
Scissors
Staplers and staples
Speech, language, and hearing
  equipment and supplies and materials
  for assessment and intervention
Stationery
Tape recorders
Tax forms and calendars
Telephone answering system
  and telephones
Telephone numbers
Tools for minor audiometric
  and office repair
Typewriter and ribbons (and
  correction materials), paper,
  carbon paper
Waiting room tables and chairs
Wall mirrors

APPENDIX 4–2
STARTER LIST: SPEECH-LANGUAGE PATHOLOGY PRACTICE

Services and Equipment

You need to determine which services you intend to offer. Will you provide

1. Diagnostic services for all disorders and all age groups, or only some?
2. Treatment for all disorders and all age groups, or only some?
3. Audiometric screening?
4. Evaluation and treatment of nonspeaking persons?
5. Consultation with teachers?
6. Contractual services with schools, home health agencies, skilled nursing facilities, and so forth?

Equipment

Although equipping a speech-language pathology private practice does not present as large a financial investment as equipping an audiology private practice, you must determine what you need and can afford in view of the services to be offered. You should ask yourself

1. Do I need a tape recorder?
2. If so, what type (audio or video or both; reel-to-reel or cassette)?
3. What make and model will give the quality I need?
4. What brand and length of tapes should I buy?
5. Should I buy a machine to bulk erase tapes? What brand?
6. Do I need an observation room with a two-way mirror?
7. If so, should it be wired for sound?
8. What kind of commercially available tests should I get? For children or adults? Both children and adults? How many do I need? How many response sheets for each test?
9. Do I need a portable audiometer for screening purposes?
10. If so, should it be fixed or sweep frequency or intensity?
11. Do I need an array of aided communication devices (electrolarynx, electronic communication board, voice synthesizer, etc.) for evaluation and intervention?
12. What other equipment/materials do I need for professional evaluation and intervention—blades, flashlight, oral manometer, books, toys and games, pictures?

From *Planning and Initiating a Private Practice in Audiology and Speech-Language Pathology,* American Speech-Language-Hearing Association, 1985. Copyright 1985 by American Speech-Language-Hearing Association. Adapted with permission.

APPENDIX 4-3
STARTER LIST: AUDIOLOGY PRACTICE

Services and Equipment

You need to determine which *services and products* you intend to offer. Will you provide

1. Routine diagnostic audiologic services (e.g., pure tone and speech audiometric services and immittance measurement)?
2. Assessment of central auditory processing abilities in children and adults?
3. Hearing aid consultation?
4. Hearing aid dispensing?
5. Aural rehabilitative services for children or adults or both?
6. Preschool speech and hearing screening services?
7. Electronystagmography?
8. Brainstem evoked response measurement?
9. Industrial hearing conservation services?
10. Consultative services to hospitals, physicians, or schools?

Equipment

Audiologic equipment represents a sizable portion of the investment in an audiology practice. You must determine what you need, in light of the services and products you wish to offer, and then prioritize them on the basis of what is immediately affordable. You should ask yourself

1. Do I need an audiometric test booth? More than one?
2. What kind?
3. Do I want a one- or two-room test suite?
4. What specifications are important for the test booth? Size? Double wall?
5. What will be needed to meet standards and accrediting requirements? ANSI? ASHA Professional Services Board? Vocational Rehabilitation? Commission on Accreditation of Rehabilitation Facilities?
6. Can the floor in my office support a test suite? A commercially built booth?
7. Are the utility and water supplies adequate and accessible?
8. Is the office large enough to accommodate such a room?
9. Can the room be locked?
10. What kind of audiometer(s) do I need?
11. Should it be single channel, channel-and-a-half, or double channel?
12. Should it have narrowband noise, white noise, speech noise, pink noise, or sawtooth noise?
13. Will it accept input and play back with true stereo fidelity for dichotic speech tests?
14. Should it have pulse switching for pulsed tone testing and binaural loudness balance measures?

From *Planning and Initiating a Private Practice in Audiology and Speech-Language Pathology*, American Speech-Language-Hearing Association, 1985. Copyright 1985 by American Speech-Language-Hearing Association. Adapted with permission.

15. Should it have a warble tone or SISI generator?
16. Do I need Bekesy-type capabilities? Should it have true frequency sweep and continuous tone features?
17. Can it sweep from high-frequency to low, as well as from low to high?
18. Do I need a unit with synchronized narrow band masking feature?
19. Do I need acoustic immittance equipment?
20. Do I need hard copy for tympanometry or reflex measurement?
21. Do I need ipsilateral reflex capability?
22. What intensity range do I need for the pure tone generator?
23. Do I need a sound field set up? One speaker or two? One amplifier or two?
24. Where should the speakers be located in the room?
25. Do I need a back-up audiometer? How much test capability should it have?
26. Do I need a tinnitus measurement unit?
27. Do I need a master hearing aid?
28. Do I need a sound level meter?
29. Do I need calibration couplers?
30. Do I need bone conduction calibration equipment?
31. Do I need hearing aid analysis equipment?
32. Do I need an electronystagmograph? Single channel or dual channel?
33. Do I need an optokinetic stimulator?
34. Do I need a calibrating device?
35. Should I have water caloric or an air caloric stimulator?
36. Do I need an evoked response unit?
37. Other?

Chapter **5**

The Office: Part II
Personnel and Operations

PERSONNEL

Just as the practitioner designs office space and furniture for maximum function, so should a practitioner design positions for office and clinical personnel. Because of the unusual combination of professional and business demands in a private practice, it is important that responsibilities of the staff are carefully considered and assigned. For example, the clinician/employee should not be involved in too many day-to-day administrative management decisions but be free to exercise professional judgment and interact with clients to meet the demands of providing quality services to the communicatively impaired. In the same way, it is important that the owner/practitioner, even though actively involved in clinical services, not get too involved in clerical work such as running errands, making perfunctory phone calls, and typing client statements. As Marshall et al. (1982) say, the most expensive person in the practice is the owner/practitioner. For that reason, it is ridiculous to spend expensive time doing bookkeeping, office maintenance, and extra typing. Although this may seem ''free'' at the time, in the long run, the depletion of resources of the owner/practitioner is much more costly than hiring other staff.

The first and last resource in a private practice is the practitioner/owner. Financial decisions, administrative policy, determination of the quality of service delivery, and personnel interaction will depend to a large extent upon the way in which the owner directs personal and professional energies. After spending so much time and energy on the goals and objectives of the practice, financial loans, management, delegating responsibilities and activities, the hardest task is yet to come—that of writing one's own job description and sticking to it.

Deciding which personnel is required for what tasks is a primary goal in office management, both clinical and clerical. When the staff is operating at what seems to be maximum production, the time has come to reconsider the direction of the goals of the practice, which may involve adding new staff and accepting more clients. Many practitioners feel that unless the professional staff increases, growth of the practice will not continue. However, a by-product of adding personnel, particularly in large numbers, may be the reduction of quality control in service delivery. Regardless of office positions that are designated and filled, the most important aspect of personnel is assigning the appropriate person to appropriate responsibilities.

Types of personnel include: professional staff, paraprofessional staff, consultants, administrative staff, and clerical or office staff.

Professional Staff

There is little need to belabor the necessity for competent, reliable professionals in any service delivery setting. A compromise in hiring will result in a compromise in services. Achieving clinical productivity while maintaining quality services is crucial when increasing professional staff. Before hiring additional employees, it is wise to consider the productivity of current staff—for example, the number of client contact hours, number of clients seen, amount of time off, and the professional's salary or commission. Productivity level must be such that clinicians are not rushed, but are seldom free to have long lunches. Many professionals feel that if a practitioner can afford to shift 20 to 25 percent of new referrals in one year to a new clinician, then addition of a new staff member is warranted.

Some practitioners become possessive of their clients and become unwilling to turn over certain clients or referrals to another clinician. In addition, the reaction of referral sources to substitute clinicians is not positive, emphasizing the need for careful introduction of new staff to the professional community.

Initially, it may be wise to consider part-time personnel who qualify as *independent consultants* or independent contractors.

In that way the owner/practitioner need not carry the professional on the books as an employee. Independent contractors or consultants must be completely independent in the execution of their professional activities and are not considered as employees by the IRS. Within certain guidelines set out in an agreement between an employer and contractor (consulting practitioner), the contractor can work without direct supervision and can work for other employers. An independent contractor is not eligible for withholding and social security, but is paid an agreed upon salary. In many instances, practitioners base the contractor's salary on a percentage of fees billed for services. Any time that wages are based on percentage of fees, the percentage the contractor receives is related to the practitioner's risk in guaranteeing payment and the bookkeeping and other services required by the additional revenue source. For example, if an independent consultant is guaranteed a fixed percentage of revenue, regardless of fee collection, then wages can be set at a lower ratio. Independent status may need to be proved by showing that the consultant receives no supervision or fringe benefits and is treated like any other licensed professional.

When a practice employs professionals on a part-time basis, but not as independent consultants, withholding taxes and social security are applicable.

Any employment agreement should be put in the form of a written contract, whether with an independent contractor or a regular employee. Not only should the contract specify wages, hours, job responsibilities, authority, fringe benefits, and term of the contract, it should also include specified policies regarding restrictions on practicing in the same geographical area once the contract has terminated. The contract should also state any desired restrictions on outside work by the contractor. Most contracts for full-time employees restrict them to employment with that one practice. Part-time employment contracts differ and are at the discretion of the employer.

It is not unusual for successful clinicians to gain experience and contract with one practice, allow that employment contract to lapse, and open their own practices with clients taken from the former practice. In some communities it can be fairly destructive for an employee-turned-competitor to set up a practice nearby. Both clients and referral sources become confused. One way to prevent this occurrence is to write a "noncompete clause" into the employment contract. It can be fairly difficult and expensive to enforce such a clause if court action is required to do so; however, the existence of such a clause is usually deterrent enough.

Supervision of Professional Staff

Administration of office procedures and management of clerical staff is an entirely different matter than supervising professional employees or professional consultants. Some private practitioners hesitate to hire a professional who needs supervision, assuming that such supervision would be unnecessary for qualified professionals. A practitioner should employ only those clinicians who have experience and an outstanding reputation for providing quality services. Supervision of interns can be extremely expensive because of the time it consumes, both in direct and indirect supervision as well as in conferences with the intern. Supervision of interns is counterindicated in private practice because of the client's expectations that he/she is paying for professional services. Most are reluctant, if not completely opposed, to paying full fees for the inexperience of a new clinician. The same argument also holds for employing paraprofessionals in private practice.

Paraprofessional Staff

Paraprofessionals can be used in many valuable ways in settings where a master clinician can supervise them in perfunctory work; they can be used in the completion of routine forms, carry-over activities, repetitive drill, and maintenance of room and materials. Use of paraprofessionals in private practice is fairly undeveloped at this time. Most practitioners feel that paraprofessionals used in private settings pose management difficulties; it is not easy to equate the skills and services of a paraprofessional with fees for services. Some professionals who work out of the office as consultants are highly successful in using paraprofessionals in certain agencies, especially those agencies with deaf, blind, multi-handicapped clients and those with severe/profound retarded clients. In these settings, paraprofessionals can perform many perfunctory tasks that do not require direct application by a master clinician. It is possible to have more than one level of paraprofessional—for example, a high school graduate who carries out nontherapy-related tasks; and a person with a bachelor's degree in the profession who can carry out many technical aspects of intervention such as scoring tests, maintenance and carry-over, certain newly learned tasks, and certain types of paperwork (see Appendix 4–4).

Consultants

The practitioner may find it desirable to enlist the services of more than one type of professional consultant. An attorney and an accountant usually are required before a practice opens and throughout its existence. Other consultants may also be necessary, including an insurance broker, computer consultant, stock broker, banker, and management consultant. It is the responsibility of the owner/practitioner to determine when and how such consultants are needed. When no direction is given with regard to consultant use, the office staff may hire unnecessary consultants.

The owner/practitioner should never presume to have all of the knowledge and skills necessary to run a professional practice. The appropriate use of professional consultants is often the least expensive way to stay out of trouble and to acquire the knowledge necessary for making decisions critical to the practice.

Attorneys

Every professional in private practice needs the advice and knowledge of an attorney. An attorney who possesses a working knowledge of small businesses as well as professional corporations should help incorporate the practice. It is helpful to find an attorney whose areas of law are appropriate to your needs.

Accountants

Accountants are the most frequently used consultants by any practice. An accountant can not only assist in setting up the bookkeeping system, train the bookkeeper and secretary, but also can assist in setting up ways for administering the business. However, neither the attorney nor the accountant has the necessary training or experience to advise one on management. The owner/practitioner must work out managerial and operational features of his/her practice once the legal and financial groundwork is laid.

Some accountants are able to provide information and experience-based advice regarding long-range financial planning. Some specialize in small businesses and related tax problems and can be of enormous value in tax planning and preparation, design of retirement programs, establishment of relationships with financial institutions, estate planning, and investment decisions. Often, management consultants are used by owners/practitioners for help in designing their practices, in setting management policies and procedures, and in formulating projections. Many management consultants also provide assistance with insurance programs, certification for Medicare vendors, and problem solving with third-party payers.

Consultants usually bill on the basis of hourly fees. In spite of what may seem to be astonishing costs for their services, it is unwise for any practitioner to substitute folk remedies and guesswork for the information and guidance of knowledgeable consultants. Shopping for bargains is appropriate when choosing consultants, but looking for the lowest fee is not the way to shop. The owner/practitioner must seek competent consultants who have experience in the area of the practitioner's need; who are prompt, accurate, reliable; and who will provide help when trouble comes along. Appropriate use of good consultants usually proves to be economical for any practitioner.

The way to reduce consultant cost is to be prepared for the contact. For example, have the secretary/receptionist/bookkeeper learn to reconcile the financial records, rather than taking the raw data for the accountant to do at a costly fee.

Office and Clerical Staff

The owner/practitioner should give high priority to the policies affecting each position and to the people employed in those positions. The office staff must understand that it is important to interact on a friendly basis with clients, but to maintain professional dignity on behalf of the office and to observe the strictist confidentiality. In some clinics, the receptionist is the person who must be in charge of the waiting room, and, when necessary, quiet unruly children. Some clinical practices require more organizational and bookkeeping skills from a secretary than other offices. Most professional offices require technical accuracy in typing, filing, billing, collecting, and keeping financial records. Sometimes the secretary can learn from the bookkeeper or accountant how to maintain financial records for the office and how to prepare the books for the accountant to reconcile and audit. Procedures regarding responsibilities, contracts, and benefits of office employees should be clear to all. Frequently, the manner and efficiency of the office staff are powerful in enhancing or diminishing the success of a professional office.

A managerial or administrative assistant is required in some large offices. When administrative office details keep the owner/practitioner from having time to plan growth, evaluate policies, and generally oversee the practice, it is probably time to consider a part-time or a full-time administrative assistant. An administrative assistant can assist the owner by developing new referral sources; recruiting good staff; producing a business plan; and overseeing the daily mechanics of running an office. The owner/practitioner must decide if, as the practice grows, it is more desirable to hire someone else to perform some of the administrative responsibilities, or to decrease his/her own clinical contact for this purpose.

Locating and Hiring Office Personnel

When hiring, it is important not to be too casual in filling positions. If using an employment agency or a university employment office, select one that screens for each particular position. When advertising in newspapers, use a blind advertisement with a box number for responses and resumes. It is helpful to discuss the job briefly over the telephone in order to do some last-minute screening, before setting up an interview for an applicant.

In the advertisements, telephone conversations, and interviews, be as specific and realistic as possible. For example, if telephone work will be an important feature of the position, be sure to talk on the telephone with the applicant prior to making a decision. If typing, writing from dictation, or using a word processor will be required, have the applicant do some short, simple work on these machines before the interview. Be specific with the applicant in terms of hours, duration of the employment contract, job responsibilities, approximate salary, benefits, and opportunities for increasing salary or benefits.

The most frequently neglected task in hiring an employee is checking references. A phone call to a former employer usually is more effective than correspondence. Inquire about job efficiency of the applicant, as well as general demeanor. An office that constantly deals with people must have office staff that is tolerant, patient, and pleasant, although firm when necessary. The office staff represents the practitioner thousands of times a month and must represent the practice and the owner/practitioner in the best possible way.

Hiring a new employee should include a written agreement that specifies fringe benefits, vacation periods, salary, and job responsibilities. Each time the contract is renewed, the written agreement can be renegotiated to the benefit of both the employer and the employee.

When hiring a new secretary, remember that an employee who is dismissed before the end of an agreed upon period may collect unemployment compensation. When the ex-employee files for unemployment compensation, the ex-employer is liable for an increase in unemployment tax insurance. It is better to take care and deliberation in hiring than to act impulsively in order to fill a vacancy quickly. When searching for a new secretary, allow at least 4 to 5 weeks to locate, interview, and hire the new employee. Remember that the person you select will usually need to give notice to the previous employer.

OPERATIONS

Redundancy in running an office provides a more efficient administrative system, just as redundancy in language provides for a more efficient communication system. In order to arrive at an efficiently redundant office system, it is necessary to establish and maintain regular procedures for every aspect of office operations, from opening the door in the morning to locking the door behind you at the end of the day. The owner/practitioner needs to sort out the various functions of office administration, clinical services, and personnel. With this categorical approach, it is easier to compose a list of items that will eventually take the form of office policy. The list is infinite, and formally written policies may never occur for many of the items on the list. However, beginning with a list that can be prioritized can be a great boon to the beginning practitioner, as well as, to the practitioner who has an established practice that he/she wants to make more efficient. Many routine procedures and policies are obvious to a practitioner but are not given formal attention until a crisis arises. Careful practitioners have formal and regularized procedures for such obviously important tasks as new client intake, billing procedures, purchase procedures, employee job descriptions and contracts, and client scheduling. Managing the office, the money, and the staff can be very deceptive for a practitioner. Even without tight management, an office can almost run itself. The difference is that clearly articulated policies produce more profit for the practice, greater client satisfaction with the services, and greater job satisfaction of employees. Some areas where the practitioner typically fails to develop clear policies include (1) initial contact with clients and families; (2) client scheduling and caseloads; (3) telephone use; (4) maintenance of time records; and (5) organization of one's desk and activities.

Initial Contact with Client and Family

Ordinarily, when clients enter a professional office, they are somewhat uncomfortable. Some families are anxious about the complete interaction, as well as about their reasons for seeking help. The client and family need direction from the moment they enter the reception area. It is important that the receptionist greet them, acknowledge that they are expected, and tell them that the professional will be with them shortly. The receptionist should then direct them to chairs and present them with appropriate information, intake forms, or case history forms. This general procedure applies to the first or second visit, but rarely applies to routine visits by clients in on-going therapy.

First-time clients need to be greeted by the professional as soon as possible after their arrival. The professional should introduce himself/herself, indicating that it may be a few moments until time for the session; the professional may then leave the waiting room, returning in a few moments for the client or the family. The initial presentation and introduction by the professional helps to relieve general anxiety about the interaction. It also gives the client and family a chance to "look over" the practitioner and time to settle down for the contact before the professional's return and invitation into the inner office. Before closing conferences—even the most routine and perfunctory—the professional should reiterate some of the major items discussed in the conference, remaining issues to be considered, and possible alternatives for resolving whatever problems are at hand. To end the conference, walk the client to the main area. (Some clients become confused in finding their way out.) Not only is this a polite termination of the conference, it also indicates to clients that your attention is still with them, and that you have not yet turned to the next task. It also keeps them from standing in the office for an extra 15 minutes asking "just one more thing."

It is of utmost importance that the client and family feel that their privacy is being respected in the interview, evaluation, or conference. Many families of people with communication handicaps are involved in frustrating home and public interactions because of the communication disorder. To some people the very fact that one is in a professional's office is compromising and embarrassing.

Client Scheduling and Caseload

A unique aspect of service delivery in private practice is the flexibility for scheduling, grouping, and arranging clients in intervention programs for their maximum benefit. A client can be seen as often as necessary and as long as maximum benefit is accomplished. Some clients can work for 2 hours at a time; others profit from only 20 minutes. Many clients are seen on varying schedules over a course of 10 to 15 years. Regularly scheduled visits are common in private practice, just as in any other practice. However, for some long-term clients it is possible to provide intensive block therapy alternating with vacation or time off. The extensive scheduling of groups provides increased benefit for many clients and also serves as an efficient form of service delivery for the practitioner. Scheduling can be arranged so that certain types of clients will not be in the waiting room or hallways at the same time. For example, some adults do not like to be in the same area with small children, and some adults are self-conscious about being seen by other adults. In these situations, appointments can be arranged accordingly. Because there are fewer time boundaries than in school or hospital programs, and because there are not as many internal contingencies that interfere with scheduling, every 24-hour period provides numerous scheduling opportunities. Of course, just as in any other setting, accommodations must be made for the clients' availability and the practitioner's own schedule and tolerance.

The size and type of caseload varies widely from one practice to another. It is not unusual for one practitioner to have 80 to 100 client contacts a week. Some practitioners choose to work 6 days a week with somewhat shortened hours—for example, from noon to 7 p.m. Other practitioners prefer intensive 3- to 4-day weeks, from eight in the morning until nine or ten at night. Caseload concerns do not arise in private practice as they do in other work settings. In private practice, the caseload problem is a double-edged sword. It is frightening to have a caseload so low that office time is unscheduled for the practitioners; at other times the same practitioners can be so busy with an exhaustive number of clients that there is little time to make a phone call. This cyclical pattern of feast or famine is fairly common to private practices and is one factor that makes expansion and future projections somewhat difficult. The search for new clients and new referrals should never stop. Even when a practitioner has a full caseload, his/her practice could decline within a few months unless active and ongoing efforts are made to obtain clients.

A caseload is affected by factors other than marketing activity and normal cycles of influx and attrition. A practice serving school-aged children can be impacted by federal policies regarding funding of public school programs. For example, in 1982, the U.S. General Accounting Office concluded that mildly speech-impaired children should not be served under Public Law 94-142 (ASHA, 1983). These children, who by law can no longer be treated in the public schools for their language impairment, become potential clients for the private sector.

The Telephone

The telephone is an essential communication tool, linking the practitioner, sources of referrals, and clients. The way the telephone is answered can leave a lasting impression on clients who may be anxious, angry, or merely in a hurry. A message from a secretary, an answering service, or a machine recording that is either too sour, too abrupt, or too pert can be offensive to a listener. Callers should not get the impression that the practitioner is having all calls screened. Identifying the caller should be handled as discretely as possible. It should be made clear that the practitioner's availability is not dependent on the identity of the caller. The reason for having telephone callers identified is obvious to anyone who has been inundated by phone calls from salesmen. One can spend the entire day talking on the telephone—to worried clients, parents, teachers, and anyone else who has time to chat. If unable to reach the client when returning phone calls, note the dates and times the calls were made (G. Smith, 10/13/86, 9:45, no answer; G. Smith 10/14/86, 2:30, line busy). If repeated attempts to return a call are unsuccessful, send a note or form letter indicating that you tried to return the call and asking that they call your secretary for an appointment. Many professionals log their incoming phone calls, as well as the times they tried to return phone calls. One efficient system for logging incoming calls is a note pad with a duplicate carbon. These can be kept in self-contained notebooks for reference. In special cases, the carbons can be filed in the clients' records and can prove to be highly valuable (i.e., in instances when a client challenges a date, or the time a referral or request was made). A few simple facts in the files can stop many arguments.

Some professionals do not like to use a mechanical answering device when a secretary is not available. They prefer an answering service or an exchange. The choice is based on personal preference, as well as the availability of high quality answering services within the city. Some practitioners feel that a self-recorded statement on a tape that allows unlimited time for messages by the caller is more effective. If a full-time secretary is available to talk with the person, to take messages during work hours, and to arrange routine matters on your behalf, then either an answering service or recorded message after hours will suffice. If a full-time secretary is not available, it may be that an answering service or exchange is the preferable alternative to a machine. Whatever the choice, anything is preferable to the practitioner's acting as his/her own telephone answering service.

Keeping Time and Activity Records

No matter what system of time-keeping and record-keeping one uses, one must have a calendar, schedule, or time schedule accessible at all times to record correspondence, telephone calls, and brief conversations with clients and parents. Be sure that all services rendered are recorded and are accessible either on the time schedule, the practitioner's calendar, or client's charts. Time records are not to be confused with billing records; but they are valuable references for ascertaining which services were rendered and chargeable. In case of litigation, time records serve as evidence for services rendered, attention to the client, and verification of statements about professional matters. Time and activity are also important for income tax deductions, such as parking lot fees, promotional expenses, meals, and other out-of-pocket expenses that later are filed and reported with the Internal Revenue Service.

Practitioners tend to forget details of client care. Brief documentation of date and topic of all conferences, phone calls, other contacts, and recommendations should be filed in each client's record for reference when necessary.

Organizing the Professional's Desk and Activities

According to Foonberg (1984), if a professional does only one thing all day, it should be the first thing on the list of important things to do. Certainly the first thing on the list of professionals who provide human services is the delivery of those services. Second in priority, for most practitioners, is any work directly related to service delivery, such as reports or calls to teachers, tutors, and other consultants or professionals. Next on the list for the owner/practitioner is paying attention to the quality of service delivery and the efficiency of office administration. If bills are not sent routinely, if collections are not made consistently, if personnel are not producing efficiently, then the owner/practitioner must make changes.

Many offices can be run more efficiently with the slightest attention to details, such as designating the proper place for things. Some pertinent examples include the following:

1. A place for incoming phone calls supplied with a log that has automatic carbons for recording those phone calls;
2. A place where recipients retrieve their messages;
3. A place at each practitioner's desk where an upright file can be put to hold files of clients who are in-process, for use during evaluations, conferences, and so forth;
4. A place for each practitioner's incoming mail;
5. A place for each practitioner to put requests and materials needing secretarial attention.

Developing effective techniques for dictating can prove to be cost effective. Some such techniques include the following:

1. Give complete instructions first.
   a. Describe the kind of paper to be used—plain, letterhead;
   b. Specify whether carbon or photocopy is to be made;
   c. Identify all persons to whom the letter is to be sent;
   d. Specify whether these names are to appear on the bottom of the original;
   e. Identify persons to whom envelopes should be addressed.
2. Indicate whether or not the letter or report is a rush item.
3. Give the address slowly.
4. Spell all names (even Ann can be Anne), unless the secretary is familiar with the name.
5. Speak distinctly and at an even rate; dictate in phrases.
6. Keep the microphone steady or put it on the stand.
7. Spell unusual terms, particularly if a secretarial service is being used, or if you have a new secretary.
8. Always proofread what goes out of the office—it represents you and your practice—even though the secretary has proofread it once.
9. A rough draft may not be necessary for short, simple, form letters, although until a new secretary is familiar with the form, the voice, and the vocabulary, it may be a good idea to use a rough draft. When in doubt, go ahead and ask the secretary to type a rough draft for you to check before the final draft is typed. This may save expensive letterhead stationery.

Almost any organizational system can be used to structure the daily routine of an office, as long as it is efficient and useful for the people who work there.

Consultation and Contracts

Many practitioners form an entire practice around consultation and contractual work outside the office. Consulting for the profession can include nursery schools, private schools, hospital out-patient services, nursing homes, and home health agencies. Many home health agencies and rehabilitation facilities must hire consultants for particular services in order to qualify for accreditation or certification. In some states there is a Private Consultant Act that rules that a state agency can use a private consultant any time there is substantial need for the consulting service and the agency cannot adequately perform the service with its own personnel or through contract with another state agency. An example of such consultation would be a private practitioner consulting with a public school program. The obvious problem with this apparently generous act is that most state agencies, such as public schools, are also mandated by law to provide adequate services to all who need them. If a program with this mandate indicates that private consultants are needed, the administration is in the uncomfortable position of admitting that its program is not complying with its mandate.

Payments and Reimbursements to Consultants

Various private agencies and schools have their own policies regarding consultant payments and reimbursements. Many state comptroller offices list exactly what should be included on the purchase voucher in order that the consultant be paid. Items usually included are the total dollar amount of the contract, any previous payments under this contract, volume and page number of the state publication in which the contract was advertised and in which the contract award notice was published. Usually the first request for payment must include a copy of the contract. In almost any situation, consultant contracts must specifically outline job duties, work responsibilities, contact dates, and payment amounts.

The broad range of activities that can be offered by speech-language pathology/audiology consultants include school systems, industry, public service, police and fire departments, courts, nursing homes, home health agencies, libraries, hospitals, the media, and religious institutions. Certain common elements in consultation can be identified. These include the following:

1. Consultation involves a system or institution utilizing the services of an expert who is not ordinarily part of the work team, in order to improve some aspect of the functioning of that team (Haas, 1983). Consultation usually provides services to individuals or groups within organizational contexts, such as those individuals who are already trained and practicing within the profession.
2. The receivers of consultation services usually apply the advice given or the skills imparted by consultants in their work with others. For example, therapy and other services in a nursing home may be directly affected by an in-service for the paraprofessionals hired in that setting.
3. Consultants frequently are forced to deal with the often unrealistic perception many people have of consultants. The ambiguous and dynamic nature of consultation requires constant adaptation to the situation and problems within the situation (Haas, 1983). Consultees frequently expect that any advice or direction given initially by consultants, particularly if the consultants are short term, will apply to the situation forever. When a consultant is hired for a longer period of time, then the changes can be used as part of the consultation role. For example, consultants who serve as short-term diagnosticians and program consultants often leave "prescriptions" that are written for specific clients for very short-term periods. The consultees frequently interpret the

original prescription to be a permanent plan and persistently adhere to it until the next consultant comes with a new plan. Some consultants work with consultees regarding unseen third parties. For example, a special education director may hire a consultant to provide an update on speech and language skills to the speech-language pathology staff, who, in turn, apply the skills to their own students in therapy. In these situations, the consultant is well advised to be judicious, particularly in regard to answering specific questions about specific clients.

4. Consultant contracts usually fall into two divisions for speech-language pathology/audiology. One has to do with direct delivery of services to clients, the other has to do with the program of professional in-service and staff development.

Whatever form the consultation takes, whatever length of time is involved, and whatever number of personnel are involved, it is imperative that a written and signed agreement precede any actual services. A written agreement is for the protection of both the hiring agency and the consultant, both of whom are liable for litigation at many levels. Whatever form the contracts take, it usually is a good idea to precede the formal agreement and signing of the contract with a written proposal. Marshall et al. (1982), suggest conditions to be included in any consultant's contract:

1. The term and conditions of the agreement;
2. Services to be provided;
3. Payment for services;
4. Managerial fees;
5. Insurance coverage;
6. Qualification of personnel to serve as consultants;
7. Specific consultant responsibilities of the consultants and designees;
8. Facilities, materials, and equipment to be provided by each;
9. Reports to be provided by consultants;
10. Authorization for access to client and other records, and to clients and families as necessary and appropriate;
11. Specified time periods, methods, and conditions of compensation;
12. Method of accounting for contingencies involving insurance companies who are responsible for payment;
13. Provisions for making change in the contract during the course of the consultation period.

The consultant must be knowledgeable about the legal rights of various groups. Many of these rights still pertain to the rights of privacy and protection or pertain to organized labor. The speech-language pathology/audiology consultant must be aware of regulations involving Occupational Safety and Health Administration (OSHA) standards, the Federal Commerce Commission, Food and Drug Administration, and restraint of trade. Legal action is rarely taken, but caution is always advisable.

As with any other situation involving professional services, the same responsibilities and liabilities apply to consultation. It is contingent upon the consultant to take steps to protect the client, as well as to engage in appropriate self-protection.

Basic professional judgement of a competent professional assumes a certain level of preparedness. The professional should implement the following:

1. Know who the client is;
2. Know the law regulating the profession, consultants, and consultees;
3. Know the code of ethics;
4. Know your own values;
5. Develop a clear contract and see that it is in writing and signed by all parties responsible;
6. Collaborate with employer and other sponsors, building reevaluation points into the consultant process;
7. Be sure that as the contracting consultant you maintain contact with all your designees and are always aware of what they are doing, being careful to obtain feedback from those involved in the entire process;
8. Be certain that informed consent of the client or legal guardian is obtained in all situations regarding records and reports and that release of information is obtained as necessary;
9. Clarify communication and information lines, including the kinds of information that are to be passed along those lines. For example, consider the following situations:
   a. A speech-language consultant in a hospital discovers that substandard care is being provided in many areas of hygiene, affecting the care of hearing aids and any other prosthetic devices necessary for basic functioning and communication; or
   b. A consultant, who is asked to help with the supervision of clinical fellows, is asked to help make the final decision regarding who will and will not be approved for certification.

These situations and many others can prove to be difficult for various reasons: (1) Such contingencies were not included in the initial contract; (2) lines of information and communication were not established; (3) the questions presented by these situations pertain in some ways to confidentiality and personal rights; and (4) the alternatives to disclosure and to whom disclosure is to be offered are unclear.

As in any other professional service delivery, consultation results cannot be guaranteed. One must function within one's realm of professional competence. A consultant must avoid being too cautious in describing possible benefits, as well as avoid being too grandiose in making promises regarding outcome of the consultation. Sometimes preventive measures for unrealistic expectations can be built in by agreeing with the employer and consultees regarding the objectives of the consultation and by building in periodic reviews to assess progress toward the agreed upon goals.

Consultation in Forensics

Some clinicians include court appearances as expert witnesses as part of their consultation package. In some situations, practitioners are called upon to advise the court. For example, public defenders and other public officials turn to professionals in the physical, mental, and allied health areas for opinion and testimony. In other situations, private attorneys need specialists to serve as expert witnesses in matters of accident, trauma, employment capability, change in communication functioning, custody, disability, and determination of the capacity to testify in court.

For some practitioners, this form of consultation can be quite intriguing. Certainly it is more intriguing to serve as a "friend of the court" and be paid as an expert witness than it is to be supoenaed by one party or the other and be put into the position of having to defend one's qualifications, recommendations, or actions. Haas (1983) and Flower (1984) suggest rules of thumb for the practitioner who chooses, or is forced, to go to court to serve as professional spokesperson. These include the following:

1. Stick to what you know. Do not bluff, and do not make statements beyond your range of experience or best professional projections for a particular client. It is not necessary to pretend to be an expert in all areas of the profession; pretense can be destructive to the area in which you are an expert. Do not give opinions about someone you have never seen.

2. Sustain your opinion by using and claiming whatever credentials and experience you have.

3. Keep all client records as if they may be subpoenaed for court evidence. Never give a court an original of a test or report. Make a photocopy, and sign or initial the photocopy as an accurate reproduction of the original. Even if subpoenaed, obtain a release of information in writing from the client in question.

4. Be sure that you obtain a copy of the deposition transcript for review, before your court appearance.

5. Whether in a deposition (a formal procedure prior to a trial and conducted under legal regulations) or in actual court appearance, remember how you answer questions and what statements you make. Attorneys frequently repeat the same questions four or five different times, trying to force contradictory statements. Do not make any statement in a deposition that will nor or cannot be repeated in the courtroom. The attorney is very likely to point out remarks made in deposition that are reversed in the courtroom. (The verbatim transcript of the deposition becomes court evidence in the case of a trial.) Admit the limitations of your knowledge, but do not apologize for conclusions drawn from nonstandard assessment. Attorneys are just as skillful in tearing down the validity of any standardized test as they are in questioning professional judgment.

6. Do not be rushed, and do not become flustered, upset, angry, or reactive.

7. Take as much time as you feel necessary to understand the questions and to frame an appropriate response.

8. When summoned for a deposition or court appearance, be certain that your out-of-office fees are understood by the summoning party, and obtain a retainer in advance.

9. If you serve as an expert witness for one of the two parties in conflict, be certain that your client's attorney understands *before the trial* what it is that you do, what your training is, how important the work is that you do, and what you have done with this particular client, including tests and intervention and what they mean.

10. If during a cross examination you find that a question or statement is based on a false premise or a false assumption, feel free to correct this assumption in your best professional manner, without appearing defensive or argumentative.
11. If an attorney reads any material, feel free to ask to see the material before responding to any questions referring to that material.
12. If your credentials, your qualifications, or the substance of your comments are attacked, do not react. It will not be appropriate, nor may you be allowed, to defend yourself. The judge will rule on that issue.
13. This is not the time to be modest. State your credentials, qualifications, and expertise.

Appendices

APPENDIX 5–1
CLIENT INFORMATION FORMS

1. New Client Information
2. Initial Intake Information
3. Insurance Information
4. Agreement to Pay
5. Agreement to Terms of Payment
6. Release of Information
7. Authorization for Release of Information
8. Sample Cover Sheet for Child's Case History
9. Sample Cover Sheet for Adult's Case History
10. Office Policies for Clients
11. Client Appointment Letter

NEW CLIENT INFORMATION

Please complete the following information. This information is considered confidential.

Client's name _____________________________ Today's date __________

Address _____________________________ Phone __________

_____________________________ Zip __________

Employed by _____________________________ Phone ______ Ext. ______

Address _____________________________

_____________________________ Zip __________

Date of birth _____________________________ Age ______ Sex: M ☐ F ☐

Single __________ Married __________ Separated __________ Divorced __________

Social security number _____________________________

Name of spouse (or parents, if child) _____________________________

Address _____________________________ Phone __________

_____________________________ Zip __________

Employed by _____________________________

Address _____________________________

_____________________________ Zip __________

Person legally responsible for account _____________________________

_____________________________ Zip __________

Relationship to patient _____________________________

Who referred you to our office? _____________________________

Name _____________________________

Address _____________________________

_____________________________ Zip __________

Client's physician _____________________________ Phone __________

Address _____________________________

_____________________________ Zip __________

Additional Pertinent Information:

____

____

____

____

INITIAL INTAKE INFORMATION

Client's name____

Parent's/Spouse's name____

Address ____

Phone number ____
            home

____
            work (self)   (spouse)

____
            work (mother)   (father)

Date of evaluation(s)/screening(s)______________________________________

Amount of time____

Date of parent/client conference_______________________________________

Charge for evaluation/screening_______________________________________

Examiner____

Recommendations____

____

____

____

____

____

INSURANCE INFORMATION

Insured's name_______________________________________ SS#_________________________

Address____

Is this your policy?_______ Spouse's?_______Parent's?_______Legal guardian's_______ Other?_______

Is this coverage:

Private? Yes_______________ No_______________ If yes, policy #_______________________

    Group #_________________________ Name of Company_______________________

Medicare? Yes_______________ No_______________ I.D.#_________________________

Medical? Yes_______________ No_______________ I.D.#_________________________

Other?

Have you previously filed a claim with this company? Yes_______________ No_______________

If yes, when____

Under what circumstances? ____

    What are your coverage and benefits?_______________________________________

    Have you satisfied your deductible this year? Yes_______________ No_______________

Do you have other insurance coverage? Yes_______________ No_______________ If yes, what

company?____

This office will prepare any necessary reports and forms to assist you in collecting from your insurance company. Any amount paid directly to this office will be credited to your account.

AGREEMENT TO PAY

I promise to pay to the order of ____ the sum of ____ , in lawful money of the United States of America, of the present standard value, plus any late charges attached because of delinquent payment. I agree to send my payment to ____ at ____ .
(practitioner's name)   (full legal address)

I promise to pay no less than ______________ per month, due and payable the ______________ day of each month starting ____ , 19 ______________ , and each month thereafter until my account is paid in full. If not so paid, the balance owing will become due and collectible at the option of the holder of this note.

In the case that legal action is instituted to collect this note or any portion thereof, I promise and agree to pay in addition to the costs and disbursements provided by statute such sum as the court may adjudge reasonable as attorney's fees in said action.

____
signed

____
witnessed

____
date

Amount of deposit $ ______________________

Diagnostic fee paid $ ______________________

AGREEMENT TO TERMS OF PAYMENT

FINANCIAL RESPONSIBILITY

I, _________________________________ , acknowledge and accept full and complete responsibility for payment of all services rendered to me by _______________ .

If eligibility is available under Medicare, I agree to pay all copayments or coinsurance amounts not reimbursed under the medical insurance part of the Medicare program (Part B) for services rendered.

I understand that health and accident insurance policies are an arrangement between my insurance company and myself, that all services rendered me are charged directly to me, and that I am personally responsible for payment. I agree to allow this office to release any information that is requested by my insurance company.

_____________________________   _____________________________
          Date   Signature of patient, parent, or legal guardian

RELEASE OF INFORMATION

No information concerning the child or the evaluation results will be released unless the following form is signed by the parent or legal guardian. Signature is required for reports to be provided for anyone other than parent or legal guardian.

I authorize the _______________________ Clinic to release information concerning _________________________________ to other professionals, agencies, or designated recipients. I also authorize _________________________________ (designated therapist) to release any information concerning _________________________________ to other professionals, agencies, or designated recipient.

____
Signature of parent/legal guardian/spouse

To _________________________________

____
Date

AUTHORIZATION FOR RELEASE OF INFORMATION

The enclosed information is sent to you with written consent from the parents/guardians
of ____
(Client)
All information in the enclosed report is confidential and should be used only by professional personnel. It is not to be given directly to parents or clients.

Questions concerning any information contained in this report should be asked of ____
____

____
Signed (Provider)

SAMPLE COVER SHEET FOR CHILD'S CASE HISTORY

Date of initial visit ___________________________

Client's name ____

Last   First   Middle   (Nickname)

Address ____

Street address   City   State   Zip

Telephone ___________ Client's birthdate ___________ Client's present age ___________

Name of parent (or guardian) _______________________________________

Address of parent (or guardian) _____________________________________

Telephone of parent (or guardian) ___________________________________

Person to contact in case of emergency if parent or guardian cannot be reached (e.g., schedule change)

____

Name   Telephone   Relationship

Who referred you to the clinic? Name ________________________________

Address or telephone ___________________________________

Relationship to client ___________________________________

Describe any concerns that caused you to bring the child to the ___________ clinic.

____

____

____

What problems in addition to speech, language, learning, or hearing does the child have that concern you? ___________________________________

____

Has anyone made a diagnosis of the problem or its cause? ___________________

If so, what was that diagnosis, when was it made, and who made it? ______________

____

____

What questions would you like to have answered about the child? ______________

____

____

____

SAMPLE COVER SHEET FOR ADULT'S CASE HISTORY

Date _______________________

Client's name ____
    Last   First   Middle

Birthdate ____ Present Age _______

Telephone: Home ____
    Business ____

Address ____
    Street address   City   State   Zip

Permanent address ____
    (Fill in only if different from above address)

Present place of employment ____

Occupation ____
    (If this has changed in the past two years, describe change on back of page).

If someone other than the client is to be contacted to schedule appointments with the clinic, give the following information:

Name ___________________________ Relationship to client _________________________

Address ____ Telephone _________

Client was referred to the clinic by ____
            Name

____
    Address   Relationship to the Client

Why was the client referred? ____

____

Has a diagnosis of the problem or the cause of the problem been made? ___________

If so, who made it? ____

What was the diagnosis? ____

____

____

____

OFFICE POLICIES FOR CLIENTS

1. At various times during the year, Dr. ________________________________ , or one of the other professional staff members, will be away from the office. You will be notified in advance of the dates and make-up sessions will be scheduled when possible.

2. Unless otherwise arranged, statements for service are sent at the end of each month for the number of sessions scheduled during the month.

3. Brief conferences between sessions, as well as brief telephone conferences, are considered a part of the regular intervention program, and no additional charges will be made. Conferences with parents, physicians, tutors, or teachers that exceed 10 minutes in length will be charged at the regular billing rate.

4. Conferences at a school, or other out-of-office visits, will be billed at the regular billing rate.

5. Each payment for evaluation and intervention is to be made directly to the clinic each month, even if insurance coverage is arranged. (The insurance company reimburses the individual and not the clinic.)

6. Although payment is the client's responsibility, we will provide assistance with insurance claims at your request. If you need to have dates of intervention, diagnosis, and/or Dr. ____________'s signature on each statement, please inform the bookkeeper.

7. Fees for intervention, evaluation, and conferences are at the rate of $ _____ per hour.

8. Bills that remain unpaid for 1 month following receipt of statement for services will be subject to an additional 5% charge on the unpaid balance.

9. Bills that remain unpaid for 2 months following receipt of statement for services will be subject to an additional 10% charge on the unpaid balance each month until the balance is paid in full.

10. Bills that remain unpaid for 3 months following receipt of statement for services will be subject to legal action for collection.

11. If you must cancel a scheduled appointment, it is necessary that you cancel twenty-four (24) hours in advance of the appointment. Except in cases of emergency or sudden illness, appointments not cancelled 24 hours before will be charged as though the session were held.

I have read and accept the policies of the ________________________________ Clinic. I understand that I am responsible for timely payment.

____
Date

____
Parent/Guardian/Spouse
of ________________________________

CLIENT APPOINTMENT LETTER

Dear
        This is to confirm the evaluation appointment for ________________________________
with ____________________ on ____________________ at ____________________.
        Unless prior arrangements are made, payment for the evaluation is due at the conclu-
sion of the conference that is set up to discuss evaluation results with you. We will be glad
to assist you in completing forms you may wish to submit for insurance reimbursement.
However, you are responsible for all charges to your account and for requesting reimbursement from your insurance company.
        We look forward to working with you.

Sincerely,

____
        Receptionist/Bookkeeper

APPENDIX 5-2
SAMPLE PROPOSALS AND CONTRACTS

1. Sample Letter to Administrator of Private PreSchool and Kindergarten
   re: Screening Offer
2. Sample Letter to Parents of Private PreSchool and Kindergarten
   re: Screening Offer
3. Items to Include in Proposals and Contracts

SAMPLE LETTER TO ADMINISTRATOR OF PRIVATE PRESCHOOL
AND KINDERGARTEN
RE: SCREENING OFFER

During the months of January and February, my associate, _________________ , and I will be scheduling speech, language, hearing, and developmental screening for private preschools and kindergartens in the _________________ area. Enclosed is a sample letter that explains the screening program to parents. In March, 19 _______ , we will schedule school readiness screening for children who are approaching first grade placement.

If you or your teachers would like to discuss either screening program in more detail, please contact me within the next few weeks. Thank you for your attention.

Sincerely,

____
                Director

SAMPLE LETTER TO PARENTS OF PRIVATE PRESCHOOL AND KINDERGARTEN
RE: SCREENING OFFER

Dear Parents:

Dr. _________________________________ , director of the __________ Clinic, and his/her associate, _________________________________ , will be at our school on _______________________ (date). They will see children over 2 years of age for screening evaluations of their speech, hearing, and visual-motor abilities. Children under 2 years will be screened for hearing and general development. The purpose of the screening is to identify children who may need complete evaluation of speech, language, or hearing disabilities.

From the screening, Dr. ____ or M ____ will make recommendations regarding the need for complete evaluation of the child in specific areas of development and/or communication and will suggest local facilities where such testing is done.

If you wish to take advantage of this unusual opportunity to have your child participate in the screening, please sign the form below giving your permission for the screening. Return the signed form to me or your child's teacher no later than ___________________ (date).

If you have any questions about the screening, please ask your child's teacher. The screening will not be unpleasant for the children, and all results and recommendations will be provided directly to the parents of each child. We suggest that all children in our school participate in this service as a routine part of their school experience. We have found that early identification and treatment of even the slightest difficulty in development and learning is vital for every child.

If you have specific comments or questions about your child, please include them for Dr. _________________________________ or _________________________________ on the form below, or in a private note.

The fee for the screening is $ ________. Checks are payable to the ________ Clinic.

Sincerely,

_________________________________ , Director

   School

Yes, I want my child, _________________________________ , to participate in the screening program for speech, language, hearing, or learning abilities.

My comments/questions for Dr. ___________________ or M ___________________ are

____

____

____________________________________   _________________________________

     Date   Parent or Guardian

ITEMS TO INCLUDE IN PROPOSALS AND CONTRACTS

This list is to be used to identify areas of consideration in proposals and contracts arranged by the practitioner with preschools, kindergartens, private schools, hospitals, home health agencies, nursing homes, and industrial firms.

1. Terms of agreement
   a. Inclusive dates
   b. Contracting parties
   c. Involved parties
      (designees of contractors, recipients of services)
   d. Other
2. Purpose and type of services
   a. Purpose and intent
      (objectives, short-term goals)
   b. Professional service areas
      (speech-language, audiological, occupational therapy, physical therapy)
   c. Types of services
      i. Direct client contact
         (assessment, screening, intervention, other)
      ii. Indirect client contact
         (observations, supervision of other practitioners, staff inservice, environmental assistance)
   d. Reports, documents, and records
   e. Follow-up and recommendations
   f. Other
3. Management and supervision of services
4. Time schedule and expectations for each area and type of service
5. Status and qualifications of service providers and other designees of contracting provider (independent consultant, employee, other)
6. Assessment of fees
   a. For services and follow-up
   b. For clerical help
   c. For management of services
7. Source and schedule of fee payments
   (contingencies, if any)
8. Insurance and indemnity
   (relationship of insurance to fee collection for contracted services)
9. Liability and responsibility to agency, to contracting provider, and in regard to service delivery
   a. Privileged communication and confidentiality
   b. Protection and contingencies in event of legal action involving contracting provider
10. Service-related features and considerations
    a. Evaluation of providers and services
    b. Staff conferences
    c. Staff travel and reimbursement
    d. Expenses related to service provision
    e. Materials and supplies
    f. Equipment
    g. Work space
    h. Access to property and employees of agency
    i. Relationship with employees and others within the school, home, or agency

APPENDIX 5–3
EMPLOYEES AND THE OFFICE—POLICIES AND AGREEMENTS

1. Items for Inclusion in Personnel Policies
2. Outline of Content for Contracting/Agreements with Employees
3. Employment Contract
4. Office Operations Checklist
    Personnel
    Management

ITEMS FOR INCLUSION IN PERSONNEL POLICY

Absences
Accidents
Attitude
Bonuses
Books and Journals
Bulletin Boards
Cleanliness
Coffee Breaks
Competition
Complaints
Computer Use
Confidential Nature of Work
Contracts
Decorum
Deductions
Disability Insurance
Discounts
Discrimination
Dismissal
Economy
Emergencies
Emergency Leave
Employee Addresses
Employee Lounge
Employee Personality
Employee-Client Relations
Fire
Fringe Benefits
Gossip
Grievances
Holidays
Housekeeping
Insurance
  Health
  Hospitalization
  Liability
  Life
Intoxication
Jury Duty
Labor Laws
Leaves of Absence
Loyalty
Lunches
Magazines
Marriage and Pregnancy
Maternity
Meal Schedules
Medical Care
Meetings
Merit Review
Military Service
Misconduct
Moonlighting

New Employees
Noise
Office Appearance
Office Supplies
Overtime
Parking
Payday
Pay Period
Pay Schedule
Pension Plan
Personal:
  Phone calls
  Bonding
  Mail
  Supplies
  Visitors
Personnel Counseling
Priorities
Privileged Communications
Privileged Information
Probationary Period
Professional Ethics
Promotions
Re-employment
Resignations
Retirement
Safety
Salary
  Calculation
  Increases
Schedules
Sick Leave
Smoking
Social Security
Soliciting of Employees
Suggestions
Supervisors
Tardiness
Telephone Courtesy
Temporary Employment
Termination of Employment
Time Cards
Time Period
Unemployment Insurance
Vacations
Work
  Evaluations
  Habits
  Periods
Workers' Compensation
Working Hours

From *How to Start and Build a Law Practice* by J. G. Foonberg, 1984, Chicago: American Bar Association. Copyright 1984. Adapted by permission.

OUTLINE OF CONTENT FOR CONTRACTING/AGREEMENTS WITH EMPLOYEES

Professional staff may be hired as part-time employees, full-time employees, or as independent consultants/contractors. With employees, the employer is responsible for withholding tax, social security tax, worker's compensation, and unemployment taxes. Independent consultants/contractors are independent agents who are paid an agreed-upon amount and who function independently in an agreed-upon manner. The contractor is not responsible for taxes for contractees.

The content of a professional staff contract/agreement should include the following basic elements:

1. Title
2. Term of employment/contract
3. Description of duties
4. Compensation
   (i.e., ______________% of payment of services rendered;
   or
   ______________% of billing for services rendered)
5. Travel expenses
6. Location of duties
7. Time schedule of duties
8. Supervision
9. Responsibilities of contractor/employee:
   a. exclusivity of services
   b. non-compete clauses
10. Benefits
11. Right of renegotiation
12. Termination
13. Use of office supplies, personnel, equipment
14. Special considerations

EMPLOYMENT CONTRACT

This contract is made and entered into this first day of September, 19 ___________ , by and between ____ , hereinafter called "employee," and ____ , hereinafter called "Corporation";

WITNESSETH:

WHEREAS, the employee is a speech-language pathologist for the _______________ , Incorporated, and has expertise in speech pathology and desires to accept employment to serve as a speech pathologist for the _________________________________ , Incorporated, and

WHEREAS, the Corporation is engaged in providing speech-language pathology services and desires to employ such employee; and

WHEREAS, the Board of Directors of the Corporation has determined what a reasonable compensation would be for the employee and has offered the employee employment in consideration for such compensation and the other benefits hereinafter set forth, and the employee is willing to accept employment on such terms;

NOW, THEREFORE, in consideration of the mutual promises, hereinafter it is agreed:

1. EMPLOYMENT

   The Corporation hereby employs employee, and the employee hereby accepts employment from the Corporation upon the terms and conditions herein specified.

2. TERMS

   The term of this agreement shall begin on September 1, 19 ____ , and shall continue until terminated as hereinafter provided.

3. COMPENSATION

   For all services rendered by the employee under this agreement, the Corporation shall pay the employee $ ___________ per annum. Such salary may be increased, but not decreased, as the Board of Directors may from time to time determine as evidenced in the minutes of its meetings.

   In addition, the employee may be paid cash bonuses, in such amounts and at such times and on such basis as the Board of Directors may from time to time in its absolute discretion determine. Not by way of limitation, but by explanation, it is understood and agreed between employee and Corporation that the Board of Directors from time to time may offer incentive bonuses.

4. DUTIES

   The employee is employed to exclusively and actively work on behalf of the Corporation. He shall not engage in any other work for remuneration unless otherwise authorized by the Board of Directors. The Corporation shall have the power to determine not only what specific duties shall be performed by the employee but also to determine the means and manner by which these duties shall be performed. The Corporation shall have the power to determine the assignment of work to the employee, and the employee must perform services as assigned to him by the Corporation. All work performed by the employee shall be subject to review by the Corporation. The Corporation shall always have the power not only to dictate to the employee what duties shall be performed and how they shall be performed, but also when they shall be performed. The employee shall work from _____________ a.m. to _____________ p.m., Monday through Friday; the employee shall not be compelled to work longer than the normal work week. The power to direct, control, and supervise in detail the duties to be performed, the manner of performing such duties, and the time for performing such duties shall be exercised by the Board of Directors of the Corporation.

5. EXCLUSIVE SERVICE

The employee shall devote his full time and attention to rendering service on behalf of the Corporation and in furtherance of its best interest. The employee shall comply with all policies and standards, and regulations of the Corporation now or hereinafter promulgated.

6. WORKING FACILITIES

The Corporation shall furnish the employee with an office, stenographic help, supplies, equipment, and such other facilities and services suitable to his position and adequate for the performance of his duties.

7. EXPENSES AND REIMBURSEMENTS FOR EXPENSES

The employee may as a condition of employment incur ordinary, necessary, and reasonable expenses for therapy materials, home entertaining, and other promotional entertainment, travel, and similar items. The employee shall be reimbursed for these expenses if the reimbursement has been approved by the President of the Corporation prior to expenditure.

8. VACATION

The employee shall be entitled each year to a vacation of two (2) weeks, during which his compensation shall continue to be paid in full.

9. INVOLUNTARY TERMINATION

This contract agreement shall be deemed to be terminated and the employment relationship between the employee and the Corporation shall be deemed severed upon the occurrence of any of the following:

a. Upon the death during employment of the employee. In such event, the Corporation shall pay to the estate of the employee the compensation that otherwise would be payable to such employee, up to the end of the month in which his death occurs.
b. The employee fails or refuses to faithfully and diligently perform the usual customary duties of his employment and adhere to the provisions of this contract.
c. The employee fails or refuses to comply with the reasonable policies, standards and regulations of the Corporation which from time to time may be established.
d. The Corporation discharges the employee for cause.

10. VOLUNTARY TERMINATION

In any event, this contract may be terminated by either party upon ninety (90) days' written notice. Unless so terminated, this agreement shall be renewed automatically on a year to year basis on the conditions set forth.

11. RELATIONSHIP BETWEEN THE PARTIES

The parties recognize that the Board of Directors of the Corporation shall manage the business affairs of the Corporation and the relationship between the Board and the employee shall be that of an employer and employee. The employee shall be considered and treated as having an employee status and be entitled to participate in any plans, arrangements, or distribution of and by the Corporation pertaining to or in connection with any pension, bonus, profit sharing, or similar employee fringe benefits for the regular employees of the Corporation.

12. NOTICES

Any notices given under this agreement shall be sufficient, if it is in writing and mailed by either registered or certified mail, return receipt requested, postage prepaid, to the Corporation at its principal place of business and to the employee at his last known residence address.

13. CONSTRUCTION

This contract shall be governed by the laws of the State of ___________. The waiver of any party hereto of a breach of any provision of this contract shall not operate or be constructed as a waiver of any subsequent breach by the party. This instrument contains the entire agreement of the parties concerning employment and may not be changed except by written agreement duly executed by the parties hereto. This contract shall inure to the benefit of and be binding upon the parties, their successors, heirs, and personal representatives. This contract shall not be assignable.

14. WAIVER

Any provision of this contract giving a benefit to the employee hereunder, may be waived by the employee by giving written notice to the Corporation ten (10) days prior to the termination date hereof or ten (10) days prior to the receipt of any benefit hereof or the date of such benefit that is to be received hereunder. Notice of waiver under this provision is to be given by sending same by ordinary mail to the address of the Corporation.

BY ____

ATTEST:

____
            Secretary

OFFICE OPERATIONS CHECKLIST
PERSONNEL AND MANAGEMENT

1. General Information for Clinician/Employees

>   Service delivery policies
>   Client billing and collection policies
>   Clinicians' schedules and client contact
>   Information regarding branch offices and relationship of branch office to main office
>   Third party payment (private, Medicare, other)
>   Leave coverage (paid and unpaid)
>
>   > personal leave without advance notice
>   > personal leave or vacation with advance notice
>   > holiday coverage
>   > paperwork
>   > clinician substitution for one on leave
>   > continuing education
>
>   Bonus and Merit Compensation
>   > salary basis plus time credit
>   > salary basis plus client visits
>
>   Diagnostic categories for use in billing and record keeping
>   Tests and resource materials available
>   Use of office equipment, telephone, copier
>   Procedures for interaction with home health and nursing home agencies
>   Termination of clients
>   Forms used for various client interaction (intake, evaluation forms, summary plan
>   forms, forms for agencies, clinician expense form, etc.)
>   Contracts for professional employees
>
>   > negotiating
>   > terminating
>
>   Relationship with clerical staff
>   > delegation of work
>
>   Communication and hierarchy

2. Speech-Language Pathology/Audiology Services

>   Provisions of services
>   Responsibility
>   Equipment
>   Financial arrangements
>   Duration of the agreement
>   Qualifications of clinicians
>   Client rights
>   Provider rights

3. Speech-Language Pathologists/Audiologists Job Description

>   Definition
>   Duties
>   Responsibilities
>   Liabilities
>   Contracts

4. Proposals and Contracts

>   For medical groups, schools, hospitals, agencies
>   Appropriate tests and intervention in various agencies

5. Records

   Clinical reports of client care
      initial
      progress
      termination
      other

   Filing
   Sending reports out of the office

      client records
      storage
      retrieval
      content
      use

6. Personnel Policies

      Attitude
      Nondiscrimination
      Hiring and firing
      Job description
      Employee health
      Employee agreement and contracts
      Orientation to the practice
      Benefits
      Compensations
      Probation assignment
      Temporary and part-time
      Dress and grooming
      Other employment
      Work schedule
      Pay day
      Overtime
      Business expenses
      On the job accidents
      Insurance
      Sick leave
      Other leave (compassionate leave)
      Jury and military duty
      Voting time
      Medical and dental appointments
      Leave without pay
      Leave with pay
      Discipline
      Termination
      Personnel files
      Employee grievances

7. Long-Range Planning

      Goals and objectives
      Philosophy of clinical services

8. Budgeting, Planning, and Borrowing

9. Billing and Collections

10. Inventory

      Purchasing

> Storing
> Maintaining
>> Contracts and leases
>> Negotiations

11. Use of Consultants

> Attorney
> Accountant
> Insurance
> Computer

12. Administrative Reports

13. Emergency Procedures and Safety Measures

14. Environmental Maintenance

> Equipment maintenance
> Preventative procedures
> Maintenance agreements with sales company
> Repair procedures

15. Office Hours

> For professional staff
> For office staff

16. Telephone Procedures

> Answering, preferred greeting
> Clinician's policy for accepting or rejecting calls
> Emergencies
> Personal calls
> Intercom system

17. Reception Policies

18. Scheduling Procedures

19. Communication with Clients

> Clinic pamphlet
> Daily procedures
> Periodic reports
> Periodic conferences
> Schedule of conferences
> Procedures for discharge
> Procedures for temporary leave of clients
> Procedures for termination

20. Mail

> Incoming
> Outgoing

21. Financial Arrangements with Clients

> Cash payments
> Insurance coverage
> Primary responsibility

22. Statistics

> Client statistics
> Professional staff statistics (number of clients seen, number of hours working, etc.)

23. Cost Accounting

    Cost effectiveness
    Cost analysis

24. Referrals

    Forms
    Practices
    Telephone referrals
    Documentation
    Referrals out of the office

25. Client Complaints

    About finances
    About services

26. Working Schedule

    Flex time
    Work days
    Work hours
    Weekend coverage
    Extended days and hours
    Staggering lunch hours
    Staggering hours to provide more client services in a longer day
    Holidays

27. Office Decoration

28. Continuing Education Policy

    Association meetings
    Volunteer work

29. Organizational Structure

    Board of Directors
      officers
      responsibilities
      reimbursements
      salary
      relationship to clinic
    Stockholders
      time of meeting
      place of meeting
      purpose of meeting

30. Administrative Positions and Job Descriptions

    President
    Secretary-treasurer
    Other

31. Administrative Records

    Minutes
    Meetings of stockholders
    Board of directors' meetings

32. Financial Records

    Books
    Ledgers

APPENDIX 5–4
PARAPROFESSIONALS

1. 1981 ASHA Guidelines for Supportive Personnel
2. 1985 Regulations for Audiology Paraprofessionals in Texas
3. 1985 Regulations for Speech-Language-Pathology Paraprofessionals in Texas

GUIDELINES FOR SUPPORTIVE PERSONNEL

The following revised guidelines, drafted by the Committee on Supportive Personnel, were adopted by the Legislative Council, American Speech-Language-Hearing Association (ASHA) in November, 1980 (LC 32-80).

In 1967 the Executive Board of the American Speech-Language-Hearing Association (ASHA) initiated discussions relative to the need to develop guidelines regarding use of supportive personnel in the profession.

DEFINITION

A variety of terms have been used to designate those individuals who have provided services in support of clinical programs in speech, language, and/or hearing disorders.[1]

The terms speech-language assistant and audiology assistant shall designate any person who, following academic and/or on-the-job training, provides clinical services as prescribed and directed by a certified audiologist and/or speech-language pathologist.[2] The audiologist or speech-language pathologist shall maintain responsibility for services provided. Individuals who are enrolled in a training program or who have obtained a professional degree (e.g., B.A., B.S., A.B. degree) in speech-language pathology or audiology could be included within the definition of the terms speech-language assistant and audiology assistant. In keeping with standards for clinical certification, however, students may not use paid work experience to satisfy clinical certification requirements.

QUALIFICATIONS OF THE SPEECH-LANGUAGE ASSISTANT AND AUDIOLOGY ASSISTANT

The following minimum qualifications should be considered in selecting individuals for employment as speech-language or audiology assistants.

1. A high school diploma or the equivalent;
2. Communication skills adequate for the tasks assigned;
3. Ability to relate to the clinical population being served.

Additional qualifications may be established according to the needs of the program and the population being served.

TRAINING OF THE SPEECH-LANGUAGE ASSISTANT AND AUDIOLOGY ASSISTANT

In keeping with local needs, a variety of traditional as well as innovative training models may be needed to prepare individuals as assistants. Whatever the training model used, emphasis should be on competency-based skill acquisition.

From ''Guidelines for Supportive Personnel,'' *ASHA*, 23(3), pp. 165–169. Copyright 1981 by American Speech-Language-Hearing Association. Reprinted with permission.

1. Examples of terms used include communication aide, communication assistant, speech technician, and audiometrist.

2. Certified means one who holds the Certificate of Clinical Competence (CCC) from the American Speech-Language-Hearing Association.

ROLE OF SPEECH–LANGUAGE ASSISTANT AND AUDIOLOGY ASSISTANT

The specific role of the speech-language assistant and audiology assistant will be influenced by the particular needs of the clinical speech, language and/or hearing program and must be determined by the professional who will be responsible for training and directing the assistant. . . . The uniqueness of the clinical setting may prescribe that the assistant could be used to either increase the frequency and/or intensity of clinical contact and/or to increase the total caseload.

The assistant should be assigned tasks only at the discretion of the professional and should not be assigned tasks for which he/she has not been trained. An assistant may execute specific components of the clinical speech, language, and/or hearing program if (1) it is determined by the professional that the assistant has the training and skill to accomplish the task, and (2) the professional provides sufficient supervision to insure appropriate completion of all tasks assigned to the assistant. It must be emphasized that the supervising professional maintains legal and moral responsibility for all services provided by the assistant and insures that such services are in compliance with the Code of Ethics of the American Speech-Language-Hearing Association.

One may engage only in those duties that are planned, designed, and supervised by the professional. Examples of such duties are given below. These are examples only and are not intended to be of a prescriptive nature.

1. Screen speech, language, and/or hearing;
2. Conduct evaluative or management programs and procedures that are:
   a. planned and designed by the professional;
   b. included in published materials which have directions for administration and scoring and for which the assistant has received the training;
3. Record, chart, graph or otherwise display data relative to client performance;
4. Maintain clinical records;
5. Report changes in client performance to the professional having responsibility for that client;
6. Prepare clinical materials, including ear molds;
7. Test hearing aids to determine if they meet published specification;
8. Participate with the professional in research projects, in-service training, public relations programs, or similar activities.

The assistant may not engage in any of the following activities:

1. Interpret obtained observations or data into diagnostic statements of clinical management strategies or procedures;
2. Determine case selection;
3. Transmit clinical information (including data or impressions relative to client performance, behavior, or progress) either verbally or in writing to anyone other than the professional;
4. Independently compose clinical reports except for progress notes to be held in the client's file;
5. Refer a client to other professionals or other agencies;
6. Use any title verbally or in writing other than that determined by the professional.

SUPERVISION OF THE SPEECH-LANGUAGE ASSISTANT AND AUDIOLOGY ASSISTANT

Prior to employing assistants, it is essential that the professional be qualified to train and supervise assistants. . . . One hundred percent of the assistant's clinical activities must be the responsibility of the professional.

1985 REGULATIONS FOR AUDIOLOGY PARAPROFESSIONALS IN TEXAS

§741.84. Requirements for a Licensed Associate in Audiology

1. The term "associate" will be used to designate those aides who provide services and support of clinical programs of audiology, who are supervised by a Texas licensed Audiologist, who have received the training specified below, and who hold a current and valid license as a Licensed Associate in Audiology. The following requirements are established as minimum requirements to function as a Licensed Associate in Audiology:

   A. A Baccalaureate degree; and
   B. No fewer than twenty-one (21) semester hours in audiology course work, at least nine (9) of which must be in the area for which license is being sought; and
   C. Transcripts shall be reviewed as in 741.81 (4); and
   D. Upon application and each subsequent renewal, a statement shall be submitted by the supervising Audiologist, acknowledging his/her acceptance of the supervisory responsibilities.

2. Although the licensed Audiologist may delegate specific clinical tasks to an Associate, the legal, ethical, and moral responsibility to the client for all services provided cannot be delegated. The Associate may execute specific components of the clinical speech, language, and/or hearing program if the professional determines that the Associate has received the training and has the skill to accomplish that task, and the professional provides sufficient supervision to ensure appropriate completion of the task assigned to the Associate. The fully licensed supervising professional Audiologist is legally and ethically responsible for the Associate and the Aide. The Audiologist must keep job descriptions and performance records; these must be current and available upon demand by the Committee of Examiners. The Audiologist must ensure that all services are in compliance with these Committee rules, particularly with the Subsection 741.41 (relating to Code of Ethics).

   A. Examples of duties which Associates may be assigned, provided appropriate planning, preparation for the task, and professional supervision, include the following:

      i.   conducting or participating in speech, language, and/or hearing screening;
      ii. conducting evaluative or management programs which may include the utilization of published materials for which the associate has received training;
      iii. maintaining clinical records of client performance;
      iv. preparing clinical materials; and
      v.   participating with the professional in research projects, staff development, public relations programs, or similar activities as designated and supervised by the professional.

   B. The Associate should *not* engage in any of the following activities:

      i.   interpreting observations or data into diagnostic statements, clinical management strategies, or procedures;
      ii. determining case selection;
      iii. presenting written reports of client information to those other than the supervisor without the signature of the supervisor;
      iv. referring a client to other professionals or other agencies;
      v.   using any title which connotes the competency of a licensed professional, as defined in Section 2 of the Act.

   C. Any references to the licensee's title shall state clearly that the license status is that of an Associate.

   D. Direct care staff in a residential care and/or treatment facility who use only the concepts of daily living in their job performance are not required to be licensed as Associates and may not assume the duties of Associates as defined in these sections.

3. Therapy/intervention:

   A. The systematic, individualized process of minimizing communication disorders, involving the dynamic interaction between the fully licensed Audiologist and client;

   B. Designed and executed on the basis of ongoing evaluation of the client's communication needs, skills, and resources;

   C. Designed and executed only by a fully licensed Audiologist; certain routine and perfunctory aspects of the intervention process, such as carryover activities, may be delegated to a Licensed Associate.

4. Carryover:

   A. The therapeutically designed transfer of a newly acquired communication ability to contexts and situations outside of the therapy situation;

   B. Designed by a fully licensed Audiologist.

5. The Associate may conduct carryover activities, language and auditory stimulation, and other activities related to intervention and record keeping as previously described in the rules and as deemed appropriate by the supervising fully licensed Audiologist;

6. The Associate may oversee activities of Aides in consultation with, and direction of, fully licensed Audiologists.

7. Direct supervision of duties assigned to the Associate shall be provided by a Texas licensed Audiologist.

   A. A Licensed Associate in Audiology shall be supervised by a Texas licensed Audiologist.

   B. Following on-the-job training, the Associate's initial client contact shall be directly supervised. Thereafter, the minimum supervision requirements for an Associate by a licensed professional shall be no less than two (2) hours a week, at least half of which is direct on-site supervision. Indirect methods of supervision such as audio and/or video tape recording, telephone communication, numerical data, or other means of reporting may be utilized.

   C. Supervisory records shall be maintained by the licensed professional which verify regularly scheduled monitoring/assessment/evaluation of Associate and client performance. Such documentation may be requested by the Committee.

8. Licensed Associates will be required to meet continuing education requirements for license renewal, Subsection 741.163.

9. Special conditions for a time-limited waiver ending September 1, 1988, are provided.

   A. The Committee on request may waive degree requirements for licensure as a Licensed Associate in Audiology for applicants who by August 31, 1988, meet the following requirements:

      i. show proof of bona fide employment as a technician, assistant, or other support services personnel directly involved with the speech-language and/or hearing handicapped on *September 1, 1984; and,*

      ii. perform their employment duties under the supervision of a Texas licensed Audiologist. Upon application and each subsequent renewal, a statement shall be submitted by the supervising Audiologist, acknowledging his/her acceptance of the supervisory responsibilities. The minimum supervision requirements for an applicant seeking license under these special conditions shall be no less than two (2) hours a week of direct on-site supervision by a licensed professional, *and,*

      iii. submit initial application forms and nonrefundable application fees for a Licensed Associate under these special conditions so that it will be received in the Committee office no later than May 31, 1986; *and*

      iv. show annual proof of pursuit toward licensing as an Associate in Audiology, by submitting original transcript(s) from the accredited institution(s) in which the twenty-one (21) semester hours of course work in audiology are taken; *and*

    v. submit by August 31, 1988, the application for Licensed Associate in Audiology indicating that the full requirements have been met.

B. Transcripts shall be reviewed as in Subsection 741.84(4).

C. Applicants, and their licensed sponsors, shall be considered subject to Subsection 741.195 of this title (relating to Violations by Nonlicensed Individuals) and Subsection 741.196 of this title (relating to Penalties).

D. Applicants, meeting the above criteria, who do not succeed in acquiring a license as an Associate by August 31, 1988, shall not be eligible for licensure under this time-limited waiver.

§741.85. *Audiology Aides.* For clarification, the following requirements and duties of an Aide are

1. A high school degree or equivalent and appropriate on-the-job training experience;

2. Accountable to a fully licensed professional who is ultimately responsible for the Aide;

3. May work under direction of Associate if approved and supervised by fully licensed professional;

4. May not singularly engage in direct intervention or assessment activities;

5. May participate in activities as described and approved by fully licensed professional such as:
    A. setting up room and equipment for evaluation/intervention/conference;
    B. clearing room and storing equipment after evaluation/intervention/conference;
    C. preparing materials for use by Associate or Audiologist in intervention, evaluation, carryover, etc.;
    D. transporting clients to and from clinical sessions;
    E. assisting with field trips and other communication stimulation situations;
    F. acting as surrogate parent;
    G. participating in daily living activities and care;
    H. applying language stimulation strategies in daily living activities as directed by Associate and approved by fully licensed Audiologist.

1985 REGULATIONS FOR SPEECH-LANGUAGE PATHOLOGY PARAPROFESSIONALS IN TEXAS

§741.64. *Requirements for a Licensed Associate in Speech-Language Pathology*

1. The term "associate" will be used to designate an aide who provides services and support of clinical programs of speech-language pathology, who is supervised by a Texas licensed Speech-Language Pathologist, who has received the training specified below, and who holds a current and valid license as a Licensed Associate in Speech-Language Pathology. The following are established as minimum requirements to function as a Licensed Associate in Speech-Language Pathology:

   A. A baccalaureate degree; and
   B. No fewer than twenty-one (21) semester hours in speech-language pathology and/or audiology, at least nine (9) of which must be in the area for which license is being sought; and
   C. Transcripts shall be reviewed as in 741.61(4); and
   D. Upon application and each subsequent renewal, a statement shall be submitted by the supervising Speech-Language Pathologist acknowledging his/her acceptance of the supervisory responsibilities.

2. Although the licensed Speech-Language Pathologist may delegate specific clinical tasks to an Associate, the legal, ethical, and moral responsibility to the client for all services provided cannot be delegated. The Associate may execute specific components of the clinical speech, language, and/or hearing program if the professional determines that the Associate has received the training and has the skill to accomplish that task, and the professional provides sufficient supervision to ensure appropriate completion of the task assigned to the Associate. The fully licensed supervising professional Speech-Language Pathologist is legally and ethically responsible for the Associate and the Speech-Language Pathology Aide. The Speech-Language Pathologist must keep job descriptions and performance records; these must be current and available upon demand by the Committee of Examiners. The Speech-Language Pathologist must ensure that all services are in compliance with these Committee rules, particularly with Subsection 741.41 (relating to the Code of Ethics).

   A. Examples of duties which Associates may be assigned, provided appropriate planning, preparation for the task, and professional supervision, include the following:
      i. conducting or participating in speech, language, and/or hearing screening;
      ii. conducting evaluative or management programs which may include the utilization of published materials for which the Associate has received training;
      iii. maintaining clinical records of client performance;
      iv. preparing clinical materials; and
      v. participating with the professional in research projects, staff development, public relations programs, or similar activities as designated and supervised by the professional.

   B. The Associate should not engage in any of the following activities:
      i. interpreting observations or data into diagnostic statements, clinical management strategies, or procedures;
      ii. determining case selection;
      iii. presenting written reports of client information to those other than the supervisor without the signature of the supervisor;
      iv. referring a client to other professionals or other agencies; or
      v. using any title which connotes the competency of a licensed professional, as defined in Section 2 of the Act.

   C. Any references to the licensee's title shall state clearly that the license status is that of an Associate.

D. Direct-care staff in a residential care and/or treatment facility who use only the concepts of daily living in their job performance are not required to be licensed as Associates and may not assume the duties of Associates as defined in these sections.

3. Therapy/intervention is:

A. The systematic, individualized process of minimizing communication disorders, involving the dynamic interaction between the fully licensed Speech-Language Pathologist and client;

B. Designed and executed on the basis of ongoing evaluation of the client's communication needs, skills, and resources; and

C. Designed and executed only by a fully licensed Speech-Language Pathologist; certain routine and perfunctory aspects of the intervention process, such as carryover activities, may be delegated to a Licensed Associate.

4. Carryover is:

A. The therapeutically designed transfer of a newly acquired communication ability to contexts and situations outside of the therapy situation; and is
B. Designed by a fully licensed Speech-Language Pathologist.

5. The Associate may conduct carryover activities, language and auditory stimulation, and other activities related to intervention and record keeping as described in these rules and as deemed appropriate by the supervising fully licensed Speech-Language Pathologist.

6. The Associate may oversee activities of Aides in consultation with, and direction of, fully licensed Speech-Language Pathologists.

7. Direct supervision of duties assigned to the Associate shall be provided by a Texas licensed Speech-Language Pathologist.

A. A Licensed Associate in Speech-Language Pathology shall be supervised by a Texas licensed Speech-Language Pathologist.

B. Following on-the-job training, the Associate's initial client contact shall be directly supervised. Thereafter, the minimum supervision requirements for an Associate by a licensed professional shall be no less than two (2) hours a week, at least half of which is direct on-site supervision. Indirect methods of supervision such as audio and/or video tape recording, telephone communication, numerical data, or other means of reporting may be utilized.

C. Supervisory records shall be maintained by the licensed professional which verify regularly scheduled monitoring/assessment/evaluation of Associate and client performance. Such documentation may be requested by the Committee.

8. Licensed Associates will be required to meet continuing education requirements of license renewal, Subsection 741.163.

9. Special conditions for a time-limited waiver ending September 1, 1988, are provided.

A. The Committee on request may waive degree requirements for licensure as a Licensed Associate in Speech-Language Pathology for applicants who by August 31, 1988, meet the following requirements:

i.   show proof of bona fide employment as a technician, assistant, or other support services personnel directly involved with the speech-language and/or hearing handicapped on September 1, 1984; and
ii. perform their employment duties under the supervision of a Texas licensed Speech-Language Pathologist. Upon application and each subsequent renewal, a statement shall be submitted by the supervising Speech-Language

Pathologist, acknowledging his/her acceptance of the supervisory responsibilities. The minimum supervision requirements for an applicant seeking license under these special conditions shall be no less than two (2) hours a week of direct on-site supervision by a licensed professional; and

    iii.   submit initial application forms and nonrefundable application fees for a Licensed Associate under these special conditions so that it will be received in the Committee office no later than May 31, 1986; and

    iv.   show annual proof of pursuit toward licensing as an Associate in Speech-Language Pathology by submitting original transcript(s) from the accredited institution(s) in which the twenty-one (21) semester hours of course work in speech-language pathology are taken; and

    v.   submit by August 31, 1988, the application for Licensed Associate in Speech-Language Pathology indicating that the full requirements have been met.

B.   Transcripts shall be reviewed as in Subsection 741.61(4).

C.   Applicants, and their licensed sponsors, shall be considered subject to Subsection 741.195 of this title (relating to Violations by Non-Licensed Individuals) and Subsection 741.196 of this title (relating to Penalties).

D.   Applicants, meeting the above criteria, who do not succeed in acquiring a license as an Associate by August 31, 1988, shall not be eligible for licensure under this time-limited waiver.

10. The requirements and duties of an Aide are as follows:

A.   An Aide is to have a high school degree or equivalent and appropriate on-the-job training experience;

B.   An Aide is accountable to a fully licensed professional who is ultimately responsible for the Aide;

C.   An Aide may work under direction of an Associate if approved and supervised by a fully licensed professional;

D.   An Aide may not singularly engage in direct intervention or assessment activities;

E.   An Aide may participate in activities as described and approved by a fully licensed professional such as

    i.   setting up room and equipment for evaluation/intervention/conference;

    ii.   clearing room and storing equipment after evaluation/intervention/conference;

    iii.   preparing materials for use by Associate or Speech-Language Pathologist in intervention, evaluation, carryover, etc.

    iv.   transporting clients to and from clinical sessions;

    v.   assisting with field trips and other communication stimulation situations;

    vi.   acting as surrogate parent;

    vii.   participating in daily living activities and care;

    viii.   applying language stimulation strategies in daily living activities as directed by Associate and approved by fully licensed Speech-Language Pathologist.

Chapter **6**

Promotion and Marketing:
A Matter of Philosophy

Promoting and marketing professional services can be a matter of education. Educating those who do not know, those who do not know how to take advantage of what they know, and those who do not believe what they know. Nonbelievers come in all varieties, but the most destructive to a profession, as well as to a specific practice, are the nonbelievers who are professionals themselves. If any professional lacks conviction about the worth of professional services, even though the doubts are not explicitly stated, promotional attempts will be diminished and the profession's public image will be affected. In the sense that delivery of services is a matter of philosophy, promoting and marketing services are also matters of philosophy.

Public image of a profession cannot be higher than the profession's self-image. Practitioners who feel that their services are unworthy of direct payment, and that their practices do not offer the highest quality of professional services, cannot promote the profession or practice. Such professionals should attempt to discover their biases that produce this outlook.

The public's image of a profession is shaped more by its *contact with professionals* than by media campaigns and promotional efforts. In a profession as young and insecure as speech–language pathology/audiology, the primary and continuous target of promotion is the profession itself. Professional pride and image are shaped by quality of professional preparation, by quality of the members as self-confident service providers, and by responsible self-government within the profession. Only members of a profession can influence these internal factors.

Promotion is offering or exalting a product—such as professional services— for general acknowledgment of its worth or value. Such promotion is directed toward the general public to increase its awareness of a product and to improve the overall image of the product. In certain instances, promotion can be considered a form of marketing when promotion is directly related to the growth and prosperity of specific services or products. For example, if one promotes the value of a certain specialty within a profession expressly for *selling* the services of a certain specialist, then marketing occurs. For purposes of discussion here, the term promotion will be used to refer to interactions that are intended to enhance the overall impression of the profession.

Marketing is the composite of activities included in the transfer of goods from the producer to the consumer. One example of this in a professional context would be transferring professional services from the practitioner to the speech-language-hearing impaired. Marketing activities are done with the intention of selling. They may address fee arrangements, various forms and types of service delivery, contractual arrangements for services, and the provision of information to consumers about potential services suitable to their needs.

The market place is the place of transaction for both buyers and sellers. Marketing, for the service provider, includes going to the market place with a promise of matching particular service needs with ideal service provisions. Marketing is usually directed toward the identified consumer and those having direct interaction with potential consumers. Referral sources, for example, have direct interaction with potential consumers and are potential targets of marketing efforts.

Promotional efforts are usually directed toward the general public, while marketing activities are usually directed toward potential consumers of services and sources of referral. Primary reasons for promotional efforts or marketing efforts include the following:

1. Informing others about the existence of a profession or a specific practice;
2. Informing others about the specialties or unique benefits of a profession or a specific practice;
3. Creating and maintaining a positive image of the profession or a specific practice;
4. Correcting distorted or negative images of the profession or specific practice;
5. Reminding a specific population of the existence and unique characteristics of a practice.

Different reasons for promotion and marketing exist at different times. The promotional goals, marketing activities, and marketing targets of a beginning practice in an unfamiliar community may be quite unlike those of a well-established practice. An established practice that intends to add a specialist to its staff might target only previous and current referral sources. An established practice that moves to a new location might use that opportunity to expand contacts with referral sources as well as refresh old contacts. Marketing activities and targets of a practice that changes ownership might include as much variety and scope as a beginning practice. Before time, energy, and money are directed toward marketing, the owner/practitioner should consider as many factors as possible in the planning process.

CONSIDERATIONS IN MARKETING

A quick way to lose money with nothing to show for it is to engage in careless marketing. A private practitioner's first consideration should be whether marketing is necessary to the practice. If the practice is working to capacity, if increased referrals would necessitate undesirable major changes in the practice, and if the owner/practitioner likes things the way they are, there is little reason to ask for problems in the form of new clients who cannot be seen immediately. In fact, unless one designs an overall plan that integrates carefully executed marketing activities and a potentially increased client load with one's present practice requirements, marketing efforts can have a negative impact on the practice. Clients and referral sources ask for services with anticipation of prompt attention. If that expectation is not met with reasonable timeliness, clients and referral sources will go elsewhere. Should the practitioner attempt to avoid losing the new clients and, instead, carelessly absorb them into the practice, then a practice that began as a well-planned operation with a good reputation can end in chaos.

If the owner/practitioner feels that more clients—or different clients—can be served and that marketing activities and expenditures are justified, then the consideration becomes ''How does the marketing plan fit into the long-range plan of the practice?'' This question can encompass such factors as:

1. How should marketing efforts change the practice?
2. What returns are desired for caseload and budget?
3. How does this marketing venture set up future promotional and marketing efforts?
4. Does this effort represent a one-shot venture? Is that desirable?
5. Which clinicians will be affected? For how long?
6. How much space will be affected?
7. How much money *should* be spent? How much money *can* be spent?

In the development of clear goals for marketing activities it is important to be realistic about what the practice is—and is not. It is not realistic, for example, to pretend that private practice is just like any other service delivery system. Each owner/practitioner must look beyond the shield of professional identity and realize that private practice places service delivery in the market place as a commodity. The realization that private practice includes the possibility of monetary success or failure can encourage one to cultivate an appreciation for a business approach to one's practice.

A business approach does not mean to plunder and pillage; it means to *develop a work plan and work toward the realization of that plan.*

Development of a realistic marketing plan involves a careful analysis of assets and limitations that address professional disciplines and specialties represented in the practice, unique aspects of the practice and its service delivery, clients best served by the practice, and financial arrangements. Listing disciplines and specialties is the easiest way to begin because the content is familiar. For example, the audiology specialty would list hearing aid dispensing, industrial consultation, and so forth. A way to avoid getting stuck after completing that list is to ask the same questions a newswriter does when gathering facts: *Who* is to be served? *What* forms of service delivery are to be selected? *Where* might the service occur? *When* can services be provided? *Why* deliver particular services? *How much* will service delivery cost?

An examination of four of these major ''facts'' to consider is illustrated in Table 6–1.

In general the tendency is to focus on assets of the practice and to give less attention to liabilities or limitations. It is, however, just as important to know what the practice *cannot* offer, as it is to know what it *can* provide. To wit—*if it's not in stock, it should not be sold.*

Liabilities and limitations include certain characteristics of the professional staff who will be responsible for providing services, as well as administrative characteristics of the owner/practitioner and clerical skills of the office staff. If staff members who are highly skilled in a few areas are not willing or able to extend their services

Table 6–1.   Ranges of Potential Services

Who is served	What form of service	Where	How much

Age:
  infants
  pre-school
  school
  adolescent
  adult
  geriatric
	Screening
	
	Assessment
	Intervention:
	  direct
	  indirect
	
	Consultation
		In-Office
		
		Out-of-office:
		  in-city:
		    homes
		    schools
		    hospitals
		    nursing homes
		Other:
		  other profession-
		    als' offices,
		  service clubs
			Amount (for each service
			  and location):
			    direct service
			    conferences
			    travel
			    reports
			    consultation
			    other

Groups
 	
Individuals
 	
Professions
 	
General Public
 	
Business/Industry
 	
Paraprofessionals
 	
Training Programs
  (i.e., practice
    sites and
    supervision)
 	
Other
	In-Service:
	  parents
	  teachers
	  other
	
	Continuing Education
	  Seminars
	
	Forensics:
	  court witness
	
	Media:
	  public information
	  news column
	  TV/Radio
	  teleconferences
	  public interest
	    magazine stories
	
	Travel:
	  short/local
	  extended/foreign
	
	Other
			Payment schedules:
			  full fee
			  sliding scale
			  direct pay
			  contractual
			  consultative:
			    by-the-job
			    by-the-hour
			    by-the-month
			
			Collection policies
			
			Insurance arrangements:
			  availability
			  requirements
			
			Contributions
			
			Other

into other areas of service delivery, then marketing goals must be appropriately tailored. For example, staff members who are skilled in intervention procedures with language/learning impaired patients may not be skilled in working with voice clients. Marketing efforts would accordingly be directed to the language/learning impaired. Although a primary purpose of marketing is to expand and maintain a flow of clients through the practice, *more* is not necessarily *better*. For example, many practices would not be able to manage long-distance consultation; others could not handle a large influx of hearing-impaired infants; most practices could not sustain a surge of low-fee clients.

The Marketing Plan

As the analysis of the practice progresses, a marketing plan begins to evolve in terms of goals, desired results, target populations, and specific activities.

The Goals

Goals of promotional efforts and marketing activities should dictate the planning and execution of the efforts. Goals must be determined in relation to the double question: *Why market?* and *So what?*

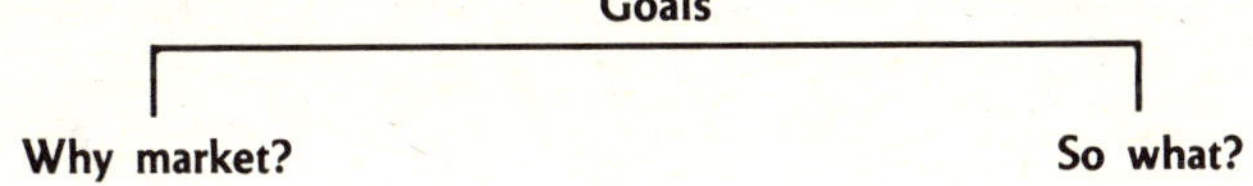

1. (For an established practice)
   Inform identified and potential referral sources of a new staff member who specializes in voice disorders:
   - to remind old referral sources of clinic's ongoing operations;
   - to elicit new referrals because of new area of specialization;
   - to introduce clinic operations to new/potential referral sources;

So That

- at least five new referral sources can be obtained for the year;
- at least two old referral sources will contact the practice with questions or referrals.

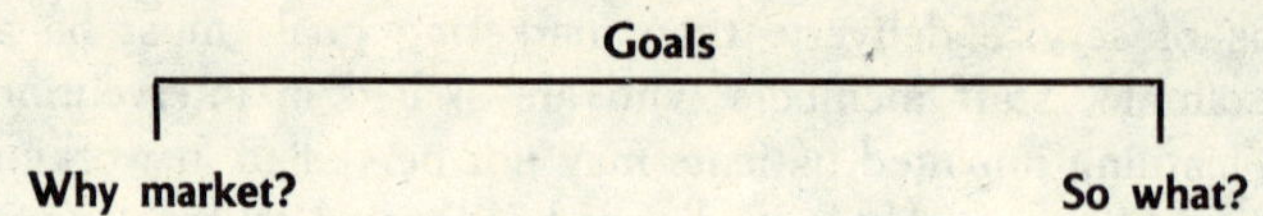

2. (For a beginning practice)
Inform the community in the immediate vicinity of the practice of availability and scope of services:
- to provide information about new services to as wide an audience as possible;
- to obtain general exposure for awareness of potential consumers;
- to provide information about unique qualities of service delivery;

So That

- at least 25 new clients will be obtained from the one activity.

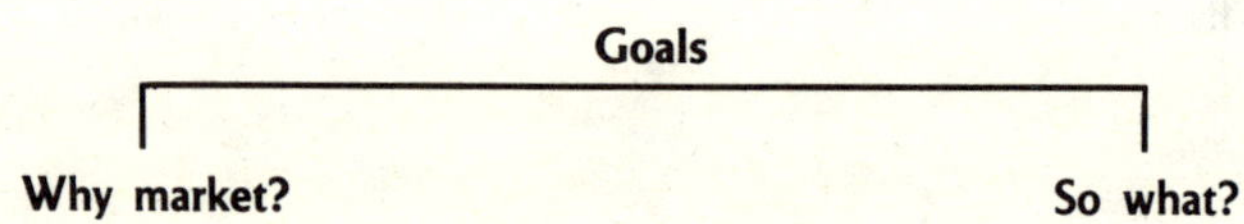

3. (For an established practice)
Inform private schools and kindergartens of new screening program for speech–language–hearing, and of consultation for teachers on individual or large group basis:
- to suggest consultation services to meet schools' needs for early identification;
- to provide alternatives to screening at school site;
- to suggest teacher in-service groups and parent education groups;

So That

- at least five kindergartens will contract for preschool screening;
- at least two kindergartens or schools will contract for teacher in-service;
- at least one kindergarten or school will contract for a two-part parent education seminar.

The Target Population

After marketing goals and desired results have been specified, the target population can be identified. Sometimes goals are so specific that recipients of marketing efforts are obvious. If the population is not clear, it may help to list possibilities before narrowing the field:

1. Active referral sources
2. Once-active referral sources
3. Potential referral sources never tapped
4. New sources of referral in the area
5. Current clients
6. Previous clients
7. Family and friends
8. Colleagues and business associates
9. Former employers and teachers
10. General public
11. Specific segment of the public:
    a. age distribution
    b. vocation
    c. income
    d. location and setting (nursing homes, private schools)
    e. geographic location
12. Professionals in general
13. Specific segment of professionals:
    a. disciplines (occupational therapists, teachers, physicians)
    b. type of practice within discipline (ENT specialists, kindergarten teachers)
14. Geographic distribution

Sometimes considering possible marketing targets generates a new set of marketing goals by highlighting certain populations who may never have had contact with the practice. By matching marketing goals with target population, marketing efforts can be more efficient than random showering of such efforts.

The Target Locations

Location of the target population can be approached in many ways. The most typical approaches are (1) to focus on a particular *type* of employment setting, regardless of location, and (2) to focus on a particular geographic area. The employment setting approach is crucial for marketing when the targeted population is setting-bound. For example, if only hospital administrators are to be targeted, then the entire city, county, or region could be included because the efforts would be directed to the persons, regardless of their hospitals' location.

On the other hand, the geographic location approach would be employed if the general population located within the vicinity is to be targeted. To ascertain the boundaries of the geographic location, one might *map* the area. Mapping is the drawing of concentric circles around the practice site in 5-mile increments. Using a city map, with the practice site as the center of the circle, draw a circle encompassing the 5 miles immediately surrounding the office. Continue to draw circles, in 5-mile increments, until at least five or six circles are drawn, representing the 25- to 35-mile radius surrounding the office site. The marketing theory on which this exercise is based holds that primary geographic targets are those closest to the practice site, with marketing effectiveness decreasing as the range of the circles increases. Twenty-five to 35 miles is considered to be the maximum physical range for most geographically based marketing efforts.

The advisability of using marketing circles depends entirely upon the type of services to be offered. A practice focusing on consultation and out-of-office work might not want to limit marketing to a small geographic area. A practice wanting to increase referrals from a certain area that is not close to the office, such as a new corporate development or housing section, might not want to bother with targeting the immediate office vicinity at all. In certain sections of the country, people are accustomed to driving long distances for shopping, medical visits, and other ordinary pursuits. A marketing target might be desirable in certain of those areas, particularly where suburban industry is booming and companies are relocating thousands of families to that area.

Matching the Method to the Market

In most communication situations, a competent communicator adjusts speaking or writing style to the conversational partner. It is not considered appropriate, for example, to address a stranger in the same way one would address a friend. When someone asks the time of day, it is not necessary to tell them how to fix a clock. The same attention to communication style is necessary for effective marketing. The message will be wasted unless it addresses the recipients' needs and biases.

Young parents may need to know how to assess whether their toddlers are developing adequate speech; professionals may want to know what special services are provided by a practice. An announcement in a professional journal would carry more technical information about a practice than an advertisement in the yellow pages of a rural community telephone directory. A proposal to kindergartens would provide specific information pertinent to the proposal, while a brochure for the general public would give information about all services. The form of the message and the information contained in the message must be relevent to the recipient if effective communication is to occur. In marketing, it is additionally important that the recipient remember *who* was responsible for the communication. The message and method of conveying the message must accomplish two things, regardless of the target population:

1. The intended message should be prominent so that the recipient will remember that which the communicator felt was important.
2. The recipient must remember who gave the message.

One way of considering style of presentation is to consider the level of contact with the practitioner. The better we know a person, the less information we have to provide in order to communicate. Total strangers are treated politely and formally, because social rules are the only basis for interaction. Good friends usually skip formalities because they are not necessary; previously shared experiences provide a basis for interaction. So it is that frequency and type of previous contact set the tone for marketing interaction. A message directed to a group of people with whom the practitioner has had no previous contact would be formal and would provide basic information about the practice. A message to a friend or colleague would be of a more personal nature, assuming knowledge of certain information while providing new information or reminders. Sometimes previous contact also helps determine the media or form of the marketing message. A personal note is appropriate for a long-time colleague, but a printed announcement or formal letter is more appropriate for a new professional contact. An announcement in the newspaper is expected for a marketing message to the general public but not to friends and family.

Both the message and the method of conveying it should be "custom-design." Attention should be given to certain characteristics of the target population, including education, interest level, and life-style. An attitude of growth and self-improvement usually is important to people who voluntarily seek help. Certain life-styles and educational levels lend themselves more easily to this attitude. Of course, many factors influence people's decisions to use available services. Professional services and related marketing activities are for people who try to take responsibility for their limitations and are responsive to information they can apply to their own needs.

Whatever the marketing *message*, there are a variety of available vehicles, styles, and media from which to select one's marketing *method*. The important thing to keep in mind when selecting a vehicle is to choose one that will attract the attention of targeted recipients and be most cost effective for that particular market. Since marketing methods and materials represent the practitioner and his/her services, they should never be done carelessly or cheaply. Materials that "go before you to make a place" should signal care and quality, not poor workmanship and bad taste. A letter, business card, or advertisement in the yellow pages may be the only tangible evidence of a professional's work that is seen by a referral source or potential client. Scrimping on consumables intended for the public is a false economy and bad advertising. Print shops usually offer a standardized format and inexpensive printing process for stationery to beginning practitioners. Many people use these short-cuts, and it looks like it. Having stationery and business cards that do not look like they are being used by every other professional in town can be an advantage.

There are, in addition to the usual brochures, printed announcements, and yellow-page ads, more personal vehicles, such as open houses, personal or professional letters on letterhead stationery, speeches to service groups and civic clubs, telephone calls, and personal visits. The choice of vehicle varies from one marketing goal to the next and from one target population to the next. The important thing is to get desired results through tasteful, ethical, and informative activities.

Guidelines

It is not possible to write a marketing recipe with step-by-step instructions that always lead to the desired result. There are too many variables that are specific to each marketing effort. Some guidelines, however, can make planning for marketing activities a little easier:

1. Based on 5-year plans for the practice, determine needs for which marketing activities might be indicated.
2. Write marketing goals for the practice.
3. Perform a product analysis; make an exhaustive list of services, noting assets and limitations.
4. Perform a market analysis and select target populations—locate the groups by geographic location or work setting; note the characteristics of the groups to help determine market strategies; select the populations on basis of marketing goal.
5. Determine fees, payment amounts, and schedules for services offered.
6. Determine the marketing message.
7. Determine the best way to reach the populations—which marketing vehicle or method to use for the message to each population.
8. Use quality materials in marketing efforts.
9. Project budget for each marketing effort before beginning.
10. Determine how to evaluate results of marketing effort.
11. Four to 6 months after each marketing activity, match results of the effort to time and money expended on the effort.

The Budget

Budgeting for marketing activities should coincide with long-range budgeting for the practice. Marketing costs money, but it does not have to cost a lot of money. Advice from print shops, advertising agencies, and marketing consultants is readily available. Sometimes it is desirable to use such advice, and sometimes it is not. Practitioners should apply the creative energy they usually reserve for clinical interactions to the intriguing puzzles of marketing. Money spent on marketing needs to be considered an investment; even if the interest rate is low, the money itself should come back!

Marketing does not stop when a practice has enough clients to stay busy for a while. Every practice has the built-in danger of becoming stagnant, and every practice experiences attrition in client load. Stagnation in a practice can result from working with the same clients week after week when the interest level and novelty that comes with each new client wears thin. Attrition, the gradual wearing down of resources, occurs in every practice as a product of dismissals, change in residence by clients, clients' failures to return, illness, death, and many other reasons. Unless a practitioner has planned some regular form of marketing to keep various populations aware of services, he/she will discover when renewing marketing efforts that his/her marketing needs are similar to those of a practitioner just starting practice.

Routine and Daily Marketing

Although we usually think of marketing as brief, concerted efforts, part of the budget in every practice must include projected expenditures for routine promotion, called ''Business Promotion,'' ''Public Relations,'' and other names that do not sound so pleasant. While the chart of accounts may show the account of ''Business Promotion'' heavy with expenses from business meals and other business entertainment items, that account is important for other marketing efforts. Some suggestions for routine market activities that are low-cost but usually high-visibility and high-return include the following:

1. Buy an occasional 2-inch newspaper announcement, particularly in a neighborhood paper or university area paper. People read neighborhood papers, while they usually scan other papers; university area people usually take more time for reading than other populations.
2. Using a 2-inch newspaper announcement every 2 or 3 months attracts more ongoing attention than one 12-inch notice once a year.
3. Acknowledge all referrals with a note on letterhead stationery. Speech-language pathologists/audiologists have not developed a high sense of gratitude for referrals—in spite of our poor self-image. We have tended to feel that if we received a referral, it was because we deserved it. We have not always taken time to respond with either an acknowledgment or a report.
4. Enclose a business card about every third time you write an acknowledgment or report, particularly if you have moved in the past year or have employed a new staff member.
5. If you send invitations to an open house or a letter to inform referral sources of a move or a new specialist, enclose a business card. The letter or invitation or announcement will be thrown away; most professionals keep a file of business cards.
6. Some professionals use printed referral pads for physicians, schools, and other referral sources. These seem to be fairly well received in some areas, although it is advisable to evaluate regional biases about techniques that could be construed as commercialization of professional services.
7. When talking with philanthropic and civic groups, leave them something in writing, preferably a business card attached to whatever handouts are distributed. All handouts should have the name, address, and telephone number of the practice; if appropriate to the situation, leave a brochure or summary of the practice and its services.
8. Buy a carefully composed section in the telephone pages, write the advertisement yourself and include the information you want readers to know about services. Use the same product analysis you use for major promotional efforts. Unless you are very well known *and* in a small, low-growth community, the yellow page advertisements can bring you as much new business as any other single marketing effort, except word of mouth. Name, address, and telephone number of a practice are usually not enough; include a brief listing of specializations and unique services.

In addition to the routine-but-special marketing efforts, there are some efforts that can be incorporated into routine client care that cost little or no money. Here are a few to consider; add to them from your own practice:

1. Return phone calls. Unless a potential client is absolutely committed to seeing you and only you, that person will call someone else. Frequently, when people see yellow page advertisements or other public marketing, they make the decision to call ''someone,'' and proceed to contact two or three different practices. They set up an appointment with the first one they contact.
2. If you cannot return the phone call immediately, have your secretary return the call promptly with suggested appointment times for an initial interview or screening. If the person insists on speaking with you before coming in, have the secretary tell them when you will call back.
3. Do not be careless with current clients.
    a. Return their phone calls immediately, or have the secretary call.
    b. Provide them with frequent opportunity to see you for a minute or two (literally).
    c. Send brief notes (i.e., on the back of a business card) with the child every few weeks or so.
    d. Offer them a chance for periodic conferences.
    e. Keep track of dates of telephone calls you have made on their behalf to teachers, physicians, and others. Put them on the bill each month, without charging unless they were longer than 5 or 10 minutes, but just to remind them that you are working for them.
    f. If you do routine re–evaluation, or write a brief note to someone about them, send the client a copy.
    g. If they ask for a report, tell them *realistically* when it will be sent. (''I can send a two-line summary tomorrow. I cannot send a two-page report until the 15th or 16th.'')
4. To avoid attrition by drop-out and client fatigue, give a client a 1-month ''time off,'' when possible. This is fairly effective after a client has been in continuous therapy for 6 months, particularly with older children and adolescents. They can be told that they must return in 1 month and therapy will resume for 3 months (for example). If they continue to make improvement in therapy and in school, they can have another month off at the end of that time. The structure helps both client and parents see that there will be some relief; that you, too, are concerned about their level of interest; and that you will provide them with time off. This permits you some control over times when the clients will be out of therapy and also demonstrates that you are not out to get ''every therapy cent'' you can get.
5. When clients have been on vacation, or have been dismissed temporarily, remind them to return when the time comes.
6. If you have dismissed clients temporarily on the contingency that they must return for routine re-evaluation, call them to remind them when the time arrives for their re-evaluation.

There is no doubt that clients want results from your services. However, they also want effort and demonstrated care from you in the pursuit of therapeutic results. Hard work in therapy and paying attention to the family by letting them know what steps you have taken in their behalf are crucial to their continuing long-term contact with you *and* their willingness to send you other referrals. Evidence of your efforts on behalf of each client will be valued almost as highly as quick results in therapy. If a practitioner tends to be careless with clients after they are in an intervention program, to ignore client calls and to take an extraordinarily long time to send reports, then the client is much more likely to drift away . . . along with any potential referrals. The perception that a practitioner is indifferent to a client is almost as damaging as the perception of malpractice.

Marketing for Referrals from Professionals

Most private practitioners encourage referrals from all possible sources. Eventually, however, successful practitioners tend to concentrate on particular referral sources, such as a core of referral sources that serve many clients with communication disorders. Familiar referral sources are more likely to know the services and quality of work and to require less complex reporting systems (Flower, 1984). Practitioners need referral sources who themselves provide high-quality services so that mutual referrals are facilitated.

Usually it is not a good idea to form exclusive relationships with referral sources, although at the time, that system seems to be a perfect arrangement for a steady source of clients. When exclusivity occurs, word travels quickly and other potential sources of referral refer elsewhere. In most situations, a broad range of referral sources is desired, including physicians, psychologists, tutors, teachers, and families of previous clients. Some guidelines can be helpful in cultivating and maintaining referrals from professional referral sources.

1. Acknowledge referrals.
2. Send a report, even a brief one, about any results pertinent to the client referred—or make phone call, if appropriate.
3. Send referrals to professionals who refer to you.
4. When sending announcements or letters to professional colleagues, enclose a business card (everyone files or throws away announcements).
5. If you have a specialty, or hire clinicians who are specialists, make professional colleagues aware of this and keep reminding them. This is a key in highly competitive markets, particularly when you may be one of several choices for the referral.
6. Offer to give lectures to professional preparation programs in areas near you. For example, if you are near a medical school, offer to provide orientation about communication disorders to residents, interns, medical, and nursing students.
7. If a referral is made specifically to *you*, not to your practice, by a colleague, be very careful about how you ''give away'' that client to one of your employees.
8. Serve on health care boards that have other health care professionals.
9. Contact potential referral sources by telephone or mail and ask for a 5-minute appointment because you are putting together a list of professionals to whom you can send referrals. In the course of getting information about them, provide information about yourself.

Resistance to Referral

Most potential referral sources are willing to refer, but many do not. The following are some of the most common reasons that referral sources do not refer:

1. They forget about you.
2. They forget about the profession and its resources for helping a variety of disorders.
3. They're not sure what you ''do,'' exactly.
4. They can't find your phone number.
5. They're not sure that you are the right professional to help someone learn (to speak, remember, read, read lips, check for hearing loss, treat learning problems, use a hearing aid, and so forth).
6. You haven't sent them anybody, but your colleague down the street has.
7. You never acknowledge referrals, so they never know if clients get to you.
8. The insurance companies are angry with you because you are unreliable about sending prompt reports.
9. You never send reports when they are requested.
10. They think you only take referrals from physicians, or from a specific group of physicians.
11. They think they can do at least as well themselves with the client, so they don't refer at all.
12. They're not allowed to name specific places for referral (i.e., bureaucratic policy in many agencies).
13. They prefer to refer to free clinics.
14. They're afraid you'll take the referral, keep the client, and not reciprocate (characteristic of within-profession referrals).
15. They made the referral, but the client didn't follow up, and the referring source lost track of both of you.
16. The schools take care of everybody, so why refer?
17. They think you moved.
18. Fill in the blank with other reasons that apply to you: _________________ .

Referrals Within the Profession

There is nothing wrong in telling your colleagues that you are in practice, that your specialty is ____________, and you would like to know what areas of service are their specialities. A personal letter announcing your presence is more effective than spending money to blanket the regional association with formal announcements. Make the letter short and concise, briefly outlining necessary information. Send the letter to all colleagues in the area, not just to those in private practices. Include those employed in agencies and hospitals. Establish and maintain contact with all colleagues in the area. Referrals come from those who know you and believe that they can trust your work. For the new practitioner, there are certain kinds of referrals from other speech-language pathologists/audiologists that are quite appropriate to solicit, for example:

1. Family and close friends with whom they do not feel comfortable working;
2. Situations/clients the other practitioners do not like to handle;

3. Low pay private clients;
4. Out-of-office consultation, contracts, and expert witness;
5. Substitute therapy for practitioners in the event of the regular clinician's illness or absence. Certain kinds of substitution therapy can be appropriate, depending on the nature of the disorder, the family's acceptance of the substitute, *and* the *substitute's* sense of integrity (i.e., not stealing the client).
6. Clients who need services the practitioner does not offer.

In many situations, practitioners within a profession complement each other, and refer clients to colleagues when situations warrant it. A problem can occur when a practitioner finds it is necessary to refer certain clients to colleagues more frequently than is desirable. For example, most clinicians have some rudimentary skills with laryngectomized clients, although many do not feel comfortable as primary service providers. An occasional referral of a laryngectomee to a colleague does not pose a serious threat to a practice, but it does focus on an issue that has ethical as well as financial implications, such as the following:

> Do I refer certain kinds of clients, losing the fees and future referrals of this kind?
>
> Do I do what I can, take the fee, and hope I don't get too many like this?

Like many issues in private practice, there is another alternative to consider; one that does not require juggling of financial concerns with ethical conduct. The most professional approach is sometimes the best business approach. In this case, hire a consultant or employee to provide specialized services. An independent consultant can be engaged on an as-needed basis with payment based on a percentage of revenue. The problems of a formal employment arrangement can be averted—such as taxes and withholding—and the client receives the services of a specialist. The owner/practitioner realizes some financial gain without compromising professional integrity. Many clinicians, employed elsewhere, welcome additional clients, particularly in the setting of private practice. It is important in this situation, as in any other situation involving people, that all parties be quite clear about the arrangements.

At some point, the practitioner will be curious about any *results* achieved from marketing efforts. Guess work is almost always involved in marketing, and sometimes it is difficult to measure the effects. One way to measure results is to have a question on the intake form or case history that asks clients how they selected the practice. Keeping records of information and comparing it to original market analysis can provide a trend for repeating or discontinuing certain marketing strategies.

Promotional and marketing activities occur daily in routine interactions with the public and with other professionals. Daily efforts include the design and quality of stationery, attention to long-term clients, and respect to referral sources. Special public relations activities occur at the beginning of a practice to announce and solicit referrals. Throughout the course of a practice, marketing efforts are exerted to maintain, change, or expand a practice. Whenever marketing occurs, all efforts must be done with the same philosophical approach that the practitioner applies to client care. Professional goals and financial realities do not have to be in opposition; each can serve the other for the well-being of both client and practice.

Appendices

APPENDIX 6–1
TO MARKET, TO MARKET . . .

1. Aim at a particular type of client.

2. In an area full of other therapists, emphasize the uniqueness of your practice, your specialty, geographic territory, and so forth.

3. Do volunteer work; serve on health care boards; give speeches to groups.

4. Go to professional meetings in the area. If there is no professional association, form one.

5. Establish core social contacts, if you do not already have some. Become active in a club, political group, church, or civic activity. Offer to provide a lecture to them about your profession or work on topics such as prevention of disorders.

6. Contact agencies in the area known for client care, such as Vocational Rehabilitation. The counselors are usually glad for new contacts, especially for their employable adults.

7. Do not expect one public relations effort to take care of the practice.

8. If you want to hand out something, use brochures, not resumes. (Your mother is the only one who isn't bored with your resume.)

9. Contact executives in large corporations in your area. Offer to provide consultation, in-service, or screening. Offer to do a workshop about communication disorders and prevention. Ask to talk to the people who buy group insurance policies for employees.

10. Contact program directors of radio and television stations. Offer to do a 5-minute call-in program where you answer questions from listeners; make contact with the talk-show hosts.

11. Contact the feature editors of newspapers in the area, especially college and neighborhood papers. Offer to do guest columns for information or for questions from readers. Offer to do feature stories.

12. Contact associations in your area, such as the American Cancer Society or the American Heart Association, to see whether joining media publicity programs would be appropriate for your practice.

13. Contact special interest and parent advocacy groups, such as the Lost Chord, Association for Children with Learning Disabilities, or the Orton Society. Offer to give speeches about communication disorders and intervention. Offer to write short columns for the local and regional newsletters.

14. Get records from the Bureau of Census about population descriptions in your area.

15. Get information from the Chamber of Commerce about new developments, new subdivisions, companies who are relocating employees, location of the companies, and persons to contact within the companies. This information might provide a new area to market. You may be able to make contact with company executives about in-service, screening, company insurance for employees, and so forth.

16. Do comparative shopping for all media and vehicles, such as cost of brochures; cost of stationery; cost of newspaper announcements by size, by number of runs, by design; cost of yellow page advertisements by size, by design, by number of lines; and so forth.

17. Obtain listing in professional references, such as the Guide to Clinical Services published by the American Speech-Language–Hearing Association. Local, commercial professional directories seem to be a waste of money. Many professionals do not use

such directories because they are expensive and cumbersome. Check this out in your community. If you do put listings in local directories, be sure that your state license number is listed.

18. Contact all private schools and kindergartens. Ask for a brief appointment with head-master or mistress or director. Offer services in general, explain communication disorders and any services specifically applicable to their program.

19. Keep careful track of results from marketing efforts, as well as of the money spent on each activity that brought returns.

20. Do product analysis. List every service and write a two or three line description of that service with its application to a population. Use wording that would be suitable for a brochure.

21. Do not forget to contact friends, family, colleagues, social acquaintances, teachers, and former students. They may be your primary source of referrals.

21. Do your best work with current clients; keep in close contact with them. Call former clients periodically to ask about status and follow-up.

Remember:
- Never guarantee.
- Never mislead the public.
- Never steal clients from colleagues.

Chapter **7**

Computer Use or Computer Useless

A clinician does not need to know how a computer works to know how to use it. Professionals do need to know how to make informed decisions about various applications of the computer to the practice. They need to ask questions and get information about hardware and software. They need to be able to evaluate that information for its relevance to office needs, and finally match office needs with computer help.

Before budgeting or borrowing for a computer shopping spree, the practitioner must answer the most vital question, "Why get a computer?" Just raising the question is likely to make many of us self-conscious about being over 35 years old. Almost everybody under 35 *is* computer-friendly . . . or even computer-intimate. However, if you are barely able to set your clock radio, you may have some realistic trepidation about spending a lot of money and time on a gadget you don't understand and whose language you don't speak.

WHY GET A COMPUTER?

Computers, or microcomputers, are most applicable to tedious, repetitive tasks, particularly those that must be done with accuracy, such as client billing and financial records, client clinical records, and form letters. Computers provide rapid storage and retrieval of numerical data, narrative descriptions, and even graphic representations, such as test data and audiograms. In addition to business accounts and client files, computers have clinical applications for evaluation and treatment.

The primary uses of computers in professional practice include the following:

1. Storing and Retrieving Records
   a. clinical records
   b. administrative records

2. Word Processing
3. Clinical Applications
   a. assessment
   b. intervention
   c. data analysis
4. Research

Storing and Retrieving Records

In Chapter 4, this book (The Office: Part I) the topic of record keeping is discussed and will not be reiterated here. Record-keeping is an area in which computers excel (unless the power goes off). The long and tedious job of recording, storing, and searching for information can be passed on to the computer in some of the following ways:

1. Clinical Records
   a. Name
   b. Family name (cross-referenced when different from client's name)
   c. Address (home and work)
   d. Telephone (home and work)
   e. Place of business (spouse, mother, father)
   f. Insurance information
   g. Diagnostic category and code
   h. Times for follow-up evaluation, callbacks, or rescheduling
   i. Treatment category or code (screening, evaluation, parent conference, teacher contact)
   j. Number of sessions in given time period
   k. Number of cancellations and no-shows in given time period
   l. Additional client-referrals made to office from client
   m. Names of professionals seeing client
   n. Test/retest results
   o. Test profiles, audiograms
   p. Summary copies of reports written, sent, received on client
   q. Summary information of various groups of clients (unilateral hearing losses, language-impaired over 15 years, and so forth)
   r. Communicative, educational, and physical status of client

2. Administrative Records
   Records may be kept of quantitative data for billing, for monitoring payments, and for accounts receivable. Software programs are available to adapt and set up specialized client files. Numerous software packages are available to handle the financial operations for running a clinic. Some schools employ computer programs to file pupil records, to display identification information, and to maintain test and grade data. Quantitative data that can be handled by a computer include the following:
   a. Identifying information for each client (name and so forth)
   b. Insurance information for each client (company, rates, pay record)
   c. Billing information for each client (fee schedule, dates seen)

d. Balance due for each client
e. Last payment by each client
f. Person or agency responsible for payment
g. Person or agency to be billed
h. Client directory (address, telephone)
i. Accounts receivable
j. Chart of accounts
k. Routine financial obligations (rent, salaries) in given time period
l. Specifically incurred debts and payment schedules (consultant fees, computer payments)
m. Current cash balance
n. Summaries of financial records for given time periods (revenue, expenses, payroll, consumables, debts)
o. Staff contracts and bonus contingencies
p. Staff absences or cancellations
q. Cost and revenue information for each professional staff member (income from fees-for-services, other income earned for office, salaries, and fringe benefits)
r. Lease agreements
s. Core form for routine letters to clients or referral sources
t. Core evaluation narratives for report writing

Word Processing

Word processing is a fancy name for electronic typing that can be composed, proofread, corrected, restructured, or otherwise modified before it is printed onto paper. The possibilities for its use in clinical practice include the following:

1. Form letters and reports with necessary data insertions for each client
2. Insurance letters
3. Insurance forms (insurance form reporting can be done on a word-processor using a format that accommodates different types of insurance forms)
4. Patient billing (statements or client billing forms are available in software packages for printing bills; some word processors and software programs can be accommodated to use office logo or letterhead)

Some professionals (Pressman, 1984) are of the opinion that any office that produces more than 10 letters or reports a week would benefit from the addition of anything from a word processor to the entire computer package. This rule should include offices that *should* produce that many letters or reports, but do not because of limited staff time or energy. When the balance between patient care and administrative care is stressed, it is time to change methods of operating.

Clinical Applications

Applications of computers to delivery of services has been the target of recent attention and some controversy. Clearly, the computer cannot replace the clinician. However, in certain situations computers can be adapted for assessment and intervention activities where clinical judgment is unnecessary. Clinical applications include the following:

1. Assessment (computerized ENG, software package for screening and assessment)
2. Intervention (interactive teaching, drill programs, facilitation of communication for severely/profoundly impaired)
3. Analysis of speech/language production (phonemic features and patterns, grammatical skills)

The use of computers in assessment includes storage and retrieval of case history information, test scores, and audiological data. Some programs automatically compare individual performance on given tests to normative data or provide test-retest analyses; others analyze performance in relation to variables such as other test scores, age, grade level, and so forth. Some software programs allow the clinician to enter raw scores from specific tests or subtests and derive scale scores or percentile ratings.

Adaptive testing for the communicatively impaired provides useful procedures (such as item selection for client ability) for assessment with hearing impaired, with attention deficits, and with clients who may be easily frustrated. Programs exist that will score and interpret results on test instruments. It is possible to use certain fully automated testing programs in which the client sits at the computer terminal (screen) and responds to test items as they are printed on the screen. Obviously certain instruments for assessing neurophysiological, psycholinguistic, psychodynamic, and intellectual functioning do not lend themselves to automation.

Two types of assessment currently exist on the commercial market:

1. Microcomputer-Administered Assessment: programs which present stimulus items, accept client responses, and, when assessment is completed, store results. Programs can be further extended to provide the clinician with reports of results.
2. Analysis Program: programs that are used by the clinician after a personally administered evaluation. The clinician enters results from the test, and the computer provides a detailed analysis of that information (Rushakoff, 1984, pp. 147–148).

Some clinicians find it possible to produce evaluation reports using computer programs. Computer scoring and interpretation have been available for a number of years for the Minnesota Multiphasic Personality Inventory (MMPI), a psychological instrument used to diagnose emotional dysfunction. More recently, software has been developed to score and interpret a wide variety of instruments such as standardized measures of intelligence, certain measures of personality assessment, including projective techniques, and certain social adjustment rating scales. Straightforward paper and pencil tests lend themselves most readily to computer scoring and interpretation. Some clinicians now write their reports directly from the interpretive statements produced by computer analysis of the data. Some school districts, as well, are using computer-generated statements to produce Individual Education Plans (IEPs) for their students. The substituting of computer-analyzed data for hands-on clinician analysis raises certain issues where complex data are involved. Can the computer be programmed to apply the clinical insight that an experienced clinician brings to the task of analysis and assessment?

In addition to administering, scoring, and profiling certain diagnostic tests, computers can be adapted to perform and assess certain types of intervention activities, providing efficiency with no loss of accuracy. When applied properly to time-consuming activities, the computer can allow more time for quality interaction between client and clinician.

The use of computers in speech-language intervention has demonstrated a dramatic application of computers that have the capability of producing speech. The computer offers a unique tool for the speech impaired with a variety of modalities, including electronic speech, graphics, and print. Some intervention programs describe specific ways to intervene with a client, to use play, and to involve peers and family members. Clients who have serious difficulty using speech communicatively can achieve expansion of interactive abilities through adaptations of computer and software programs.

In addition to the basic computer components, some intervention may necessitate peripheral devices. One such device is a speech recognition unit that allows the computer to receive sound and convert it to visual displays or printouts (Rushakoff, 1984), or even to convert the input to computer-speech output.

Computer-assisted intervention may provide tutorial drill, stimulation, problem solving, and other combinations of text and content for normal or impaired learners (Pressman, 1984, pp. 8 and 9). Programs can be adapted to the specific needs of each individual, providing each with self-paced activities, immediate feedback, and varying presentations of text, graphics, or speech. They are designed to accept the client's response, evaluate it, and provide cues for improving partially correct responses.

Research

Research in clinical environments is more feasible through the use of the computer to collect and store data, compare populations, and predict future performance. Previously, tedious storage and analysis of data have been so time consuming that most clinicians have not attempted research. The longitudinal study of speech-language-hearing impaired during the course of intervention has long been neglected, as have other aspects of clinical research. With the availability of the computer, clinical activities need no longer be limited to whatever one can do with paper, pencil, and the free time provided by a client who fails to keep a therapy appointment.

Summary

If office operations yield the need for extensive records, data charting, record books, and endless accounting of clinical and administrative information, consider borrowing or budgeting for a computer. If the computer and its software are selected properly to fit the needs of the practitioner, if the practitioner and the staff take the time to become properly trained to use the computer and, if the limitations of the computer are understood, then begin learning how to speak ''Computese.''

Jargon and Jabberwocky

Computer jargon, or technical terminology, can be the greatest obstacle to learning about computer use and can increase the fright factor by several degrees. Current manuals and salesmen are much improved over earlier versions, although neither are much help until some hands-on experience with the computer is obtained by the potential user. In conversations about computers the following terms are likely to occur:

hardware: All the equipment, including wires, cables, and plugs connecting the components of the computer (Lasky, 1984, pp. 2–3). Hardware needs, or the main components, for a basic clinical system should consist of the following (Rushakoff, 1984):
1. Microcomputer with 256K RAM (memory)
2. Dual Disc Drives: There are many programs which require two disc drives. Some programs operate with the program disc in one drive and the data selection disc in a second drive.
3. The Monitor: A color monitor is used to enhance program effectiveness because it is more interesting to watch than black and white. Color monitors are not as useful for software that utilizes only written text.
4. The Printer: Data can be viewed on the monitor and then printed out as required or desired.

communication hardware: Devices that allow the computer to communicate with other computers. For example, the modem is communication hardware. The word itself is an acronym for a modulation or demodulation unit that permits computers to communicate over telephone lines.

software: The instructions necessary to govern activities of the computer. Software, or programs, can be bought commercially or may be composed by a consultant (i.e., a computer programmer) or by the practitioner for specialized purposes. Technological advances influence the type of software used for programming (floppy discs, hard discs, cartridges, and so forth).

program or programming: The design and technical writing of instructions to the computer for carrying out its tasks. It is *not* necessary to know how to program instructions before one uses a computer. Package software programs are available for administrative tasks, such as record keeping, and clinical tasks, such as assessment or intervention programs. The professional market has been deluged with packaged software programs designed for clinical application (see Appendix 7).

compatibility: Assures that software designed for one brand of computer can be used on another. Different brands of computers use different jargon, or language, or dialect. A program written in one computer language for a particular computer system may not be understood by another system.

word processor: A term for the cycle of writing and dictating, typing and correcting, retyping and printing. Word processing provides text correction and modification with a final product rapidly produced on paper.

Other bits of information pertaining to computer use and computer systems are referenced in the Annotated Bibliography.

Shopping

If you have determined that you want a computer for your practice, and if you know a few words from having visited a computer store, then you must decide which computer and what software you need. In addition to talking with computer representatives and salesmen, talk with your colleagues who engage in professional practice of the same type as yours—teaching, group practice, solo practice, corporate practice with employees, and so forth. Find out their mistakes and learn from them.

You may decide to buy your computer system through what is called a *turn-key operation*. A turn-key operation is one in which a consultant (usually a company representative) determines your computer needs, provides the equipment, software, training, support, and maintenance for the equipment.

The alternate method of selection is good old American do-it-yourself. This approach usually involves less initial cost than the turn-key operation, and may cost in the vicinity of $5,000. As most do-it-yourself buffs know, however, the lower initial outlay may not be the savings it appears to be when time, frustration, and the undoing of mistakes are considered.

Turn-key operations are not trouble-free. Some companies offering their services may not be legitimate, although competition and user sophistication are reducing the number of fly-by-night computer companies. Software and programming problems may occur in any operation, even the guaranteed turn-key system. The professional sometimes has to add a computer consultant to the list of consultant specialists required for efficient operation of the office.

Costs of computer systems have declined sharply in the past few years. Automated systems are available at all levels and in all price ranges. Computers no longer have to be considered the major investment they once were, but neither are they cheap. A small office should be able to acquire a system to meet its needs for about $5,000; some operations may need services ranging in cost up to $15,000. The addition of a word processor usually adds $2,500 to the cost of the system.

Except in the hands of novices, there are minimal hazards for loss of records or problems in locating records. However, Rushakoff (1984) points out that it is possible to lose computer records. He advises clinicians not to replace standard paper records even when computers are used for primary client record storage.

Novices in computer use often are concerned that it will be necessary for them to learn one or more of the computer languages to prepare programs for the computer. This depends on the needs and interest of the user. Although entering information into computerized systems may require more training than is desirable for all staff members, most of the staff can learn to access whatever information they need.

Start-up and Training

With the purchase of a computer, it is necessary to allocate office time for training, practice, and routine use. Learning to use the computer's operating system and the chosen software may be accomplished through self-study, consultant help, formal instruction, or a combination of these methods. Pressman (1984) indicates that word processing takes about 10 hours of formal instruction. Training time varies for learning programs for handling financial records, and storage and retrieval processes. Pressman (1984) also indicates that training usually takes three times as long for self-instruction as it does for formal instruction. After one has learned the procedures, it may take three times as many hours to master the various techniques and commands. A novice should allow at least a month to learn any computer system. Program modification or design need not be attempted by the practitioner and is not necessary for his/her use of the computer.

Almost any office will find that the first 30 to 90 days after a computer is purchased the workload and time required for office management is increased rather than decreased (Pressman, 1984). Data must be entered into both the old system (paper records) and the new system (accounting software on the computer). Many software programs are not designed to replace commonly used ledger sheets, and use of both systems can go on indefinitely. Even the time-saving word processor can increase work-load because of the temptation to produce more correspondence or reports with the time-saving process.

Regardless of the preparation for the introduction of the computerized system, the change is time-consuming and costly. Only after the computer and its users can produce rapid and accurate client billing, information retrieval, and insurance form completion, does the computer finally show its strength. The practitioner should anticipate that the changeover to a computerized system will initially be stressful to the staff and disruptive to the office operation (Pressman, 1984).

To avoid disappointment, one should be realistic about the computer's capabilities and expect no more from it than it is programmed to do. An orderly plan for entering various types of information into the computer should be followed, as well as an orderly sequence for buying software and changing paper records to computer records.

If a practice cannot yet justify purchasing a computer, but the work load is almost to that point, some alternatives are available.

One Alternative

Some companies provide out-of-office computer services based on information from paper records kept by the office staff. For example, payment is taken and recorded in a one-write system (such as Safeguard Business System). This system allows for a single entry to record on the daily income ledger, patient payment card, and client receipt. This system is also called a pegboard system because of the way the ledger sheet and payment cards fit into pegs or posts. At the end of the day, week, or month, the bookkeeper can balance the receipts and expenses by hand and determine current cash balance. If it is desired, the bookkeeper can mail daily receipts to the Safeguard office. These receipts are returned several days later with a packet that includes a weekly financial management report, which may contain completed patient billing statements, or monthly financial status reports. The packet can include a missed-payment report for each patient, cash flow report, gross cost analysis by specified category, and an accounts receivable ledger. In some instances, insurance reports can be included in this packet. Quarterly and annual financial summaries can also be obtained from out-of-office computer services.

By using out-of-office computer services, it is possible to minimize expenses, the training period for the office staff is fairly routine, and little time is required to transfer data from paper to computer output. Trouble shooting is done by the computer company. Out-of-office computer services also have disadvantages, however. Custom programming is unattainable, turn-around time from original data to corrected computer output can be as long as 10 days—and whatever software the company has in stock is what must be used. Usually word processing is not available with out-of-office computer services, and insurance statements are not automatically printed by computer directly onto the payment form, requiring that they be done by hand.

Other Applications of Computers in the Practice

In addition to storing and retrieving one's own data, it is possible to tap into other data bases—particularly medically oriented data bases—for information regarding statistics and development in health and allied health fields. Interactive services are currently developing that provide assistance to medical practitioners by allowing communication with certain specialty centers for confirming diagnoses. At the time of this writing, very few data bases and interactive systems are available in speech-language pathology and audiology. However, many institutions are designing computer-accessed programs for continuing education experiences. It seems likely that traditional lectures with pre- and post-tests will be accessible with certain computer systems and, certainly, independent study can be designed at many levels through computer use.

There is no shame in not owning a computer, even if you are under 35. However, you should know whether you need one or not, and implement what you know.

Appendices

APPENDIX 7–1
COMPUTER SOFTWARE SOURCES AND INSTRUCTIONS

Various publishing companies participate exclusively in computer software development for education and special education needs. Traditional publishing companies now have divisions devoted to software and its marketing. Some materials available include various programs for linguistic analysis, assessment of grammatical skills, vocabulary inventories (in several languages), articulation screening and analysis, and interactive teaching designed to provide for progression through language-skill stages. Because of rapidly changing software, and the highly competitive commercial market, no specific examples are listed. Almost every mailout from publishing companies contains a section of currently available software for speech, language, and hearing.

The American Speech-Language-Hearing Association and the American Speech-Language-Hearing Foundation, as well as various other professional associations, offer computer conferences that usually feature two forums: commercially available programs and noncommercial materials of speech-language-hearing professionals. Frequently such conferences provide software directories to participants. Sample conferences include formal teaching sessions in the following areas:

1. Futuristic and high technology (artificial intelligence, robotics, multi-dimension operating systems), the integration of microcomputers into college level curriculum for speech-language pathologists and audiologists, and special education
2. Hardware labs (hands-on opportunities for using various computers) and software labs (hands-on opportunities for exploring software as well as information about new and unpublished software)
3. Workshops by professionals who have adapted, converted, or initiated various computer devices in their own practices or teaching situations

Some seminars assume no previous personal computer experiences. The emphasis is on introduction to vocabulary, hardware, and software. Other seminars range from learning how to operate and care for the computer keyboard, display, and disc drive to advanced programming for esoteric needs.

Chapter **8**

Insurance: For the Practice
For the Client

The practitioner finds that two different kinds of insurance concerns must be addressed. One form of insurance protects the owner/practitioner, the office space, and the employees. The other provides reimbursement for services to the client. Insurance for the practice and the practitioner is the responsibility of the owner/practitioner; insurance coverage for professional services provided to the client is the responsibility of the client. The practitioner may provide assistance to the client in this area by forwarding reports, diagnostic statements, and other information to the insurer at the client's request.

INSURANCE PROTECTION FOR THE PRACTITIONER

The owner/practitioner should consult an insurance agent or broker periodically in order that comprehensive insurance plans can be designed and updated to meet the varying and specific needs of the practice. Insurance protection that is usually considered necessary and desirable includes the following:

1. *Liability insurance* protects the firm from financial loss due to any claims of bodily injury or property damage in connection with business operations. This should not be confused with malpractice or professional liability insurance.
2. *Crime and vandalism insurance* reimburses for losses due to robbery, burglary, employee dishonesty, or vandalism.
3. *Fire insurance* covers damage to the premises, equipment, and inventory that is caused by fire, explosion, wind, riot, or smoke.
4. *Automobile insurance* encompasses both physical damage and liability insurance for company-owned vehicles or vehicles used for business purposes.

5. *Worker's compensation insurance*, mandatory in some states, covers injuries and loss related to employee accidents on the job.
6. *Business-interruption insurance*, sometimes called income protection, compensates the business for revenue loss during a temporary halt of business caused by fire, theft, or illness.
7. *Disability income insurance* compensates the individual during an extended period of illness or disability.
8. *Employee health and life insurance* (major medical insurance) provides workers and dependents with financial benefits in case of illness or death. In states that are unionized, employers are usually required to set aside benefit funds for workers who belong to labor unions.
9. *Key person insurance* compensates a business when a partner or person essential to management becomes disabled or dies. This type of insurance is frequently acquired by partners or corporation directors.
10. *Product liability insurance* protects the business from claims against defective merchandise.
11. *Fidelity bonds* are purchased for employees with access to cash receipts and other company funds, in order to provide protection against loss from embezzlement.
12. *Professional liability or malpractice insurance* is designed to provide coverage for legal defense in litigation and for any resulting damages awarded to clients for professional misconduct. (See Chapter 12.)

No one likes to pay insurance premiums. Insurance is an investment designed to minimize a loss; regardless of the compensation, it is never as good as not needing it. Insurance payments, and the principle behind them, seem to be contrary to most other uses of cash for investments or acquisition of possessions. However, for personal and professional protection, it is absolutely mandatory that one maintain various forms of insurance coverage. Because a professional practice is so closely aligned with the owner's personal estate, it is also important for the practitioner to acquire various types of personal insurance. At a minimum, this should include life insurance, equal to at least all of the indebtedness of the practice, and homeowners' coverage for the structure and content of one's home.

Premium deadlines and dates for coverage expiration should be closely monitored so that one does not allow important coverage to lapse. It is preferable that all insurance premium payments not fall due at the same time. One should also take time, prior to renewal, to review all existing policies and to consider modification of policies and companies.

It is possible to get caught in a time lag during which one insurance policy has lapsed and another policy has not yet become effective. Such a period is not only frightening, it is potentially dangerous and expensive.

Usually it is necessary to use more than one company. However, some insurance brokers represent multicompany organizations. These brokers are in the position of offering the most extensive coverage. Remember when dealing with insurance brokers that, like stock brokers, their advice can be expensive. Most insurance needs for the practitioner can be categorized according to the *office* (structure, contents, and possessions), and the *personnel* (owner and employees).

Office

Structure, contents, and possessions of the office are usually insured for the cost of replacement. Most businesses depreciate office furniture and equipment. Sometimes insurance coverage is based on the depreciation schedule; however, if damage or loss of furniture or equipment occurs toward the end of the depreciation schedule, insurance payments for such losses may be inadequate. Policies should always be carefully read before purchase. This is especially true in the case of liability coverage. In many parts of the country ''rising waters'' are specifically excluded from liability coverage. That is, following a hurricane, heavy rains, or prolonged rains, water back-up or drain-off resulting in damage to the office would not be covered by insurance.

Keeping accurate inventories of property covered by insurance is crucial if it becomes necessary to file a claim. To keep complete and current records for both home and office, existing property should be described by content, dates of purchase, cost, serial numbers, and any other important information relating to equipment, appliances, and furniture. New property should be added to the records as it is acquired, and records should be updated to reflect changes in the status of previously recorded property. Pictures of property, especially furniture, art work, and jewelry, are helpful in substantiating claims and in locating property that has been stolen. Some items require a special rider and appraisal to be insured. Records should be stored in a safe place, with duplicate records filed in a separate location.

Hazard insurance, such as fire insurance, should be reviewed annually, regardless of whether the office is owned or rented. Sometimes inflation drastically reduces the value of fire coverage, and improvements made to property frequently have not been updated in the fire insurance policy.

If it becomes necessary to file an insurance claim, do not rush into settlement. Be sure that actual cost of replacement and all expenses of repair are included in the final settlement. In the event of a large loss (over $5,000) it may be beneficial to enlist the assistance of a public adjustor who is a claims specialist. This specialist can assist one in determining the extent of the loss and in negotiating the largest possible settlement from insurance companies. These specialists are usually accredited by the National Association of Public Insurance Adjustors.

Things to remember after the damage and before the settlement are the following:*

1. Do not just call the insurance company, but also provide written notification of the damage, its assumed cause, and any special problems encountered.
2. Be sure that you observe the time limit for submitting proof of loss after the damaging event. Many policies have 40-, 60-, or 90-day limits for submitting such evidence.
3. An office damaged by fire or other cause may attract vandals. Be sure that even partially damaged property is protected by locks or security guards.
4. Before considering rebuilding after a total loss, consider changing sites. Sometimes insurance companies charge increased premiums for insuring a same-site

---

*From *Guide to Private Practice* by Ridgewood Financial Institute, 1984, Ho-Ho-Kus, NJ: Author. Copyright 1984. Adapted by permission.

property that may potentially have the same problems leading to the first damage. Rebuilding is costly and time consuming. If a total-loss fire has occurred, it may be better to find a new office ready for immediate occupancy. Then settle with the insurance company at the old site.

5. In case of partial loss, determine exactly what the limits are on any future coverage if the property is repaired.

6. Use your own specialist to repair smoke, water, and other damage, and not a contractor recommended by the insurance company. They may cut corners because they are working for the insurance company, not for you.

In initial negotiations for fire and hazard insurance, be sure that protection includes coverage for income loss that may result from the damaging event. Should the fire and hazard insurance not cover income loss, an income protection policy is necessary.

Insurance designed to cover office and home equipment and contents should include coverage of valuable papers and documents. Client files and financial records can be reproduced. However, original manuscript drafts and other valuable papers cannot always be duplicated. An insurance policy can help recover at least some of the dollar value assigned to these papers.

Automobile Insurance

Whether the practice owns the vehicle or the office staff uses their own vehicles to run errands, the practitioner is responsible for insurance coverage for those vehicles. Various types of automobile coverage include the following:

1. *Liability coverage* is designed to protect you if someone is hurt in an accident. It covers situations where you (or your policy) pay for damages done to someone else's property or person which resulted from your negligence or misjudgement.

2. *Collision coverage* refers to situations in which you hit a fixed or inanimate object, and your policy pays. This coverage may be the most expensive part of a policy; the amount that may be recovered in case of an accident is usually restricted to the current book value of the car. If the car is over 3-years-old, one may consider dropping collision coverage altogether.

3. *Comprehensive coverage* provides protection in case of major losses, such as those from fire and theft. A higher deductible can reduce premiums substantially. For example, the difference in premium can be more than $100 if the deductible is $500 rather than $100.

4. *Uninsured motorists coverage* protects the policy holder in case he/she is involved in an accident with an uninsured driver. The policy holder's company is responsible for the claim.

5. *No-fault coverage* refers to the situation in which your insurance company pays for an accident after it is determined that the accident was not your fault. For example, you hit a telephone pole that was left lying in the middle of the road due to telephone company negligence. This type of coverage may also cover claims resulting from accidents involving uninsured motorists.

Some insurance companies have started providing discounts on auto policies. Be sure to check whether you are entitled to any such discounts. Umbrella policies may cover all automobiles owned or used by a business, but only up to a fixed rate in liability claims, and they only apply after regular liability coverage is exhausted.

Liability

Liability insurance is protection against accidental injury to anyone entering your premises or operating within the physical boundary of your office structure. Be certain that the liability insurance policy covers the parking lot, elevators, bathrooms, and all common areas of the property, as well as your specific inner office complex.

Life Insurance

Considerations of the private practitioner with regard to life insurance are similar to the considerations of any professional.

Term insurance allows the maximum amount of insurance protection for premium dollars, but it never accumulates cash value that can be borrowed against or redeemed. Cost of the policy is usually determined by age; the premium is usually increased with every renewal. Whole life insurance is designed with a premium that is set when it is bought and that stays the same year after year. Whole life premiums are at least twice the cost of term insurance premiums. Sometimes it is possible to choose convertible term insurance, which allows one to switch to whole life insurance at a future date, usually before 60 years of age. At that point, premiums are calculated at the rate applicable to a comparable age group.

Group insurance is almost always less expensive than an individual policy. In some instances it would pay the practitioner in solo practice to incorporate, or join with others as a consultant in a group practice or business enterprise, in order to qualify for a group insurance policy. Most corporations buy insurance through the corporation with pretax dollars.

Consider dropping insurance when it no longer serves you. For example, if you have two whole life policies with about the same value, cash in the newer one. Since you were older when you bought it, the premium is higher. However, the newer policy may have a waiver of premium clause if you become disabled; whereas, the older policy may not. If the mortgage is paid off or a child has just graduated from college, certain types of insurance can be dropped. If one owns both whole life and term insurance, the term insurance should be dropped first because rates increase as one gets older. Deciding between two policies bought by an individual at about the same age may depend on whether the insurance company is a mutual or a stock company. The mutual company's premium may be higher, but increasing dividends can make new cost lower over the years. It may not pay to drop a mutual policy that is over 10 years old. The stock company policy usually should be held up to 10 years, then dropped if one has other types of policies.

Disability Income Insurance

When one becomes injured or ill and no income is forthcoming, bills and other financial obligations do not abate. Disability insurance usually provides a choice of various plans for income supplementation. Most plans base payment on average income of the insured. The best ones continue payment as long as the disability exists.

Income protection, which pays income loss due to hazards such as fire or vandalism, may or may not be included in disability insurance policies. If not included, this is important insurance for any professional to consider. Many practitioners have found that in the course of a long career, one or two fires or an occasional flood can cause serious interruptions to a practice. Even smoke or gas fumes resulting from fire in other offices in the same building can force the cancellation of many clients with respiratory problems.

Buy–Sell Agreement

In certain situations insurance coverage can be used for this purpose. For example, buy-out in the event of permanent disability can be covered by a buy–sell agreement and funded by disability buy-out insurance. Buy-out in the event of premature death can be covered by a buy–sell agreement and funded by a life insurance policy on any partners involved.

Worker's Compensation

Liability insurance covering those persons who enter the premises and are injured does not cover employees working on the premises.

Some personnel protection should be automatic with the employment of the first employee. Hiring one secretary may place the employer within the minimum premium category for worker's compensation. Regardless of cost, this type of insurance cannot be ignored. Insurance for professional personnel is considered a direct expense of office operations, and often it can be used as a fringe benefit for the professional employee.

Worker's compensation usually provides benefits in at least three categories:

1. Reimbursement for income lost during recovery from job-related physical impairment, or the form of lump-sum payment for irreversible physical impairment
2. Medical benefits to cover diagnostic and treatment of impairments
3. Rehabilitation to ameliorate the effects of irreversible impairments

The profession of speech-language pathology/audiology is most concerned with those worker compensation programs related to occupationally induced hearing loss, although occasionally speech-language disorders are related to job-incurred injuries. Some variables affecting workmen's compensation coverage for nonphysician providers include:

1. Setting in which service is provided:
   a. hospital:
      in-patient unit
      out-patient department
   b. private practice:
      provider's office
      clinic
2. Provider of services:
   a. licensed professional
   b. certified professional
3. Kind of services provided:
   a. diagnosis
   b. treatment (type)
4. Need for services:
   a. injury
   b. illness
   c. acquired
   d. developmental
   e. organic
   f. nonorganic
5. Role of provider to beneficiary:
   a. treatment
   b. supervision
   c. referral

Health Insurance

Health insurance for owners and employees can be categorized by at least five types of functional insurance: (1) hospital, (2) surgical, (3) major medical, (4) disability, and (5) dental.

Different organizational insurance patterns include: (1) individual plans, (2) group plans, and (3) health maintenance organizations (HMOs).

The latter plans, called HMOs, are characterized by prepayment for health care services from specified providers, rather than by reimbursement for fees. These usually cover medical care from groups of individual practitioners who agree to provide specified services to HMO subscribers at agreed-upon rates.

Coverage is usually defined in insurance policies according to the following categories:

1. Type of service rendered.
2. Method of payment:
   Health insurance carriers adhere to one or more of several methods for determining the amount to be paid for a particular service. These include the basis of usual and customary fees, fee schedules, or relative value scales.

3. Assignment of payment:
   Assignment is made directly to the client in most cases, who is billed for the services by the provider with the provider's own fee schedule. According to this arrangement, the client is responsible for payment of fees, but he/she is reimbursed by the insurance carrier for all or part of that payment beyond the deductible. In some situations, however, the insurance carrier pays the professional directly for service with adjustments for the deductible and assigned rate of payment. Some professionals accept whatever the carrier allows as full payment, except for the client's responsibilities and deductibles. In some instances, when insurance covers only a portion of the charges, clients tend to accuse professionals of charging exorbitant fees.
4. Co-payment: Co-payment is a plan in which a flat amount or percentage is specified for each unit of service. The insured is responsible for a certain portion of any charges.

All health insurance coverage should be updated periodically, particularly on major medical policies to reflect current costs of room rates and hospital schedules.

Professional Malpractice Insurance

The personal assets of each professional who practices with other professionals in a partnership are exposed to any liabilities resulting from the malpractice of any partner. Noninvolvement is irrelevant. In a professional corporation, each professional is personally liable only for his/her own acts or omissions, or the acts or omissions of others for which he/she had some supervisory responsibility or participated in in some way. All assets of the corporation are exposed to claims against any professional employed by the corporation, but the personal assets of all uninvolved professionals are secure from suit.

Discussion of the specific malpractice insurance policy should be undertaken with an insurance advisor. Most malpractice insurance agrees to pay damages arising from ''malpractice, error, or mistake.'' These terms obviously are subject to legal interpretation and simply indicate the type of legal responsibility covered by the insurance policy. Insurance coverage is more satisfactory when the company agrees to pay damages for the claims of suits arising out of services rendered or services which should have been rendered, because it broadens the coverage and provides greater protection for the insured. Many companies obviously are reluctant to write policies with this kind of terminology because exposure for the company is increased with the increased protection of the professional.

Malpractice insurance policies that agree to pay claims arising from a list of specific professional services require careful examination. Omissions from the list are as important as inclusions. It is virtually impossible to write a list of all claims that could arise from a practice. A practitioner's professional responsibility lies in areas additional to provision of direct services to clients. The practitioner is also exposed to claims for damages by reason of his/her activities as a member of professional committees, boards, or consultations. Coverage for professional liability needs to include claims arising from acts performed by employees, assistants, and associates. When a practitioner relies on the services of interns and paraprofessionals designated as ''subordinates,'' in legal terms, the professional who is responsible for the subordinate is liable for his/her actions and for risks or harm which these actions may engender. A liability policy may cover the employee, as well as the supervisor, but coverage must also be provided for the owner who is usually named along with the employee or supervisor in claims for wrongful acts.

Many professional associations provide access for their members to reputable companies offering professional malpractice insurance coverage. Usually this is group coverage that extends several options. It is fairly inexpensive for maximum coverage. The most desirable policy will pay claims arising from acts or omissions by employees for whom the insured may be legally responsible. The insurance company should also agree to defend the owner/practitioner against any claim or suit based on services rendered that should not have been rendered, and to defend against the claim when the suit is false, fraudulent, or groundless. The insurance policy should cover court appearances, when necessary, at a rate commensurate with the consultant rate charged by the practitioner.

Under some conditions, certain insurance premiums are tax deductible. State and federal regulations change frequently and should be reviewed by the practitioner periodically. Sometimes an accountant, when preparing a tax return, will check current regulations in order to deduct costs for premiums.

Limitations of Malpractice Insurance

1. Some insurance policies only cover the damage portion of a lawsuit and may exclude legal fees. Even if the professional is found to be perfectly innocent of allegations in the lawsuit, legal fees can be quite expensive. If there was any legal justification for the suit, the court may disallow payment of legal fees by the person who has brought suit against the professional and may order each party to pay his/her own legal fees.
2. Many professionals are poorly equipped to defend themselves against formal accusations of malpractice. Many professionals, particularly in a field as young as speech-language pathology/audiology, tend to be open and even confrontive toward the accuser. In some situations the therapist almost supports the opposition's statements or feelings, which can lead to a judgement against the therapist. Most attorneys advise any human services professional to enlist the aid of a qualified attorney whenever legal action is brought against the professional.

When seeking employment with any agency, institution, or hospital, the professional should obtain a written statement regarding the employer's responsibility for providing legal representation and malpractice insurance. Many professionals assume their employers automatically accept such responsibilities. They discover too late that such was not the case. Professionals in any work setting—not just in private practice—should be aware that employment by an institution, even a public institution, does not ensure protection from litigation.

INSURANCE PROTECTION FOR THE CLIENT

The term *third-party payment* refers to any plan in which payment of fees comes from someone other than the recipient of services, and it may include private insurance, private foundations or gifts, and public (nonprivate) third-party payers, such as governmental health care programs. Difficulties over third-party payment can outweigh many other problems in professional practices, and many practitioners allow these difficulties to affect their fees, their service delivery, and their time. Most practitioners are keenly interested in facilitating third-party payments for their clients, but they often find the related problems of delays and red tape a source of irritation and frustration. Decreases in federal support, tightened restrictions by third-party payers, and growing competition for money by the expanding number of health and allied health care providers make for a tough market.

Health care coverage is paramount in most insurance programs, but the relationship between speech, language, and hearing disorders and health or medical care is unclear. Insurance guidelines for claims approval differ from company to company, vary with state insurance codes, and are inconsistently applied from one branch of a company or agency to another branch of the same company or agency. Policies are often written in such a way that interpretations can change from one claim to the next. This problem of inconsistent interpretations is further complicated by claims reviewers' lack of sophistication about professional services. The latter is not helped by the fact that the profession of speech-language pathology/audiology has no clear taxonomy for labeling services and disorders and no universal licensure requirements. Without even completing the list of problems related to insurance payment and professional services, one may wonder how *any* speech-language pathology/audiology services qualify for third-party coverage without compromising professional autonomy by becoming subservient to physician domination.

A major trend in both private and public insurance programs is toward the provision of coverage for speech-language-hearing services without requiring prescription or supervision by a physician. This change has opened many possibilities for speech-language-hearing practitioners, but it has also increased the confusion among insurance companies. The opportunity for independent practice, as well as the need for clarification of services, emphasizes the profession's responsibility for self-regulation and monitoring.

Self-Regulation and Monitoring

Certainly the minimum requirements for speech-language pathologists/audiologists are state licensure and/or certification by the American Speech–Language–Hearing Association. Some state licensing laws for speech-language pathologists/audiologists also require the continuous updating of professional knowledge and skills with mandatory continuing education requirements. Those regulations that do not mandate continuing education emphasize the need for members to participate in such activities on a voluntary basis. The setting of minimum standards and regulations for continuing professional education are part of the profession's attempts to perform ongoing review of service delivery. Included in this effort is the review of patterns of care in speech-language pathology/audiology programs, documentation of appropriate patterns of service delivery, and identification of areas in which improvement is necessary. These attempts at review of standards for service delivery are referred to as peer review and involve audits of client records and client care. This approach to quality assessment of clinical services was given formal impetus in

1976 when Peer Standard Review Organizations (PSRO) were set in motion by federal regulation (PL 92-603). This regulation required that services provided by health care practitioners, other than physicians, were to be included under the aegis of PSROs. Several disciplines providing allied health care services, including speech-language pathology/audiology, are covered by this regulation.

The profession of speech-language pathology/audiology has acted slowly in defining standards of care for broad application to clinical programs of diagnosis and intervention. Some efforts have been made to regularize client records and client care procedures through committees of the American Speech-Language-Hearing Association and the attempts of some member states to provide model state-wide peer review programs. The Iowa Quality Assurance Program is one example of such a program. However, for the most part, models of client care have not been widely adopted by the profession. It is clear that some usable system of self-monitoring and self-regulation must be applied by the profession to help insure the quality of speech-language pathology and audiology services. The impact of self-assessment within the profession will bolster the profession's resistance to accepting prescriptions from physicians as sometimes demanded by insurance programs.

Prescriptions and Payments

The persistent requirement of some insurance companies that physicians prescribe and/or supervise professional activities of nonphysician professionals, has forced many nonphysician professionals to pit their ethics against their pocketbooks. In countless situations, speech-language pathologists and audiologists have succumbed to the mighty sword of physician signature on a prescription or supervision treatment form; when in reality the only relationship with the physician was referral and occasional communication regarding a mutual client. In other situations speech-language-hearing professionals have refused to play the signature game and have lost a client, third-party payment for services, or both. Unfortunately, this situation persists, presumably with support from some physicians. However, in several states, the insurance code regulations are being modified to include nonphysician professionals as free-standing recipients of insurance payments, including speech-language pathologists and audiologists in states where the profession is licensed. Once licensure has been granted to a nonphysician profession, the trend has been for that profession to gain additional professional recognition and income from third-party payers through formal agreements or legislative mandates.

Legislation and Court Ruling

Legislation that has been used to affect insurance coverage for nonphysician providers has taken three major forms, *mandatory coverage*, *freedom of choice*, and *required option*. Mandatory coverage statutes require insurers to provide coverage for certain services as mandated by law. The intent of the freedom of choice provision has been to neutralize the insurers' insistence that covered services be rendered only by physicians. This provision declares that when other health care professionals are licensed to perform a service, that service need not be performed by a physician. The required option legislation requires that insurance companies offer certain benefits to be accepted or rejected by the policy holder. For example, an insurance code could state that insurers must offer to major medical policy holders the option of coverage for speech, language, and hearing services as part of the major medical policy. The purchaser of the policy could elect to purchase the option or could reject that part of the coverage.

Several cases are now pending in various state and federal courts regarding attempts of nonphysician professionals to achieve third-party reimbursement. As the result of court decisions favoring nonphysician professionals, certain private insurance companies, health maintenance organizations (HMOs), some Blue Cross-Blue Shield Plans, and other insurance companies have been mandated to offer as benefits services that legally could be provided by nonphysician professionals. Government third-party payers, under such programs as the Federal Employees' Health Benefits Program (FEHBP), CHAMPUS, Medicare, Medicaid, and Workman's Compensation, have recognized and reimbursed a variety of nonphysician professionals. Although federal insurance programs vary by state, this trend toward nonphysician service reimbursement may have an influence on commercial insurance programs that have been fairly cautious in allowing nonphysician recognition and reimbursement.

Most nonphysician professionals are concerned about reimbursement practices and whether or not third-party reimbursement will continue to expand for the nonphysician provider. Some of these concerns discussed by Thompson (1982, pp. 10–12) include:

1. The conditions under which reimbursement is granted (physician supervision, progress reports);
2. The method of reimbursement (direct or indirect); and
3. The reimbursement schedule, or the way in which reimbursement amounts and limits are determined.

The increase in number and type of nonphysician providers seeking and obtaining third-party compensation is likely to result in an environment in which both physicians and nonphysician professionals will compete for control of compensation provisions, as well as control of the economic marketplace. A 1980 court case (Virginia Academy of Clinical Psychologists vs. Blue Shield of Virginia) illustrates the point. A 3-judge federal court considered the legality of Blue Shield's refusal to pay for services of a clinical psychologist except when services were billed through a physician. The critical issue for the court was whether the Blue Shield policy requiring psychologists to bill through physicians was in restraint of trade and a violation of the Sherman Act. The courts eventually ruled against the Blue Shield requirement that psychologists' fees be billed through a physician.

With increasing frequency, state legislation, court ruling, and federal regulation tend more toward recognizing the nonphysician professional as an independent economic entity. The increasing number of professionals in human services and the increased cost incurred by some insurance companies have led to some variations on the insurance theme.

Preferred Provider Organizations and Health Maintenance Organizations

Preferred Provider Organizations (PPOs) are a mechanism by which payers of health care services, such as insurance companies, can contract directly with a provider for services. The insurance company, being the payer, acts through the employer to direct clients and patients to specified providers. Theoretically, the purpose is to limit what health care providers can charge, thereby putting a ceiling on escalating health care costs. Various forms of PPOs can occur. For example, a comprehensive rehabilitation and diagnostic clinic can contract directly with the payer, becoming the only recognized provider of certain services. In some situations, an entrepreneur signs up health care providers for a fee, contacts the payer of insurance company, and serves as the administrative intermediary. Proponents of PPOs state that many large companies have been self-insuring, negotiating with health care providers for many years. In some states specific professionals, such as psychologists, have contractual agreements with particular insurance companies, such as Blue Shield. The same practice of contracting with specific providers has also been observed by Health Maintenance Organizations (HMOs).

Health Maintenance Organizations are insurance mechanisms by which participants pay a flat, up-front fee to the HMO, which then covers the cost of necessary care. In this way a participant's health care costs are predictable and stable, regardless of the use of services.

Some professionals feel that the expansion of the PPO and HMO systems, in which contractual arrangements are made with specific providers, will reduce the quality of health care services. However, some professionals are pursuing alliances with various health care groups and organizations. At the very least, a practitioner in private practice should remain informed of changes in insurance arrangements and systems as they become available to the consumer.

Insurance Coverage by Private Health Insurance Organizations

In general, most basic policies will reimburse hospitals for speech-language pathology/audiology services provided on an in-patient basis. Services are likely to be reimbursed on an out-patient basis only under major medical policies. The policies vary from company to company and from one state insurance code to another. Many companies require evidence that the speech-language–hearing disorder is related to medical cause, or that the intervention is performed with a physician's approval, supervision, or prescription.

Blue Cross and Blue Shield plans tend to be less flexible in their reimbursement policies, and many do not reimburse speech-language pathologists directly. Blue Cross and Blue Shield central organization coordinates the Blue Cross and Blue Shield plans within the various states, each of which is a separate, nonprofit organization. Most plans in the Blue Cross and Blue Shield organizations tend to be limited to medical or surgical care and require a prescription from the physician which indicates that the disorder results from some disease or physical ailment.

Other Insurance Programs

Various federal and state insurance programs exist for certain populations such as CHAMPUS and CHAP, the Federal Employees' Insurance Programs, Vocational Rehabilitation, Crippled Children's Division, Social and Health Services Administration, and Public Health Services. These programs usually are administered within a division of the state bureaucracy or through a private insurance company. Vocational Rehabilitation Services is a state-administered program that provides or reimburses for the provision of services designed to prepare the adult handicapped for gainful employment. Crippled Children's Services is a federal health program administered at the state level. CHAMPUS is the Civilian Health and Medical Program for Uniform Services. It is a medical benefit provided by the federal government to help pay for civilian medical care that is rendered to spouses and children of active duty uniform personnel, retired uniform services personnel and their spouses and children, and children of deceased active duty and retired personnel. The Federal Social and Health Services Administration (FSHSA) is designed to provide services to the elderly, through state and county Area Agencies on Aging. Several states include audiological and hearing aid services for low-income elderly through their Health Services Agencies (HSA) or Public Health Services programs. Usually the services are contracted and require formal bids for acceptance. Most programs in state public health service agencies also include programs for the indigent.

Medicare and Medicaid

Medicare is a provision of the Federal Social Security Act that offers hospital and medical insurance protection for people aged 65 and older and for certain groups of people under age 65. Medicare consists of two parts. Part A is hospital insurance and covers in-patient hospital care, in-patient care in a skilled nursing facility, and home health care. Part B is medical insurance and covers physician's services and certain out-patient services, including rehabilitation services, laboratory tests, some appliances, and medical supplies. Part B, for which participation is voluntary, requires subscribers to pay monthly premiums. To receive reimbursement under either Part A or Part B, services must be delivered by a qualified provider, and with few exceptions, it must be provided in a facility that is certified to provide Medicare services.

Fiscal intermediaries usually provide the administrative functions for Medicare, processing claims and disbursing payments. Audiology services are sometimes covered in various Medicare programs, although they are not specifically provided for by law. Hearing aid selection and fitting, and all associated services, are specifically excluded from Medicare. Speech-language pathology services may be reimbursed if provided by a (licensed or certified) speech-language pathologist, if the services are performed under *initial physician's referral*.

Medicaid is a federal medical assistance program for low-income and otherwise needy individuals or families who are eligible to receive monthly cash payments under various welfare programs, including Aid to Families of Dependent Children (AFDC) and Supplementary Security Income (SSI). Medicaid benefits may also extend to people who have enough money to cover basic living expenses but not to cover medical care. These benefits may apply to people with moderate income who encounter catastrophic health care problems that are not covered by health insurance.

Mandatory services under Medicare include (1) physician's services, (2) skilled nursing facilities (with provisions for some home health services for adults), (3) out-patient hospital services, and (4) laboratory and x-ray services.

Included within several of the mandatory categories are speech-language pathology services, incorporating ''early and periodic screening, diagnosis, and treatment.'' Although speech-language–hearing screening may be included within mandated services, speech-language pathologists/audiologists are not necessarily reimbursed separately for the service.

Medicare Coverage of Speech-Language Pathology/Audiology

Audiology services, although not specifically mentioned within the Medicare statute, are reimbursable under certain conditions. For example, both diagnostic and rehabilitative audiological services may be covered in part A of Medicare Benefits for hospital in-patients when they are provided by an audiologist and when the services are requested by a physician. Part B benefits reimburse diagnostic audiology services for an audiologist in private practice who has obtained a Medicare provider number. With both speech-language pathology and audiology out-patient services, the plan for furnishing such treatment may be written by either the speech-language pathologist/audiologist or by the physician. It is no longer necessary for a physician to ''prescribe and supervise'' speech-language pathology and audiology services for Medicare reimbursement, although the physician still possesses authority for specifying that such speech-language/audiological services are necessary for the patient within the context of the overall health profile. In this respect, speech-language pathologists/audiologists are responsible for functioning as completely independent professionals in the development and education of their intervention plans (ASHA, 1981).

Medicare regulations require that speech pathology services be provided by qualified speech-language pathologists within a rehabilitative program that is approved as an agency within Medicare guidelines. A rehabilitation program must include, in addition to speech-language pathology services, social or vocational adjustment services to all patients in need of such services, with a qualified staff consisting of psychologists, social workers, and qualified vocational specialists as defined in the Medicare guidelines. Services may be provided by qualified professionals who are employees of the agency, or by professionals with whom the agency contracts and supervises. Services provided under the supervision of a rehabilitative agency may be performed in the patient's home, in the facilities of the rehabilitation agency, or in a hospital or skilled nursing facility.

Speech-language pathology services, which include diagnostic as well as therapeutic services, cover a wide variety of formal and informal procedures. The following therapeutic services are examples of common communication deficits related to medical disorders frequently covered by Medicare:

1. Neurological Diseases (dysarthria, dysphagia, voice disorders)
2. Cerebral Vascular Diseases (dysphagia, dysphasia, dyspraxia, dysarthria)
3. Laryngal Carcinoma Requiring Laryngectomy (aphonia, dysphonia)

Frequently speech-language pathology services are required, but not included in categories clearly related to medical disorders. For example, carry-over and maintenance activities for the patient are usually not covered under the Medicare reimbursement program. The reason frequently given for the denial of such services is that these procedures do not require performance by, or supervision of, a qualified speech-language pathologist.

Medicare provides a high degree of coverage for speech-language pathology and audiology services. For this reason, hospitals may need to keep speech-language pathologists and audiologists as employees or consultants in order to remain competitive with other recipients of Medicare reimbursement. Medicare guidelines, including the amount of coverage for services, change from time to time. The *Governmental Affairs Review,* published by the American Speech-Language–Hearing Association's Governmental Affairs Department, provides continuing information and is available by subscription.

Claims Reviewers

Claims reviewers often are clerks or technicians who follow a prescribed checklist for processing claims. Rarely are claims reviewers members of the profession undergoing scrutiny for claims approval. Claims reviewers for speech-language pathology and audiology claims are not available to third-party payers, nor is there a registry of qualified speech-language pathologists and audiologists who can serve as reviewers or as consultants for claims review. This neglected feature of third-party payment continues to affect reimbursement patterns even in companies with the clearest guidelines and in states with optimum insurance codes.

Changing and Clarifying Insurance Regulations

Members of the profession must take particular care to provide insurance companies and other third-party payers with information regarding the range of communication disorders and the duration and frequency of treatment. The profession already tends to blend with other nonphysician providers seeking money from third-party payers. This lack of clarity surrounding the scope of the profession extends from the general public to lawmakers to third-party payers. Employers who purchase group policies for employees have minimal understanding of the importance of accepting an option coverage of speech-language–hearing services. Communication necessary for the public's understanding of the profession's unique contribution to health care is crucial. The economic potential of the speech-language–hearing profession depends on its differentiated status as an independent health service provider. And, in turn, that status demands persistent advocacy, particularly in the following areas:

1. Appropriate responsibility must be directed to the speech-language pathologist/audiologist without the requirement of physician prescription and/or supervision.
2. Appropriate qualifications must be pursued by speech-language pathologists and audiologists, through American Speech-Language–Hearing Association Certification, state licensure, or some other form of accreditation.

3. Use of terms such as ''therapy'' limit the scope of coverage and frequently are interpreted in ways that overlook major responsibilities of the speech-language–hearing profession.
4. Reference to speech-language–hearing services should include reference to audiological rehabilitation services.
5. Within the profession, the development of appropriate means of self-assessment and regulation must be pursued.
6. Appropriate taxonomy must be developed specific to communication disorders and ensuing services by speech-language–hearing professionals.

While advocacy for third-party coverage continues at the level of regulation and legislation, everyday submitting of claims continues. Managing third-party coverage in a practice can be somewhat eased by following certain procedures.

Procedures for Managing Third-Party Coverage

1. Collect fees directly from clients. Be certain that clients are aware that they are responsible for all charges. When insurance remits its portion, the client is responsible for whichever portion insurance does not cover, including a deductible and services beyond the coverage of their insurance policy.
2. Help clients file insurance claims for reimbursement and encourage them to question and challenge denials of reimbursement claims.
3. Make clear to clients which third-party payers cover speech-language–hearing services in their reimbursement guidelines. Sometimes just pursuing clarification of guidelines for reimbursement can obtain coverage for speech-language–hearing services which might not otherwise be obtained.
4. Use diagnostic and intervention terms that are compatible with diagnostic codes or taxonomies, particularly when it is possible, relate the speech-language–hearing disorder to a medical condition.
5. Understand and follow both public and private guidelines for helping clients file claims reviews. The various governmental programs such as CHAMPUS, Medicare, Medicaid, Federal Employee Plan, and others differ from each other. Private insurance payers also have different requirements for filing claims.
6. Cite professional credentials including certification and licensure. Some insurance companies require that license numbers of the provider as well as the provider's signature, be on every statement for services.
7. Complete all boxes and lines and mark the ones that are not applicable. The clerks who process claims can hold up the reimbursement process and reject an entire claim because one small item was left undone.
8. Observe guidelines regarding time limitations. Both governmental and private insurance programs often have strict time limitations. Claims filed outside the allowable time period usually are not honored.
9. Encourage clients to test eligibility for reimbursement as soon as possible—at the end of the first session or first conference following the diagnostic session. Have the secretary provide the client with a signed and dated statement of fees for services and urge them to pursue the filing of the claim immediately to test

eligibility for reimbursement, as well as to clear up any problems with the guidelines.

10. Do not use an openly stated sliding fee schedule. Sometimes insurance companies factor in a reduced fee schedule and set reimbursement levels for professionals. A private agreement can be arranged with clients who clearly cannot afford to pay the full amount.

11. Do not accept the first rejection of a reimbursement claim. Encourage clients to ask an insurance reviewer to appeal any automatic rejection of a claim. Send a protest letter, or have the client send the protest letter through the employer if necessary. When possible, have the employer write a letter for the entire group policy on behalf of the professional services that have been disallowed. When new insurance codes have been adopted by legislatures within states that may affect the processing and approval of claims, send the insurance company a copy of the change in statute that may affect their responsibilities under the new law.

12. Be sure that the client knows what diagnosis and generally what information you are providing the insurance company. Make sure that you have their informed consent in writing, even though their signing of an insurance form usually waives the confidentiality requirements for the provider.

13. When an insurance carrier consistently does not provide coverage for speech-language–hearing services, inform local, state, and national professional associations of this fact to encourage lobbying efforts with those companies. Make sure that the insurance company is informed of such notices to professional groups and clients regarding their lack of coverage.

14. Avoid using the word ''therapy.'' Instead, use words like intervention or treatment or rehabilitation.

15. Do not use terms like ''habilitation'' when it would be more appropriate to use ''rehabilitation,'' implying a relationship with a medical disorder. Use diagnostic and treatment codes from recognized indices when appropriate and possible.

16. Indicate improvement when appropriate, relating accomplishments within the intervention session to functioning in everyday life.

17. In descriptions of treatment/intervention, describe procedures, goals, and outcomes.

18. When seeing a client with a degenerative or terminal illness, indicate stabilization, maintenance, or improvement as it relates to therapy, when appropriate.

19. Do not hesitate to ask your state insurance commissioner to take action to familiarize a company with current insurance codes.

20. Be persistent, but not punitive, with reluctant third-party payers. Anger and rudeness can halt appropriate insurance reimbursement almost completely.

21. Be sure that all your clients are informed about current state insurance codes, how to pursue insurance claims, and how to question rejected claims.

22. When the claim form calls for a diagnosis, supply the medical diagnosis given by the physician as the primary diagnosis to which the speech-language pathology/audiology services are applicable. Then list the associated speech-language–hearing diagnoses. When clients are contacting insurance companies

for information about coverage, they will need to know, in addition to whether coverage is possible or not, the following:

a. Whether coverage is possible for speech-language pathology/audiology;
b. What the deductible is;
c. What percentage of coverage they provide;
d. Whether there is a maximum amount of services covered;
e. Whether there is a maximum number of visits covered;
f. Where there are different classifications of participants for the insurance policy (sometimes certain family members are not qualified for benefits for which the employee is qualified);
g. What procedures are necessary to acquire the provider's status. (Most insurance companies merely require the license number, name, address, social security or employer I.D. number. Sometimes they require other information. Some companies require specific forms or will allow the practitioner's own billing forms. Some insurance companies also have a time limit after when they will not honor claims for services. Some companies require copies of evaluation forms, treatment plans, or status reports, and periodic progress reports regarding client's progress in the intervention program. Some companies also require information from the referring source for claims for services.)

23. When possible, establish a person-to-person relationship with individuals who process claims in the insurance office. Frequently this makes a difference in the attention that a claim form gets and in the amount of harrassment that the insurance company can give the service provider before honoring a claim.

Appendices

APPENDIX 8–1
POSSIBLE AREAS OF INSURANCE PROTECTION FOR THE OWNER/PRACTITIONER

Accounts receivable
Advertising liability
Automobile: owned, nonowned, hired
Building: structure damage or destruction
Building: contents damage or loss
Deferred compensation
Dental
Disability
Employee bonding
Equipment and furnishings
Extra expenses due to interruption of practice
Fire
Flood
Health: group, personal, family
Homeowner's
Key-man life
Legal and contractual liability
Legal expense
Liability on persons entering the premises
Life: term, group
Loss of rental income
Major medical payments
Maternity
Miscellaneous fiduciary liability (when managing a pension fund)
Optical
Owner's liability
Pension or profit sharing plan
Personal injury
Pharmaceuticals
Professional liability
Rehabilitative therapy
Retirement plan
Tenant improvements
Theft or vandalism: office equipment, special equipment, and instruments
Valuable papers
Wills, trusts, and contracts

APPENDIX 8–2
A LETTER TO CLIENTS FROM THE PRACTITIONER

In order to prevent misunderstandings about insurance coverage for services, the policies of this clinic are the following:

1. All professional services are charged directly to the client.
2. Clients are personally responsible for payment of bills.
3. Agreements regarding fee schedules, late cancellation charges, and charges for no-shows are between the client and this clinic and are unrelated to potential insurance coverage.

When you have insurance coverage, a contract exists between you and your insurance company. It is the policy of this clinic that the client pays for services rendered in this office; following this you may be reimbursed by your insurance company for the amount of money to which you are entitled under the policy.

My office will help prepare necessary report forms to aid you in collecting benefits from insurance companies. If insurance companies mail checks to this office, unless otherwise arranged with you, I will credit these payments to your account or immediately refund any overpayment.

Professional services rendered in this office are done with the understanding that clients are responsible for payment for services. Services are not rendered with the expectation that insurance companies will pay for all or part of the charges.

Please feel free to discuss fees with me prior to any services.

Sincerely,

____
Speech-Language Pathologist, CCC

APPENDIX 8–3
INSURANCE INFORMATION

Name of Client ____

Birthdate ____

Age ____

Party responsible for payment _______________________________________

Home Address

    Number ______________ Street ________________________________

    City __________________________ Zip code ___________________

Home Telephone ____

Name of Husband/Wife (if applicable) ________________________________

Employer ____

Occupation ____

Business Address

    Number ______________ Street ________________________________

    City __________________________ Zip code ___________________

Spouse's Employer ____

Business Address

    Number ______________ Street ________________________________

    City __________________________ Zip code ___________________

Insurance Company ____

Group Number __________________________ Certificate Number _______________

Party Insured (Subscriber) ____

Effective Date ______________________ Coverage Code _________________

Social Security # ____

Driver's License # ____

APPENDIX 8–4
ASSIGNMENT OF INSURANCE BENEFITS

I hereby authorize payment directly to ____ of the insurance benefits otherwise payable to me. I understand I am financially responsible for charges not covered by this authorization. I also authorize that a photocopy of this authorization is as if such copy were the original. If it becomes necessary for the account to be referred to an attorney for collection or suit, the undersigned shall pay reasonable attorney's fees and collection expenses.

Date ____________________   Signed ________________________________

Chapter 9

Cost Analysis, Cost Containment, and Cost Efficiency

Rumor has it that the private practitioner ''makes,'' that is, takes home, the amount of the fee.

Of course, there are some bills to pay, but after that it's supposed to be all gravy.

Well . . . where's the gravy?

If you have heard the siren call of private enterprise, you will be keenly interested in learning the whereabouts of all that gravy, and you should know. In fact, it is your responsibility to know. Realistic money expectations are based on knowing where the money comes from, and where it goes. Practitioners in work settings other than private practice find that they also must know where the money goes. In a hospital or agency, the practitioner must justify costs of services to administrators, who, in turn, must justify insurance claims to Medicare, or other third-party payers. In public school settings, if costs are not contained, children either do not get served at all, or only the most profoundly impaired receive funding. Public Law 94-142 requires that all children who need services receive them. However, the schools must justify the needs of their students in order to receive public monies to provide necessary services. Professional preparation programs in universities are finding it increasingly difficult to justify the enormous amount of professional time and supervision required to prepare students. Many university practicum programs find that fees-for-services are necessary to supplement support for expensive student preparation.

The process used to describe sources of revenue and expense is called *cost accounting* or *cost analysis*. For the purposes of this book, the term *cost analysis* will be used to describe this process. Determining what money is necessary for the provision of quality services and how unnecessary spending can be controlled is called *cost efficiency*. Passing cost efficiency on to clients through quality services at the lowest reasonable cost is called *cost containment*. These terms need not strike terror to the heart of the professional. They are merely ways of describing what happens with one's money in order that financial decisions have some basis other than impulsive reactions to crisis.

Qualitative judgements based on quantitative data are the core of professional practice. In our respective disciplines, we learn to perform intricate analyses involving the influences of speech, language, and hearing and the relationships among them. We are not turned to jelly by the thought of juggling numerous contingencies in the dynamics of intervention, nor in performing the necessary problem-solving tasks of assessment. We rarely flinch at our monumental professional efforts until we are confronted with the reality that services cost money, and that someone, somewhere, pays the cost of such services. When we are required to analyze the costs of our services and account for them, professional rationality turns to fiscal fluff.

Whatever the emotional or intellectual cost to the professional, cost analysis of service delivery will result in benefits for both client and practitioner. If the practitioner overprices his/her services, the consumer may not be able to handle the cost, and the services will go unreimbursed. If the practitioner underprices his/her services, the overhead of the practice cannot be paid, and the personal income needs of the practitioner cannot be met. Ultimately, the practitioner will be unable to afford to extend services to clients.

The practitioner must separate price from cost and cost from value. No professional service is so invaluable as to be beyond the scrutiny of cost analysis. Nor is a professional service so inexpensive that it has no cost.

COST ANALYSIS

Two considerations are basic to *cost analysis:* (1) sources and amount of income; and (2) sources and amount of expenditures.

Income is money brought in, regardless of source. *Revenue* is a source of income, carried on the books as gain. *Expenditures* are the actual monies paid to satisfy costs. *Expenses* are the costs that are directly or indirectly attributable to the provision of services (see Appendix 9–1).

Income and Revenue

Sources of income can be classified into two general categories—money from the private pocket and money from the public pocket. A private corporation (or proprietor) usually is not eligible for money from the public sector. Revenue accounting of both source and amount is important for many reasons, including taxation. For purposes of financial planning, untapped revenue sources should be identified and pursued. For example, many private practitioners depend solely upon fees-for-services. They rarely explore private foundations or philanthropic organizations, which might be potential sources of funding for a variety of services to the communicatively impaired. In similar fashion, practitioners paid with public (charitable or governmental) funds, rarely seek donations of time, money, office space, therapy materials, or volunteer services from the private sector.

Revenue accounting obviously is important for comparison to expense accounting. For example, if the owner/practitioner discovers, through his or her own revenue accounting, that therapy is a significant revenue source, and that assessment services contribute very little revenue, such a finding would have to be taken into consideration when making decisions about expenditures. It would seem to be fiscally unwise to increase expenses in the assessment area by purchasing new test instrumentation or raising the salary of the diagnostician. When revenue and expense accounting does not justify certain expenditures, the practitioner must justify those expenditures on some other basis. For example, an item that could not be justified on the basis of its potential for revenue generation might be justified on the basis of its contribution to aesthetic charm of the surroundings.

Expenditure and Expense

Expenses can be classified into general categories: *direct costs* attributable to a specific service or person; and *indirect costs* that are shared by all services and persons in the maintenance of the practice (see Appendix 9–2). In many programs it is important to separate direct from indirect costs, particularly when there is a need to demonstrate that the direct service costs are equal to the income from direct services. For example, some programs are required to be self-supporting, with fees-for-services balancing the costs of the program. In many situations, the fee schedule is so low that it is impossible for a program to pay for direct and indirect costs from fees alone. This is particularly true when secretarial pools, building utilities, and elevator repairs are figured into costs for a specific program.

Allocation of costs to either direct or indirect categories may vary, depending on one's interpretation and bookkeeping system. For example, if a room is used exclusively by one clinician for one type of service, the costs of that room (percentage of rent, utilities, and janitorial help) may be directly attributable to that service and that clinician. However, if a room is shared by various services or clinicians, such as a waiting room, the cost must be evenly divided among all clinicians and services using it. Costs allocated to clerical and receptionist services are usually divided among the services and clinicians, even when one clinician may use the typing skills of the secretary more than another clinician.

Allocation of expenses can be very difficult. One approach is to make an exhaustive list of every item paid for by the practice within a specified time period. Usually expenditures are more easily interpreted when described by quarter than when described for shorter time periods. Categorize costs into groups that can be sub-categorized, such as personnel, office, consumables, and so forth. From this categorization, a Chart of Accounts can be developed where expenses can be itemized by category.

Delineate sub-categories of personnel, such as Direct Services in Speech-Language Intervention, Direct Services in Speech-Language Screening and Assessment, and Direct Services in Speech-Language Consultation. For example, note the following schema.

Expenses: Personnel

Direct Services for Speech-Language
   Intervention:
      Pediatric
      School-Age/Adolescent
      Adult

   Assessment/Screening:
      Pediatric
      School-Age
      Adult

   Consultation:
      Pediatric
      School-Age
      Adult

Direct Services for Audiology
   Intervention:
      Habilitation/Pediatric
      Rehabilitation
         School-Age
         Adult

   Assessment/Screening

   Consultation:
      Industry
      Service Agency

Do a similar breakdown for other personnel, such as supervisory, administrative, paraprofessional, clerical, consultative, janitorial, and so forth. Designate the persons in each category, their various functions or duties, the percentage of time spent in each duty per week, and the actual hours spent per week in each duty or capacity (see Table 9–1). Note whether each person contributes to direct provision of client services and the percentage and amount of time spent in direct services. Note the percentage and amount of time each staff member devotes to indirect and general support of the practice.

Professional personnel in direct services deliver such services to clients through screening, assessment, consultation, intervention, and other. Although professional personnel also spend time in delivery-related activities, such as report writing and in-service, their time is still considered 100 percent direct. An exception to this would be professionals employed specifically to carry out other responsibilities that include administrative or clerical duties. Owners/practitioners frequently spend part of their time in direct delivery of services and part of their time executing administrative responsibilities necessary to manage the entire practice. Time allocations for personnel whose responsibilities are divided between direct and indirect responsibili-

Table 9–1.   Breakdown of Personnel Expenses

Person	Job Description/Function	Hours/ Week	Percentage of Time/Week
Jones, T.	*Speech-Language Services*	*40*	*100% Total*
	Type of Service		
	Intervention	30	75
	Assessment	2	5
	Screening	2	5
	Consultation	4	10
	Administration		
	reports	2	5
	record keeping		
	Other		
	Location		
	In Office	38	95
	Out of Office		
	hospital	2	5
	agency		
	other		
	Age Group		
	Infant/Pediatric	18	45
	School-Age	20	50
	Adult		
	Geriatric		
	Disorder Type		
	Voice	4	10
	Language	18	45
	acquired		
	developmental		
	Articulation	6	15
	Other	10	25
	Etiology		
	CVA	2	5
	Cerebral Palsy	2	5
	Cleft Palate	2	5
	Hearing Loss	6	15
	Other	10	25
	developmental	16	40

ties are usually recorded on an estimated basis. Clerical personnel, although assigned to a particular service division such as audiology, are usually included in the indirect costs category for purposes of cost analysis.

When the personnel description is as complete as possible, list office items using sub-categories such as Space and Structure, Equipment and Furnishings, and Office Protection. For example

Expenses: Office

Space and Structure

Buying, renting, adapting, and maintaining or remodeling any of the structures (shells) of the office, including rental payments or mortgage payments.

Equipment and Furnishings

General office equipment:
  (list)
General office furnishings:
  (list)
Service equipment:
  audiometer
  other test instruments

Office Protection

Insurance payments may include both structure and contents insurance:
  (list)

Some practitioners like to consider office space and structure separate from furnishings and equipment when doing cost analysis, particularly when trying to justify the cost effectiveness of changing offices. In some instances, tax supported facilities describe their space payments as ''bond retirement,'' or ''construction bond payments.''

Within the sub-category of office equipment and furnishings, a distinction can be made between general office equipment and professional services equipment. For example, office equipment usually includes typewriters and copying machines, while professional equipment and supplies include items such as audiometers and test instruments. General office equipment and furnishings are fairly universal to most small offices; professional equipment and furnishings are discipline-specific. All equipment costs usually are treated as a combination of initial expense and life of the item, including its maintenance. Outright purchases may be amortized over the expected life of the item so that cost allocations are spread over the number of years of use. Outright purchases may also be treated by an accounting method that considers replacement cost, thereby allowing for inflation.

Replacement accounting allows for the allotment of cash toward replacement of equipment as it wears out or becomes obsolete. A replacement fund is set up as a separate restricted account to be maintained regularly and consistently. The amount to be charged annually to equipment replacement is either based directly on projected needs for equipment to be purchased, or is figured from a formula for depreciation of present equipment plus an allowance for increased costs. This method takes into consideration current cost, price increase due to inflation, and price increase due to technological advances. When predicting replacement cost, one should add no less than 50 percent to the current cost.

Many short-term lease options are now available for computers and other office machines. These allow a practitioner to try various types of equipment before purchasing or leasing on a long-term basis. Lease purchase plans are the most expensive form of acquiring equipment, because the interest for the lease period must be added to the original price of the equipment. However, capital is often a concern for beginning practitioners, and a lease purchase allows one to avoid a large initial outlay of money. In addition, some lease purchase arrangements include free maintenance of the equipment for the duration of the lease.

Supplies and consumables are those items that have a life expectancy or usefulness of less than one year. They are allocated to either direct or indirect costs of an office, depending upon their function in the practice.

Other items within the office expenses category can include maintenance and repair, which are self-explanatory, and protection. *Protection* of the facilities—both structure and contents—is usually achieved through insurance. As discussed in Chapter 8, several different types of insurance coverage are necessary for the professional office, including insurance for the structure, contents, hazards that a client may encounter on a visit to the office, and health of office personnel.

The expenses discussed thus far are predictable and stable, within limits. Insurance premiums, rental and lease prices, replacement costs of consumables, and so forth, may fluctuate to some degree, but in general their range is predetermined by negotiation. Some expenses, however, are less stable and less predictable and depend on the practitioner's establishing and enforcing minimum and maximum cost expectations. These expenses reflect the working philosophies of the practitioner and include such items as telephone, travel, entertainment, continuing education, consultation, public relations, and marketing expenses.

Taxes, while predictable in their regular arrival, can change form drastically through legislation, particularly during nonelection years. Another dramatic but unpredictable expense to an office is catastrophe caused by illness, fire, accident, or economic disaster. These factors are possibilities in every career, but they cannot be predicted from past experience and are very difficult to include in cost analysis.

Productivity of Personnel

In private practice, fees-for-services provide the majority of income. This income is generated through the productivity of professional personnel. In a quantitative analysis, such as that required for cost analysis, it is necessary to subject professional personnel to stringent assessment on the basis of what he or she does, or in accounting terms—what he or she is *worth*. Remember, in cost analysis, the object is to determine whether expenses are justified. Personnel salaries and benefits constitute one of the greatest expenses of any office. It is not difficult to compute what each professional receives in salary, benefits, vacation, and other compensation and to compare that with what each professional produces for the office.

In the time-honored tradition of using an expensive garage as a storeroom for junk is the equally sacred tradition of using the computer as a table-top for stacking old files. A parallel can be drawn when one begins to assess what employees or consultants actually *do* to earn the wages they are paid and to keep the space they occupy. In cost analysis it is easy to determine who is *useful* to the practice and who is *using* the practice. Obviously, all employee contributions are not quantifiable. But in an office where income means survival and personnel means income, the owner/ practitioner cannot afford to ignore the productivity of the personnel.

Professionals in different employment settings have different ways of describing and analyzing expenses and revenue related to service delivery, different ways of discussing the results, and different reasons for engaging in fiscal analysis at all. The purpose of describing professional productivity is to be able to compare the ratio of income from individual employees to their total services with the ratio of expenditures for individual employees to their total services.

Financial descriptions are a valuable source of information with regard to expense and revenue of one service versus expense and revenue of another service within the practice, expenses versus revenues of each service, and expenses versus revenues of each employee (see Table 9–2).

The difference between what the office pays an employee and the income produced by that employee can be valuable management information for considering raises, job requirements, and even fees charged for services. The amount of money a practice spends on a service area must be offset by revenue from that service area. If it is not, that service area deserves owner scrutiny.

Another method for analyzing available data in a practice is a slight variation of the previous illustration. This method considers rate of payment compared with amount of service delivery.

> Clinician *X* provides *service delivery* at the rate of $30/hour. In one month, Clinician *X* spent 80 hours providing that service which equals $2,400/month *revenue*.

> Clinician *X* receives salary and benefits at the rate of $15/hour.

> In one month of full-time employment (160 hours), Clinician *X* spent 80 hours *not* providing services, which equals $1,200/ month *expenses*.

> To Clinician *X* indirect costs are attributed in the amount of $540/ month (allotment of rent, utilities, janitor, security, secretary, con- sumables, supplies, and so forth).

> Net loss from Clinician *X* equals $1,740/month.

Certain group personnel functions are especially difficult to assess by cost analysis. A good example of this is the staff meeting. Some staff meetings can be avoided if they are merely housekeeping in nature. Calling a group meeting usually takes more time than the content deserves. Some types of staff meetings, such as case conferences, can vary dramatically in their value. Some clearly waste time and satisfy the administrator's need to have them. Some are clearly instructive and educational for staff; some may be productive for the client who is the subject of

Table 9–2. Comparison of Revenue and Expense between Services, for Individual Services, and for Individual Employees

Subject of Analysis	Revenue/Month	Expense/Month	Difference/Month
1. T. Jones, clinician	_____________ (From Fees-for Services)	_____________ (From Salary and Benefits/Month)	(+ or −) _____________
2. Audiology (2 audiologists)	_____________ (From Fees-for Services)	_____________ (From Salary, Benefits, Equipment, Supplies)	(+ or −) _____________
3. Service Compared with Service a. Audiology	_____________ (Total Audiology Revenue)	_____________ (Total Audiology Expense)	(+ or −) _____________
b. Speech-Language Pathology	_____________ (Total Speech-Language Revenue)	_____________ (Total Speech-Language Expense)	(+ or −) _____________

Difference = _____________ Service _____________ (+ or −)

consideration in the conference. Some private practitioners are relatively isolated from contact with other professionals, and their need for the case conference is greater. However, the owner/practitioner should assure that meetings satisfy the condition of measurable productivity for the practice and not merely satisfy social needs. In many instances, a brief observation and hallway consultation with a colleague may replace the professional's need for a case conference. In too many employment settings, social and professional interactions occur that are rationalized by the content—''What should I do about Johnny?''—when the client is actually much less served than the needs of professionals seeking personal and social interactions under the guise of staff meetings.

The functions and concomitant costs of individuals and equipment should receive periodic attention, particularly in terms of who is least costly, yet most qualified, to perform a specific function (Marshall et al., 1982). Professional personnel are the easiest to quantify because of the revenue they produce for the practice. It is more difficult to assess the contributions made by clerical staff, administrators, and equipment. The most expensive and least expendible person in the practice is the practitioner/owner. Every other employee should provide the skills and support necessary to facilitate the functioning of the practitioner/owner at his or her highest level. For example, the owner/practitioner should not be spending his or her time typing address labels or filing charts. With an earning power of over $50 an hour, the owner/practitioner who performs a $7 an hour function incurs potential loss of over $43 an hour. By doing it yourself, the "savings" gained from not hiring a clerk to do the filing can become expensive. Even if the owner's time is not filled with client services, the energy and physical drain eventually take their toll on the practice. Qualified and productive clerical staff are just as important to the practice as qualified and productive professional staff. Cheap help is worth it.

Small programs may find it sufficient to determine average cost per service (or client contact) for the year. The formula for computing that data is

$$\text{Total Annual Program Costs} \div \text{Total Number of Client Contact Hours Per Year} = \text{AVERAGE COST PER SERVICE}$$

Other information that may be computed includes.

1. Cost of each clinician per year = Total direct and indirect expenses minus total revenue ÷ Total number of clinicians.
2. Cost of each staff member = Expenses charged against each staff member.
3. Cost of equipment by service = Expenses charged against equipment ÷ Revenue attributed to that equipment.
4. Cost of administration per year = Expenses charged against administration compared against the considered worth of the function of the administrator.
5. Cost of supervision per year = Expenses charged against supervisors compared against their contributions to the program and the importance of those contributions to the practice.
6. Cost of furniture and equipment per year by area of specialty = Expenses charged against each area of specialty for purchase/lease of equipment and furniture specific to that area.
7. Cost of protection to whole practice per year = Cost of insurance considered in relation to risk.
8. Cost of each area of specialty per year (audiology, speech pathology, intervention, etc.) = Total cost per service minus total revenue per service.

Different types of services require different accounting procedures, utilize different equipment, supplies, space, and contribute differently to the practice. Average-cost-per-patient receiving cleft palate team services may be much greater than average-cost-per-patient for hearing screening. This differential should be considered first by analysis of fiscal data, upon which qualitative judgements must then be made. Continued scrutiny of cost efficiency is as important to the survival of a practice as is continued scrutiny of professional effectiveness.

Analysis of service costs does not diminish or taint the quality of service delivery. The intention is to enhance services while minimizing waste. This function is crucial to analysis of staff performance, salary changes, merit bonuses, fee determination, and other important management decisions related to cost effective service delivery.

COST CONTAINMENT

Attempts at cost containment vary widely within the profession. Cost containment is affected by numerous factors outside the control of the practice and the practitioner. Variables that influence cost and cost containment include:

1. *Administrative Philosophy:* Philosophy of service delivery affects program emphasis and, therefore, spending emphasis. This includes the determination of how much administration and supervision is necessary, how clerical time and efforts are used, how much profit margin is considered acceptable for program survival, and so forth.
2. *Regional Influences:* Rental costs vary from one part of the country to another and from one part of town to another. Insurance costs also fluctuate with geographic differences and with the physical condition of the office structure. Liability factors are more prominent in some regions than in others.
3. *Type of Program and Service Delivery Model:* Some programs necessitate more expense by virtue of their defined services. For example, a program that includes interns and their supervision is more expensive per service hour than a program involving only experienced clinicians. Programs that require team work-ups, programs that neither reward nor require certain levels of productivity from personnel, and programs that necessitate the use of up-to-date technological equipment all keep costs high without necessarily yielding commensurate revenue.
4. *Economic Factors:* The general state of the economy including tax changes, inflation, and political climate influences wages, fringe benefits, insurance payments, and availability of grants.

These factors, as well as other self-contained features of the employment setting itself, affect cost containment, which in turn affects charges to the consumer and margin of profit for the provider. An important aspect of cost containment is the cost efficiency of service delivery.

COST EFFICIENCY

Whatever the circumstances surrounding the practice, there are usually ways in which efficiency and productivity can increase without jeopardizing quality of service delivery. Specific suggestions for increasing professional productivity and office efficiency are as follows:

1. Engage in periodic cost analysis:
   a. Describe all expenses as completely as possible—equipment, furnishings, space, personnel, insurance—and identify current sources and amount of revenue.
   b. Define functions and activities of all aspects of the practice—clerical and professional personnel, equipment, space, furnishings, insurance, travel expenses, in-service, and so forth.
   c. Use all identified factors of the practice to determine cost of one unit of service delivery.
2. Increase productivity:
   a. Realize that many children and many types of disorders benefit by being grouped with clients of similar age and/or disorder. Some clients and their communication disorders are more easily grouped than others; frequently it is extremely beneficial to clients with language disorders, certain articulation disorders, or hearing impairment, to participate in group work. To

see five 8- or 9-year-old children with spoken and written language impairment in a series of individual client contacts is not only a waste of valuable professional time and energy, it deprives clients of the opportunity to learn and function in group communication.

b. Eliminate unnecessary staff meetings. Scrutinize the benefits of using potential service delivery time for unnecessary administrative lectures, social conversation, and client staffings that have no real benefit for either staff, parents, or clients.

c. Eliminate unnecessary report writing and record keeping. Determine exactly what records are necessary for administrative management, such as billing and files. Have each clinician determine which professional records are necessary for maintaining quality client care and for communicating necessary information to other professionals and to families of each client served. Do not engage in any other record keeping, writing, charting, or other paper work superfluous to service delivery. Writing daily lesson plans for each 30-minute session for all 20 or 30 clients usually is unnecessary for an experienced clinician. A brief record of every client telephone conversation and weekly, succinct therapy notes probably are necessary.

d. Eliminate unnecessarily long telephone and hallway conversations with parents and teachers. If a conference necessitates more than 5 to 10 minutes, the clinician should schedule an appointment, which then becomes part of the child's intervention, and consequently is charged to the client.

e. Employ paraprofessionals if they can increase contact time for clients. This allows the professional to direct the program and supervise work with two or three times as many patients as would be possible if the professional were to provide all direct intervention. Obviously some programs lend themselves to such arrangements more easily than others. Paraprofessional services may be considered to be one means of satisfying cost analysis requirements by
    i. reducing client costs, and
    ii. maintaining quality services, as long as adequate supervision and direction are provided.
    Use of supportive personnel can often increase client services without increasing cost to the client, and can also provide the master clinician with the means for directing, supervising, and sometimes providing services to a greater number of clients.

f. Do not employ cheap help. Mistakes in letters, errors in telephone messages, forgetting or ignoring important features of the job, can be more costly than paying a qualified person a respectable wage.

g. Do not use expensive, specialized employees for mundane, perfunctory jobs. This includes the owner/practitioner who often engages in a little janitorial work, a little errand running, or a little typing of form letters in order to get something ''free.'' The energy demands eventually catch up. The specialized professional owner/practitioner who is too fragmented by extra little jobs will be unable to provide quality services that are demanded by assessment and intervention.

h. Be sure each employee knows his or her responsibilities and does what is expected. If an employee, from secretary to professional, is not completely aware of employer expectations, the gaps will gradually reduce efficiency.

3. Be sure that clients are completely informed about policies, fees, services, vacations, substitute clinicians, groupings, and so forth, before they begin intervention programs. Remind clients, periodically, of policies.

4. Scrutinize costs considered to be stable and predictable to see if they might increase without your knowledge. One example occurs in many lease contracts where a built-in cost-of-inflation increase occurs yearly without reminder to the tenant.

5. Scrutinize insurance on office contents and personal liability to reconfirm the necessity for the amount of insurance carried and its cost.

6. Periodically reevaluate office policies regarding use of telephone, postage, copier, and other equipment. The staff may consider them an important fringe benefit and use them judiciously or there may be abuse of the opportunity to make ''free'' calls.

7. Periodically, review travel and vehicle expenses of staff. Consider encouraging independent study plans rather than routinely reimbursing travel to conferences for continuing education.

8. Consider flex-time for employees. Both clerical and professional employees may be delighted to have a chance to choose their own hours. This should not be interpreted as permission to come and go as they please. The owner may find that client needs are served better by one professional working from 8 a.m. to 5 p.m., while another works from 12 noon until 9 p.m. This can eliminate the need for hiring additional professional help for late afternoon and early evening demands of certain clients.

9. Provide bonuses, merit payments, or a percentage of profits-over-base to professionals who exceed certain minimum productivity levels. Provide parallel incentives to office workers who tend to take on extra loads or work overtime on their own initiative. Buy Certificates of Deposit (C.D.s) or mutual funds (for pension plans) for productive employees as yearly merit raises.

10. Encourage professionals to provide client services during certain blocks of time, while saving blocks of time for uninterrupted work. The efficiency of both tasks (patient-contact and paper or telephone work) will probably increase, and the tasks, themselves, are less fragmenting to employees.

11. Charge clients when they fail to cancel appointments, except in cases of emergency.

12. Improve bill collection procedures. Do not allow overdue payments from clients to run more than 6 weeks without adding penalties, such as finance charges, personal discussion about the bill, cessation of therapy.

13. Use your own time and that of your employees efficiently.

a. Learn to dictate patient reports, conferences, and memos; handwritten information is a waste of time.

b. Use dictating equipment when travelling from one setting to another; for example, dictate screening reports on children just screened as you travel to the next screening site.

c. Have staff learn to dictate when possible. Use inexpensive typing paper, not expensive stationery, for first drafts.

    d.   Take a small electronic typewriter and dictaphone on airplane trips and to conferences. You may be surprised by what you can retain away from the office that you will forget by the time you return.

    e.   Be sure you and all employees have pencils/pens and notepads at every desk and by every telephone. Tie them down if necessary.

14. Be sure someone other than yourself is in charge of keeping supplies in stock and in place whenever they are needed (notepads, pencils, test forms, and so forth).

15. When a client is late for an appointment, there *are* things you can do, even if you have only 2 or 3 minutes. Make a note; place a call; ask a colleague a question you have been meaning to ask. If you cannot think of anything to do for the office, then do something for yourself—get a soft drink; lie down for a short rest and have your secretary call you when your appointment arrives. Use the time to save yourself—not to walk around in frustrated circles. Revise a form; make a list; start an analysis of untapped sources of revenue.

16. Do not buy something just because you have the money. Do not buy equipment or machinery or hire another staff person if you cannot make the numbers pay for it before you buy it. The need will expand to fit the supply when the need may never have existed without the supply. This rule does not necessarily apply to space or personnel needs. These are such large expenses, the need usually is pretty obvious before money becomes available. It is the small dollar items that are frequently tempting. When the need grows to fit the supply, cost is no longer contained and not always predictable. For example, if you do not have a copy machine in your office and decide that it is too inconvenient to have your secretary travel to another location for copies, the tendency will be to purchase a machine. But, consider the numbers briefly. If you do not have a copy machine, you will use carbons, except for some copies that must be better quality than carbon paper produces. Count the number of copies you make a week. Suppose you now pay a copy service 7 cents per copy, and you make no more than 400 copies per week. At $28 per week, 52 weeks per year, you are spending roughly $1,500 on copying costs. Your secretary's time in making and correcting carbons and traveling to obtain copies will cost at least $500 per year. In that situation, buy a copier for $1,500–$1,800 whose own operating cost is only 3 cents per copy. If, however, you were making no more than 100 copies per week, the numbers would not justify the purchase.

17. Avoid late charges and penalties, and minimize finance charges by keeping your credit payments and tax payments timely.

18. Be sure that any financing you have to do has a clause allowing early payoff of the debt without penalty.

SUMMARY

Cost analysis is a basis for policy, client services, agency evaluation, and program change. It can be used as a tool for program assessment, regardless of job setting. For example, public school programs incur indirect, as well as direct costs that have some bearing on the policies of the program, budget, type of service delivery offered, and retention, replacement, or addition of staff, such as speech-language pathologists. Direct and indirect costs of a school speech-language–hearing program affect taxpayers through school taxes; they provide one form of data for program comparison within and across school districts; and they offer one measure for determining how many children can be served.

Efforts to achieve recognition and reimbursement for provision of quality services may not succeed unless we are sensitive to the economic issues of accounting for expenses and containing costs. An important feature of an autonomous profession is the right to set fees for services. But professionals must act responsibly in the area of cost efficiency and cost containment, or they risk having others impose cost regulations upon them.

A word of caution in the midst of encouragement for counting money, clients, and time. As Seigel (1975, p. 797) reminds us — *in the provision of professional services, what is countable is not the only thing that counts*. Although quantifiable data provide crucial information, they do not replace the qualitative value of good clinical judgement.

Appendices

APPENDIX 9–1
REVENUE AND EXPENSE

REVENUE

	Private	*Public*

Fees and Tuition
   Private Payment
   Private and Public Insurance
Consultation
   Grants and Foundations
   Donations (formal; private)
   Gifts (free office space, other)
   Barter
   Volunteers

Tax Appropriations

Other (i.e., feature stories in newspaper = reduced expenses for public relations)

EXPENSES

	Direct	*Indirect*

Personnel
Office Space and Structure
Office Contents (depreciation or replacement)
   Furnishings (purchase and maintenance)
   Equipment (purchase and maintenance)
Operational
   Supplies and Consumables
   Public Relations
   Continuing Education Meetings
   Travel, Time Off
Other

APPENDIX 9–2
DIRECT AND INDIRECT EXPENSES

DIRECT EXPENSES:
Allocated directly to delivery of professional services:

PERSONNEL

Professional Salaries
   Direct Patient Contact
   Supervision Time (if directly attributable to specific service and professional)
Professional Fringe Benefits
   Professional Liability Insurance
   Vacation Time
   Continuing Education Time and Expenses
   Travel Expenses
   Major Medical Insurance
   Pension Plan
   Professional Dues

OFFICE SPACE AND STRUCTURE

Office(s) and Test/Therapy Room(s)—used specifically and only for delivery of professional
   services (designate which service and which professional)

OFFICE CONTENTS

Furnishings—used only by designated professional
Equipment—used only by designated professional and particular service (can include test
   kits, therapy materials, other)

OPERATIONAL

Supplies and Consumables—such as postage and stationery (useful life of less than one
   year; used only by designated professionals and for particular services)
Vehicle Maintenance—designated to specific professionals and particular services
Uncollectable Accounts—bad checks, money spent on bill collection
Public Relations—money spent only and specifically by and for a designated professional
   and a particular service
Time Off and Expenses—professional meetings and continuing education (allocated to des-
   ignated professional and particular service)

OTHER

INDIRECT EXPENSES:
   Shared by all professional and operations components of the practice:

PERSONNEL

Clerical Salaries
Clerical Fringe Benefits
   Vacation
   Retirement or Pension Plan
   Major Medical
   Merit Pay or Bonuses
Administrative Salaries—percentage of owner/practitioner time used for management and
   administrative duties

OFFICE SPACE AND STRUCTURE

Offices and Space Shared by All Staff and Clients—such as waiting room, hallway, bathroom, coffee area, other
Insurance—on space and structure and common building area

OFFICE CONTENTS

Furnishings—used commonly by all staff and clients, such as secretarial furniture, waiting room furniture, and conference room furniture
Equipment—used commonly for entire practice, such as typewriter, recording machine, and copier
Insurance—on contents

OPERATIONAL

Supplies and Consumables—used for general operation of office, useful life of less than 1 year
Public Relations Money—on behalf of entire practice
Staff Meetings, Case Conferences—unless regarding specific client
Fund-raising
Library

OTHER

Telephone

APPENDIX 9–3
COST ANALYSIS

FORMULAS FOR ANALYSIS

1. Calculating percentage of scheduled visits to actual visits:

$$\frac{\textbf{No. Scheduled Visits (per child/month)}}{\textbf{No. Actual Sessions}} = \textbf{Percentage}$$

Using a time span of 2 to 3 years, one can observe the cycles in his or her practice of heaviest absences and/or cancellations. These observed trends make it easier to predict income by month or season and to provide information about staff vacations and other scheduling needs.

For example, my heaviest no-show and cancellation periods are June and July, and December and January. The months in which I come closest to a predictable 100 percent attendance are March, April, August, September, and October. These are also the months that are most heavily scheduled.

2. Calculating percentage of bill collection:

$$\frac{\textbf{Amount Billed}}{\textbf{Amount Paid}} = \textbf{Percentage Collected}$$

This can be calculated by service, such as audiology; by clinician; by age of client; by method of payment; and for the practice as a whole, both in current billing terms and in cumulative terms, to derive total amount outstanding and collected.

This should be done every quarter to assess changes in collection patterns and to help determine changes in collection procedures, initial agreement letter concerning fees, and so forth.

3. Calculating revenue and expenses for each professional staff member:

Revenue/Month for Clinician X

Fees Billed (or Fees Collected) + Other Revenue Attributed to X = TOTAL

Expense/Month for Clinician X

Salary + Benefits (insurance, + Indirect Costs (prorated— = TOTAL
travel, release time, utilities, rent, consum-
sick pay, dues, vaca- ables)
tion)

Questions to consider in relation to staff:
a. Are the salary and benefits of each clinician more/less than the clinician's cost to the agency? How much? Does this allow for owner's profit? For emergencies? For a raise? For no-pay clients?
b. How does an agency handle the inequities of nonrevenue producing activities performed by staff on agency time? Unequal productivity from one staff member to another?
c. If the staff is not generating enough revenue, how does the agency create or encourage change so that more revenue is produced?

4. Calculating total revenue and expenses for the agency:

Total Expense

Total Personnel Costs + **Total Personnel Costs** = **Total Expenses**
Direct (salary and   **Indirect (rent, utilities,**   **for Agency**
benefits)   **and so forth)**

Total Revenue

Total Revenue from Fees + **Total Other Revenue** = **Total Revenue for Agency**

Net Income

Revenue − Expenses = Gravy before Taxes

5. Calculating average cost of services per client:

Average Cost

$$\frac{\textbf{Total Expenses}}{\textbf{Number of Clients Served}} = \textbf{Average Cost per Client}$$

6. Calculating average income per client:

Average Income

$$\frac{\textbf{Total Revenue}}{\textbf{Number of Clients Served}} = \textbf{Average Income per Client}$$

Chapter **10**

Professional Autonomy and Private Practice

Almost all of us want to be in charge of ourselves, but find that difficult to accomplish. As a friend of mine once said, ''If I could be in control of 15 percent of what happens to me in my life, I would feel successful!''

THE 15 PERCENT SOLUTION

Clearly, there are circumstances over which we have little or no control; sometimes such circumstances are unavoidable. However, in other situations where we have the opportunity to exert a measure of control, we sometimes allow ourselves to become victimized and give up whatever autonomy we could have. It is not the concern of this book to discuss factors that lead us to lose control in our personal lives. Rather it is to discuss how, as professionals, we unnecessarily relinquish our autonomy and control over our professional practice, and how we might recapture some of what we have relinquished.

Autonomy is a term that means self-regulation. Autonomy in professional terms refers to governance of a specific profession by its own members. The Ad Hoc Committee on Professional Autonomy (ASHA, 1985), adopted the definition that

> An autonomous profession is one in which the practitioner has the qualifications, responsibility, and authority for the provision of the services which fall within the scope of the practice. (p. 2)

Determinants of professional autonomy include the *qualifications* of the professional, professional *authority*, professional *responsibility*, *economic factors*, and *cultural factors*. (ASHA, 1985).

Qualifications

The profession must continue to develop standards for the provision of its services. Standards of the profession and qualifications of professional personnel acting through professional preparation programs and facilities to provide services affect the degree to which we are autonomous. Criteria for standards of care must be generated, and the profession must respond when it is misrepresented by individuals and/or groups.

The incorporation of professional standards in requirements for state licensure and voluntary certification should be done with care so that exemptions do not erode professional autonomy. Exemptions, which are of particular concern, include members of the profession practicing in certain employment settings and members of other professions who provide services that fall within the scope of practice of speech-language pathology/audiology, such as physicians. The exemptions suggest that services provided are of standard quality because of the nature of a specific job site, or because of the appropriateness of ancillary professional training. In reality, such exemptions did not arise from any presumption of quality, but rather from legislative compromises required for securing passage of a professional licensure bill. The existence of exemptions presents a long-term source of erosion to the autonomy of a profession that should be setting its professional standards of preparation and qualification by design, not by default. These exemptions are regrettable because they may award the right to practice this profession to individuals who do not meet entry level standards established by this profession (ASHA, 1985).

A resolution (LC-53-83) passed by Legislative Council, the policy making body of the American Speech-Language–Hearing Association, called for ASHA to adopt the position that state laws establishing licensure standards for speech-language pathology/audiology should not provide for exemption of any unqualified individuals; and further, it called for ASHA to adopt the position that state laws establishing licensure for speech-language pathology/audiology should provide for licensure of all qualified individuals. David Yoder (1984), past president of the American Speech-Language–Hearing Association, explained the policy as follows:

1. A licensure law is to protect the consumer of services. Exemptions confuse consumers as to who is, and who is not, qualified to provide services.
2. Exemptions can lead to development of a dual delivery system. This is especially true in states which allow bachelor-level persons to work in schools.
3. When we speech-language pathologists/audiologists permit exemption in our licensure laws, state legislators and officials find it difficult to accept us as a bona fide profession.
4. If the legislature intends to protect the consumer by specifying standards for obtaining a license and defining the scope of practice, then the licensure law should apply to all providers of services regardless of employment setting.
5. Administration of the licensure law will be simplified and enhanced when all professionals working with communicatively disabled are licensed.
6. Laws should be universal; therefore, all exempted categories weaken the law. If some exceptions are allowed, it sets a precedent for other exemptions, and soon only a few providers of service are covered by the licensure law.

7. Professional identification and image of speech-language pathologists and audiologists will be enhanced, and professional autonomy will be strengthened by nonexempted licensure (ASHA, 1984).

In addition to basic qualifications for professional preparation and practice, qualified professionals must supplement and update their skills and knowledge in areas in which they provide services. Some form of continuing education, whether traditional format or independent study, is imperative to maintain the highest quality of service delivery. Autonomy is a status derived from the degree of specialized knowledge and expertise demonstrated by a profession and its members. The public and other professions need assurance that professionals maintain a high level of continuing education.

One means of assuring quality professional preparation programs is through universal accreditation. At this time, only 60 percent of graduate preparation programs in speech-language pathology/audiology are accredited by the Educational Services Board of ASHA. It is important that all graduate education programs that prepare students to enter the profession strive to achieve formal recognition of accreditation as established by the profession.

Institutions in which services are provided should also have formal recognition of standards for service delivery. Institutional qualifications have been established in the standards for accreditation by the Professional Standards Board of the American Speech-Language–Hearing Association, but not all agencies and institutions adhere to them.

The Professional Services Board (PSB) of the American Speech-Language–Hearing Association is the accrediting body that evaluates and recognizes service programs for the purpose of assuring high quality of speech, language, and hearing services. Two other accrediting agencies that evaluate quality of clinical services, including those available to communicatively impaired, are the Joint Commission on Accreditation of Hospitals (JCAH) and the Commission on Accreditation of Rehabilitation Facilities (CARF). The Professional Services Board offers a higher level of quality assurance within our profession than the other two, which have only minimal references to speech-language–hearing services. Recently, however, both JCAH and CARF have cited PSB standards to employers when more information was necessary to qualify applicants. Institutions that provide speech, language, and hearing services, such as hospitals and rehabilitation facilities, should be directed by the profession toward standards of peer scrutiny and accreditation in order to ensure acceptable delivery of speech-language and hearing services.

Professional Authority

Exercise of autonomy requires authority over areas of practice for which the profession is responsible. For example, members of the profession:

1. Define at what point a client enters services (i.e., point of entry for clients);
2. Select appropriate candidates for services;
3. Select appropriate assessment and intervention approaches and duration;

4. Refer appropriately within the profession, as well as to other professions (ASHA, 1985).

Traditionally, physicians have been the point of entry into almost all health care and allied health care programs. Many laws and policies still in operation reflect that tradition, and many public and private insurance programs base their reimbursement programs on physician authority. Although physician attention and cooperation is warranted in instances of direct health care, supervision and prescription of speech-language or audiology services by a physician is not generally applicable. Physician interaction and acknowledgment regarding speech-language–hearing services is appropriate; physican approval for insurance claims reviews is not acceptable. Usually individuals outside the profession of speech-language pathology review claims and make decisions regarding reimbursement, when only members of the profession should have authority to decide the scope or duration of speech, language, or hearing services for communicatively impaired. Peer review is a system that advocates evaluation of quality in professional services by professional peers. With ever-increasing concerns about cost and quality, the profession of speech-language pathology/audiology will find it mandatory to participate in peer review at a formal level. If, as a profession, we do not choose to police ourselves, we forsake a crucial element of self-government. If self-regulation is not defended, it is replaced by regulation from others.

As outlined in a position paper drafted by the Ad Hoc Committee on Professional Autonomy (1985), it is crucial for the autonomy of the profession that professional associations and members of the profession of speech-language pathology/audiology begin to

1. advocate that decision making rest with qualified speech-language pathologists/audiologists with respect to treatment and referral for the speech, language, and hearing impaired;
2. oppose health plans and physician-dominated programs which require that type, frequency, or duration of services be established by prescription of an individual who is not a qualified speech-language pathologist/audiologist;
3. generate public information materials which reflect the position that entry into the health care system may appropriately be made through the speech-language pathologist/audiologist.

Responsibility

Inherent to professional authority is the legal and ethical responsibility that the profession must carry. The speech-language pathologist/audiologist always bears individual responsibility for services delivered, and sometimes shares responsibility with the employing institution. The practitioner, who supervises paraprofessionals and students, also carries ultimate ethical and legal responsibility for supervisees. In practices that are incorporated, the owner/practitioner usually shares, by law and by ethical prescription, responsibility for services provided by employees.

As a profession receives the recognition of autonomy, it also receives recognition of the risk and responsibilities inherent to that autonomy. The professional must bear responsibility for:

1. Providing the highest quality of services to each client at all times.
2. Referring the client to a colleague or another professional when it is in the best interest of the client.
3. Providing information necessary for the client to make an informed decision about available choices.
4. Maintaining current information about legal and ethical responsibilities.

The professional, whether paid directly for services or not, also has a fiscal responsibility toward each client to provide cost effective services.

Economic Factors

Richard Flower (1984), ASHA past president, suggests that an incongruity exists between our insistence on professional independence and our substantial dependence on public institutions. Feldman (1981) points out that the majority of our professional services are performed in sheltered settings, either governmental or institutionally supported agencies, such as public schools and hospitals. He notes that although our profession is constituted primarily of practitioners, the practitioner in speech-language pathology/audiology is rarely engaged in independent practice. It is a fact that when professionals become employees, fiscal autonomy, as well as other forms of self-government, are diminished. The employer decides how much services will cost clients, how much professional employees will receive for delivering services, how insurance claims will be submitted, and numerous other policies that will affect the professional employee. Thus, decisions that are professional in nature are made by administrators who rarely understand clinical issues. The realities of employment automatically compromise certain positions of professional autonomy; and, the two largest employers of speech-language hearing service providers—public schools and health care systems—usually demand the greatest compromises. Adverse effects resulting from these compromises impact consumers of services and the public, in general, which in turn serves to reduce the profession's image and potency in the public mind.

Resisting compromises within employment settings is important to the self-image and public image of the profession of speech-language pathology/audiology. Refusing to accept the cafeteria or auditorium stage for office space, resisting physician control of treatment decisions regarding communicatively impaired, and exhibiting competence and professional self-esteem are all important. Professional autonomy is limited, however, in arenas that require one to accept a compromised position. It seems apparent that growth of our professional autonomy is almost completely dependent on private practice.

Only in the position of a practitioner/entrepreneur is it possible to determine policies for payment, service delivery, and self-evaluation and regulation, and to exercise complete authority, while assuming complete responsibility, for the liabilities of such decisions. In a financially successful practice, the professional has the freedom and the responsibility to offer the communicatively impaired population the most direct access to professional services. In this setting the professional may come close to having 15 percent control.

The other 85 percent belongs to clients, taxes, and insurance companies.

Private practitioners who seek financial help for clients through third-party payers may find that autonomy is once again abridged. Decisions regarding insurance payment sometimes appear in written policies requiring physician approval; other decisions are sometimes made on a case-by-case basis, almost randomly. Problems with terminology related to assessment and intervention in our profession compound difficulties when dealing with insurance companies. Such companies frequently have no guidelines from state or national professional associations for reference to taxonomic classifications. In these confusing situations, insurance companies usually resort to medical terminology, which places the nonphysician provider in a dilemma. Practice medicine and use medical diagnoses, or don't get paid. Claims reviewers usually are clerks, and guidelines for intervention profiles for speech-language–hearing services are almost nonexistent. It is indeed a rare practitioner who can remain completely autonomous and still maintain relationships with insurance carriers.

Cultural Factors

Preferences, biases, and prejudices of the American public become apparent in the social acknowledgment of professional autonomy. The profession of speech-language pathology/audiology is particularly vulnerable to several societal biases such as deference to:

1. Professionals with doctorate degrees;
2. Professionals who are male;
3. Professionals who make money in their profession;
4. Professionals who do not work through the public education system.

Because of our cultural and socioeconomic teachings, we have grown up with the opinion that someone called ''doctor'' is a person of quality and knowledge. Thus, a person who has such a title is to be held in greater esteem than one who does not. As a society, we have been hesitant to accord autonomy and responsibility to females. To upwardly mobile America, an indicator of professional worth is professional wealth. Although public education is considered to be basic to society, there is a tendency to diminish autonomy of the professional employed in the education system.

It does not take close scrutiny of our profession to note that the greatest percentage of clinicians are masters-level females employed by public schools or by a male called Dr. Someone. Most do not make much money. No matter how narrow the view of society, public opinion is influenced by that view when considering whether to acknowledge our profession's autonomy. These biases of society are hard to change, and they pose one of the greatest deterrents to professional autonomy. The profession must become aware of the need to devote serious effort toward changing the low-prestige and low-income image we project by demanding appropriate recognition and compensation for the worth of our services.

Burn-out

Everyone has heard of burn-out—that used-up, thrown-out feeling that makes Friday fatigue feel refreshing by comparison. Sometimes work-related stress converts to problems at home, physical ailments, and emotional unpredictability. None of these characteristics are desirable for someone who earns a living helping people in need.

The constant exhaustion, negativism, and depression associated with job stress, or burn-out, may be directly related to the degree of professional autonomy one possesses, *not* merely to the amount of work one must do. It is entirely possible, even enjoyable, to work many years for long hours in a job that is demanding at every level, *if* that job is a position in which one has control commensurate with responsibility.

If a practitioner finds that in spite of heavy responsibility, he or she has little authority to change any aspect of the position, then the job can become unbearable. When an employee makes efforts to provide quality services in the face of unrelenting (and perhaps mindless) barriers to service delivery, burn-out is born.

Consider the employment settings in our field where burn-out is most rampant. These are usually settings where a superior manifests absolute rigidity and control. Even in settings where intensive services are provided to clients with little or no interest in improvement, or to clients who make minimal change after years of intervention, the burn-out rate is less than in work settings where the practitioner is helpless to control his own service delivery.

Miller and Potter (1982) investigated reports of burn-out by speech-language pathologists. They found that burn-out was not related to case load, but was related to negative effects that job position had on the personal lives of clinicians. Respondents who experienced burn-out also reported job ineffectiveness and dissatisfaction. Results were not sorted by employment setting or position of authority in the job.

The absence of authority and control as an isolated factor is not a problem in some job settings. Assembly-line workers rarely experience burn-out. There is simply no need for them to have autonomy. Problems with burn-out occur when a professional who has the idea that judgment is part of his or her professional obligation must operate in a situation where his or her judgment is overridden. Autonomy with regard to one's professional work is a distinguishing factor between an occupation and a profession.

THE 100 PERCENT SOLUTION

Total autonomy for the profession is many years away. Certainly efforts of professional associations and our special-interest lobby groups for legislative changes in licensure and insurance regulations will have a positive effect. Continued education of the public and other professions regarding the purview of communication disorder specialists will change certain aspects of the profession's public image. Continued development of standards programs for the profession is also necessary. The most important contribution toward acquisition of autonomy for the profession, however, is the daily effort of each member of the profession. Without service delivery of the highest quality from competent speech-language pathologists/audiologists, and without professional demand for fiscal recognition and public regard for those services, our struggle for autonomy is doomed.

Chapter **11**

Taxes and Tax Deductions

Organizational structure of a practice is a primary factor in the determination of taxation of that practice. This structure further determines what IRS forms must be completed, what type of payments are due, and when they fall due. This section is designed to provide a summary of some of the tax information with which a practitioner should be familiar, so that when the accountant and bookkeeper ask questions and give advice, their counsel and work will be more easily tolerated and properly applied.

Due Dates

The Internal Revenue Service publishes a tax calendar every year, which includes a general tax calendar, an employer's tax calendar, and an excise tax calendar. The three calendars explain when to file tax returns, when to pay estimated tax, when to apply for extensions, and when to do the other things required by federal tax laws. The calendars cover tax laws that apply to individuals, sole proprietorships, partnerships, and corporations. (See Annotated Bibliography.)

Dated lists in the calendars are due dates. If a due date set by law falls on a Saturday, Sunday, or legal holiday, it is delayed until the next day that is not a Saturday, Sunday, or legal holiday. Federal holidays are adjusted in the IRS publication, but state holidays usually are not noted.

Caution No. 1: Whenever possible, take action before the due date; late payments incur a late penalty and interest on overdue taxes.

Caution No. 2: Take every precaution to follow all tax laws that apply to you. There are both civil and criminal penalties for intentionally filing a false tax return, for intentional failure to pay taxes, and for filing no return at all.

Accounting Periods

Every taxpayer must figure a taxable income and file a tax return on the basis of an annual account period (a tax year or fiscal year). Corporations establish their tax year when they first file an income tax return.

1. *Tax Year:* A tax year is usually 12 consecutive months and may be a calendar year or a fiscal year (including a period of 52–53 weeks). A tax year may be less than 12 months, but it may not be more than 12 months unless a 52 to 53 week year is used.
2. *Calendar Year:* A calendar year is 12 consecutive months ending on December 31. If you are a calendar year taxpayer, your sole proprietorship would be on the calendar year basis.
3. *Fiscal Year:* A fiscal year is 12 consecutive months ending on the last day of any month other than December, or a 52 to 53 week year. To report on a fiscal year basis, books must be kept on that basis.

A short tax year is a tax year of less than 12 months and can occur when a taxpayer is not in existence for an entire year, or when the taxpayer changes tax years. Each of these situations necessitates special ways of figuring taxes for the short year.

Employment tax periods are the calendar quarters for figuring and withholding income tax and social security tax.

Self-Employment Taxes

Self-employment tax is a social security tax for individuals who work for themselves and is parallel to that withheld from employee wages. Someday we may recover some of this income in the form of retirement benefits such as social security checks, and insurance benefits such as Medicare.

There are *income limits* such that if you have net earnings from self employment of $400 or more, you must pay self-employment tax. At the time of this writing, there is a maximum amount of earnings that can be taxed as self-employment for self-employment tax purposes. Self-employment is not subject to self-employment taxes if one has also received a certain amount of wages as an employee that were subject to social security tax.

Self-employment *tax rates* change yearly as do formulas by which they are fixed. Obtain the latest revision of the IRS publication regarding self-employment tax for the newest rate and formula up-date.

You are *self-employed* if you are a sole proprietor, an independent consultant or contractor, a member of a partnership, or otherwise in business for yourself. The ''otherwise'' includes ventures such as writing research grants, administering continuing education programs for profit, and serving on boards of directors of corporations, bank boards, and so forth. A *limited* partner in an investment venture figures self-employment income by excluding the distributive share of partnership income or loss. Guaranteed payments, such as salary and professional fees received for services as the limited partner, are included as self-employment. An *inactive partner* figures income from self-employment by including the distributive share of partnership income or loss and any guaranteed payments. A *retired partner* pays no self-employment tax on retirement income received from the partnership as part of a written retirement plan.

For income tax purposes, the term *partnership* includes (in addition to an ordinary partnership) a syndicate, group, pool, joint venture, or other unincorporated organization that is carrying on a business that may not be classified as a trust, estate, or corporation.

Employment Taxes

If you have employees, whether you are incorporated or not, you will probably be required to withhold federal income tax and pay social security (FICA) and federal unemployment (FUTA) tax.

Common-law employees: Every individual who performs services that are subject to the will and control of an employer, both as to what must be done and how it must be done, is an employee. Two of the unique characteristics of an employer–employee relationship are that the employer has the right to discharge the employee, and the employer supplies the employee with tools and a place to work (IRS Pub. No. 539).

If you have an employer–employee relationship, it makes no difference how it is described. It does not matter if the employee is called an employee, or a co-adventurer, agent, or independent contractor, nor does it matter whether the individual is employed full time or part time. Superintendents, managers, and other supervisory personnel are employees. Individuals are employees for FICA tax purposes if all the following conditions apply:

1. The service contract states or implies that almost all of the services are to be performed personally by them.
2. The investment in facilities used to perform services is not substantially that of the individual.
3. The services are performed on a continuing basis (IRS Pub. No. 539).

The amount to be withheld is figured from gross wages before any deductions are made for social security taxes, pension, and so forth. Ways of figuring withholding are contained in Circular E, provided by the IRS.

Corporate Employee: Even if you own most or all of the stock of a corporation, your income as an employee or officer of the corporation is not self-employment income.

Social Security Taxes: The Federal Insurance Contributions Act (FICA) provides for a federal system of old age, survivors, disability, and hospital insurance. The system is financed through social security taxes (FICA taxes).

Liability for Tax Withheld: You are required by law to deduct and withhold income tax and social security tax from the wages of employees, even if you do not collect them from your employees. If, for example, you deduct less than the correct tax from your employees' wages, you are still liable for the full amount of correct tax (IRS Pub. No. 539).

Payroll Taxes

Payroll tax costs for staff employees of a professional practice are the same, whether or not the practice is incorporated. The difference lies in payroll taxes on the principals themselves. To evaluate the difference, remember that taxes paid by the professional corporation are all deductible by the corporation, which in effect reduces their cost by the difference between the corporation's tax bracket and the principal's tax bracket. However, the incorporated professional pays unemployment tax and workers' compensation insurance, which is not required of unincorporated employers.

Estimated Tax

Estimated tax is the method used to pay tax on income that is not subject to withholding, which includes income from self-employment (i.e., sole proprietorship and partnerships), interest, capital gains, and so forth. You may also have to pay estimated tax if the amount withheld from your salary or other income is insufficient to meet your tax obligation. If your total tax paid through income tax, or self-employment, or through estimated tax payments is insufficient, you may be charged a penalty (IRS Pub. No. 505). Estimated tax is paid in four payment periods during the year; each period has a specific due date (April 15, June 15, September 15, January 15 the following year). Beginning in 1985, the estimated tax laws changed to deny previously allowed exceptions. Other changes seem imminent (Davis, Kinard, & Co., 1984).

Business Taxpayers

The IRS has an automatic data processing system to process returns of taxpayers. Central to this system is the taxpayer identification number, which is either a social security number or an employer identification number. The social security number is familiar to all of us.

Employer Identification Number: The EIN is a 9-digit number issued by the IRS. The EIN issued to a business will remain the same even when that business moves to another IRS district. Some individuals and most organizations and businesses need an employer identification number, even if they do not have employees. Everyone who pays wages must have an EIN; all partnerships, corporations, and trusts need an EIN. Sole proprietors must have an EIN if they have one or more employees. A nonprofit corporation, which receives income reported on an information return, also must have an EIN.

A new employer identification number is required if the form (corporation, sole proprietorship, partnership) changes or ownership of the business changes. For example, if one buys an existing business that one plans to operate as sole proprietorship, a new EIN is required.

Apply for an EIN with File Form SS-4, Application for Employer Identification Number, with the IRS Center for your area (see IRS Pub. No. 583). File the form in sufficient time to receive your EIN before it is necessary to file a return or statement or to make a tax deposit. Allow at least 4 weeks for receipt of this number. Penalties are imposed for failure to obtain or to use an employer identification number.

Records

The law does not require any particular type of records for tax purposes; records must be kept, however, for preparation of accurate tax returns. Pay only the amount of tax owed. In addition to ledger entries, it is advisable to keep any other records and dates that might be necessary to support entries in your books and on your tax and information returns. The form your business takes—sole proprietorship, partnership, corporation—affects the type of records that are necessary for federal tax purposes.

Capital Expenditures

Some costs incurred by a business in the course of a year are counted as part of the investment in the business. These investments must be ''capitalized'' rather than deducted, and are known as capital expenditures. Capital expenditures are distinguished from other costs. Generally, three kinds of costs must be capitalized; those related to the process of (1) establishing oneself in business; (2) purchasing business assets; and (3) making improvements.

You cannot directly deduct a capital expenditure. Usually you can recover the cost by subtracting it from income, one part at a time, over a number of years. This is done in the following ways:

1. *Depreciation:* used to recover capital expenditures for most tangible assets;
2. *Amortization:* used to recover only certain kinds of capital expenditures, such as some research costs and business start-up costs;
3. *Depletion:* used to recover the cost of an economic interest in natural resources; for example, lumber, minerals, other (see IRS Pub. No. 334).

Income Averaging

Beginning in 1984, income averaging laws changed. For tax returns that were due on April 15, 1985, income averaging was available only if the year's taxable income was greater than $3,000 plus 140 percent of the average of the 3 preceding years. This change narrows eligibility for income averaging and reduces its benefits for those who qualify.

Tax Audits

Preparing and filing a tax return is not necessarily the last step in determining one's tax bill for the year. Taxpayers must also know how to defend their own assessment of taxes due against a possible IRS audit.

The odds of being chosen for audit are fairly small. There is approximately a 10 percent risk of having an audit (*Guide to Private Practice*, 1984). Audits generally occur when one or more deductions is far above the average for one's income level; when a major deduction was claimed for something that is frequently reported in error; and when the return was randomly selected for audit. If an individual or company has been audited once, the chance of another audit is better than average. Statistics, however, become irrelevant when your own return is selected for audit. Some ways to prepare in case an audit is required include the following:

1. Prepare your tax return as if you were required to prove and defend each item it contained. Keep records, receipts, sales slips, vehicle maintenance slips, mileage charts, expense journals for trips, and anything else you can think of. Having check stubs, sales receipts, and bills to cover business charges is not enough, however. The IRS seems more interested in whether the money was spent for business-related purposes than in whether the money was spent at all.
2. Don't take the chance that you might avoid audit and risk padding your deductions or use questionable tax-saving devices.

If you are selected for an audit, let a tax consultant, such as an accountant, handle the entire audit procedure. The IRS agent will ask you to support your deductions, to verify that you have not omitted income, and to justify your claim for dependents. Providing the necessary records and documents will help validate your claims. An *office audit* is one in which the IRS agent works in his or her own office and asks the audited person to either send in data or to bring in his or her records. Provide only the information requested. Contact the auditing agent in advance to get permission to send specific documents rather than personally take them to the agent's office.

A *field audit* usually means the auditor will set up an appointment to visit your office. A professional often is audited both personally and professionally. In some instances, if an accountant maintains the records, the audit can be held at the accountant's office. The agent will spot-check records, ledgers, books, and documents to see how income and expenses were managed and may ask questions for clarification regarding certain items.

During the audit:

1. Keep answers factual and to the point;
2. Do not concede anything while the audit is in progress;
3. Avoid signing anything you do not completely understand;
4. Maintain a business-like approach (*Guide to Private Practice*, 1984, p.13).

At the conclusion of the audit, should the agent indicate that additional tax is owed, it would be wise to try to reach a compromise agreement on the amount and agree to pay. If you feel that amount is too high, or, that it is unfair, you may want to challenge the audit. Remember, you could spend months trying to justify your argument. You would probably want your accountant and attorney to help you prepare your appeal. Even if you win the appeal, you could spend more money on legal and accounting fees and in time lost from your practice than you would have had to pay originally. In addition, as a result of the appeal, your complete return could come under scrutiny, increasing the chances that the IRS would find other things to question.

TAX DEDUCTIONS AND FRINGE BENEFITS

We pay taxes to the federal government on the basis of our income. This income may be received in the form of cash, property, or services from numerous sources, including dividends, compensation for services, distributions of partnership or corporate holdings, profits, interest earned on savings, and other. Gross income to an individual or company is adjusted to allow for certain deductions to which the individual or company is entitled. Income tax is paid on the basis of the adjusted income. Everyone who pays taxes is interested in deducting all items allowed by law that will reduce the amount of income on which taxes must be paid.

Taxable income is figured by using a fixed accounting period and a specified accounting method. The accounting method is a set of rules used to decide when and how to record income and expenses, and how to prepare a profit and loss statement for the accounting period.

The same method must be used from year to year to figure taxable income.

Among the records necessary to support entries in the bookkeeping system (''the books'') are the following:

1. Inventory records in business in which the production, purchase, or sale of merchandise is an income-producing factor (probably applicable in some form to audiologists dispensing hearing aids) and;
2. Disbursement records to properly classify all expenditures as a current expense, a capital expenditure, or an improvement (IRS Tax Guide, No. 334).

The accounting methods that can be used to figure taxable income are (1) cash method; (2) accrual method; and (3) other methods that clearly show income, including a combination of (1) and (2), or other special methods.

Cash method of accounting is used by most individuals and many small businesses with no inventories. With the cash method, you include in your gross income all items of income actually received during the year. In other words, income is taxed when cash is received. Generally, expenses paid in advance are deductible in the year you actually pay them. There are certain exceptions, such as rent, interest, and so forth, which must be paid in the year to which they apply. The U.S. Treasury Department has proposed to do away with this method for all but the smallest businesses (Seidman & Seidman, 1985).

Accrual method is designed to match income with expenses for the correct year. Under the accrual method, all items of revenue are included in gross income in the year revenue is *earned*, regardless of whether *payment* is received in another tax year. All events that fix your right to receive the income must have happened, and you must be able to figure the amount with reasonable accuracy. In other words, you pay tax on revenue that has not yet been received. Business expenses are deducted when you become liable for them, whether or not you pay them in the same year. This system can present cash flow problems for service providers.

Some expenses incurred in the course of running a business or private practice are not allowable as deductions, but many are. It is the owner/practitioner's responsibility to know the difference. Some categories of deductible expenses include the following:

Employees' Pay

Salaries, wages, and other forms of pay to the employees may be deductible business expenses. The term ''employee'' includes a sole proprietor or partner. Employees' pay must meet these tests: (1) It must be ordinary and necessary, (2) it must be reasonable, and (3) it must be paid to the employee for services rendered.

Rent

Rent paid on office space or property that is used for the business or practice can be deducted. If the property has ever, or will ever, result in your receiving equity in or title to the property, then rent is not deductible. Rent on personal residence may not be allowable under current rules (see ''home-office'' section later in this chapter). Leased property may be deducted as rent, as well as taxes that must be paid to the lessor. Deduction of real estate taxes paid on leased property depends on the accounting method used:

1. *Cash Method:* You may only deduct taxes as additional rent for the tax year in which you pay them.
2. *Accrual Method:* You may deduct taxes as additional rent for the tax year in which you can determine that you have a liability and the amount of liability. This is usually set by state law and the lease agreement.

Improvements, Replacements, Repairs

What you spend to keep your office and practice in ordinary and efficient operating condition is deductible. If what you spend adds to the value of your property, or significantly increases its life, the cost is considered a capital expenditure and must be capitalized. Capital expenditures must be depreciated over time.

Costs of repairs, including labor and supplies, is deductible. Improvement, however, is usually considered a capital expenditure.

Depreciation

Many different kinds of property, tangible and intangible, can be depreciated, that is, taken as amortized deductions. Tangible property is any property that can be seen or touched, such as furniture, equipment, and buildings. Intangible property includes items such as copyrights or franchises.

Property is depreciable if (1) it is used in business or held for the production of income; (2) it has a determinable life, which must be longer than one year; and (3) it is something that wears out, becomes obsolete, loses value from natural causes, and so forth.

Bad Debts

If you cannot collect money owed to you, you have a ''bad debt.'' Generally, you can deduct the amount owed if there is a true creditor–debtor relationship between you and the person or organization who owes you the money. There must be a legal obligation to pay you a fixed sum of money, and you must realize a loss because of your inability to collect the money. You also must show that the debt is worthless and is not collectible. For example, bankruptcy on the part of the debtor is usually considered evidence that an unsecured debt is worthless. The deduction must be taken in the year the debt becomes worthless. It becomes worthless when it is determined that there is no chance of its being paid.

A bad debt deduction is possible only if there is an actual loss of money. A practitioner cannot deduct as bad debt money that is not collected from fees for services. The clinician, according to IRS, is not a creditor because services have no intrinsic monetary worth as does the extension of credit through loans or sales of products. Practitioners may consider unpaid bills a loss, but the IRS does not consider them deductible as a bad debt loss.

Travel Expenses

Travel expenses incurred in the conduct of business, or in the production or collection of income, are ordinarily deductible for tax purposes. The taxpayer must keep fairly precise records in order to ''prove'' that such expenses were ordinary and necessary expenses primarily for the purposes of business. Deductible expenses include (1) air, rail, and bus; (2) car expenses; (3) taxi fares; (4) meals and lodging while away from home (''away from home'' means *overnight*); (5) handling of luggage; (6) telephone; (7) tips; and (8) other charges incurred as a result of qualified travel.

Documentation is required for any expense of $25 or more. Keeping a daily record is the best source of proof, in addition to receipts; record amount paid and for what purpose, dates of departure and return, and the business reason for the trip. Travel to business or professional seminars or conventions must be documented in the same way as other travel expenses, but they should also specify the professional benefit or reason for attending and number of hours spent on business. The IRS recently reminded employers, including state agencies, that they must *report certain travel expenses paid to their employees as taxable income*. Specifically, employers must report travel reimbursement if employees are paid more than 20.5 cents per mile for that travel. If an employee travels more than 15,000 miles per year, taxes are due on any reimbursement over 11 cents per mile (Business Deductions, 1984).

Education Expenses

Usually any costs of education to maintain or improve skills as a professional are deductible. The educational costs incurred for the purpose of qualifying for licensure or certification are not deductible because they are considered to be necessary to enter the field. Other educational costs beyond that point are deductible. Educational expenses may include tuition, books, materials, trips that involve overnight stay, and expenses incurred from those trips, as long as the primary reason for the trip is business related.

This same documentation is necessary for foreign travel for the purpose of education, except the taxpayer must also show that the same educational experience could not have existed separate from its setting. In other words, it was reasonable and justifiable for the meeting or seminar to have been held in the specific foreign setting. Cruises are usually difficult to justify for educational or professional deductions. Deductions must be particularly well justified when (1) a spouse travels and attends the meeting; and (2) business is mixed with pleasure.

Documentation with complete records will be of help in maximizing the deductions.

Entertainment

Entertainment expenses may include the cost of furnishing food or beverages, a car, or motel to a business customer, or paying the costs of night club visits, hunting trips, and other. In order to be considered deductible, the expenses must be

1. Ordinary and necessary to the purpose of carrying on a business or for the production or collection of income. You must show a valid reason that some income or other benefit will be realized from the entertainment; that the principal reason for the entertainment was business; and what the relationship of the recipient was to the business as well as the identity of the recipient.
2. For entertainment conducted in a setting conducive to business, such as a quiet meal. A meal and drinks for generating good will in a night club may not be viewed as a setting conducive to business discussion. Having lunch with the same person over and over, so it appears that you are alternating in paying for nonbusiness lunches would also be suspect. Large deductions for a cocktail party or entertaining extravagantly at home might also arouse suspicion (Research Institute of America, 1984).

Social or athletic club dues might be considered deductible if the taxpayer uses the club more than 50 percent for business purposes. The portion of dues allowable by the IRS for entertainment is that which is directly related to the active conduct of business.

When an employee incurs unreimbursed expenses in carrying out his duties, the employer must make it clear that the expenses are part of the employee's job and both employee and employer may be required to prove that the expense was ordinary and necessary. This can be done by including an appropriate resolution in corporate minutes.

Deductions are not allowed for approximations or estimates, nor for expenses to the extent of extravagance. If travel and entertainment amounts are used for employee's or employer's personal expenses, the penalty can include a 50 percent civil fraud penalty in addition to supplementary tax payments.

Business Gifts

Business gifts may be deducted for no more than $25 per person during one tax year. A gift to a company, if not eventually intended for personal use of an individual, is not usually considered a gift. For a business gift deduction, record the cost, date, description, and business reason for each gift. Other payments or larger gifts to referral sources are usually considered kickbacks and are not deductible.

The $25 limit does not apply to

1. Any item costing less than $4 on which the giver's name is printed and which is one of a number of identical items distributed generally (pens, cases, matches, and so forth);
2. Signs, display racks, or other promotional material to be used on recipient's business office or premises;
3. Any tangible personal property awarded to employees because of outstanding service, productivity, and so forth.

Interest Expense

Interest is the charge made for the use of money. You may deduct all interest you pay or accrue during the tax year on a debt that is related to your practice. The interest must be on a debt for which you have a valid obligation to pay a fixed or determinable sum of money. To deduct the interest paid, you must be liable for its payment. For example, you may not deduct interest paid on a corporation's debt on your individual return.

If you borrow against your life insurance and use the proceeds for business purposes, you may take a business interest deduction. If you use the proceeds for a nonbusiness purpose, you may deduct interest only as an itemized deduction on Schedule A (Form 1040). Cost of insurance for your business or profession may be deducted as a business expense. You generally may not deduct the cost of life insurance. Premiums ordinarily are deductible in the tax year to which they apply.

You may not deduct premiums paid on a policy that reimburses you for earnings lost due to sickness or disability because the proceeds from the insurance are not income.

Home Offices

Recent changes in tax laws have resulted in more stringent regulations for offices in homes as an allowable tax deduction. A home office must: (1) be exclusively and regularly used for business; and (2) be the principal place of business, or a place where you see clients.

If client services are your primary revenue source, then you must see at least 20 percent of your clients in your home office in order to deduct use of the home office. This requirement holds regardless of your use of the home office for writing books, preparing seminars, studying, and so forth. Some advisors claim that earning a few thousand dollars in a home office would justify deduction of the home office, but use caution.

Automobiles

Many professionals have an automobile which is used primarily for business but partly for personal purposes. New deduction guidelines for automobiles limit the depreciation deduction and investment tax credit available for automobiles acquired for business use after June, 1984. If the automobile is used less than 100 percent for business, then depreciation and investment tax credit are reduced accordingly (Business Deductions, 1984).

The same 1984 tax act also tightened laws on record-keeping requirements for deductions involving business use of cars, computers, and other property. A few rules of thumb about use of automobiles for deductions include:

1. Travel to work from home and back is not an allowable deduction;
2. A log book must be kept in the car to record mileage to destinations travelled in the course of professional pursuits, or the percentage of the car's annual use for business-related mileage can be calculated and used for all car expenses;
3. Car use (business or personal car) is deductible if it is used for job-hunting in another city, driving to do charitable work, and so forth.

Fringe Benefits

Fringe benefits are those benefits provided for employees by employers that may not be taxable as income to the employees and that *may* be deductible for the employer who bestows them. Fringe benefits that fit these criteria and, therefore might be provided to employees in place of salary increases that would be fully taxed include:

1. Malpractice insurance premiums;
2. Professional dues;
3. Subscriptions to professional journals;
4. Reimbursement for certain regular expenses such as books, business cards, parking costs related to business trips;
5. All or part of the costs incurred in attending professional meetings;
6. Health or disability coverage; and
7. Retirement plans: Keogh for employers and employees, contributions to an IRA plan, any form of tax-sheltered contributions or profit-sharing plan; see accounting or investment firm or other advisor for choosing retirement plan (Seidman & Seidman, 1985).

It is important to stay abreast of legislative changes that affect the tax situation of a practice and its employees. For example, fringe benefits made available to employees in 1985 and thereafter are subject to income tax with certain exceptions. If subject to income tax, the employer will have to withhold payroll taxes and income tax even on non-cash benefits. Exceptions to taxable treatment include: (1) benefits provided by an employer at minimal cost; (2) certain employee discounts; (3) working condition benefits, such as use of demonstration cars by auto sales person; and (4) benefits of minimal dollar value.

Pensions for Professionals

Recent tax reforms have changed the rules on pension plans for many professionals.

Professional Corporations (PC) face the greatest level of changes. Their pension plans will provide less of a tax shelter for many professionals, will be less flexible, and will be more expensive in terms of benefits that must be provided for non-shareholders. In many cases, PCs may choose to dissolve rather than live under the new rules (Seidman & Seidman, 1985).

Self Employed Professionals who want to set up Keogh plans gained higher maximum tax deductions for pension contributions and more flexible plans. And as of 1984, Keogh plans are operating under the same rules as corporate retirement plans, with a few exceptions.

Individual Retirement Accounts remain basically as they have been for the past few years. In many cases, professionals who feel that other plans do not give them enough contributions will find that their IRA is becoming relatively more important in overall retirement planning.

Tax Reforms

Tax reforms that will cover many areas and take many years in evolving are on the verge of occurring. The primary changes affecting businesses and practices will probably include corporate tax rates, corporate dividends, cash methods of accounting (limited to certain types and sizes of businesses), and investment tax credits. Changes in tax rates that affect service professionals are very likely to occur (Seidman & Seidman, 1984).

An accountant or financial advisor should be consulted concerning tax planning, corporate tax rates, deferred income, and the cash method of accounting. Whether a professional practice is newly established or is well under way, tax reforms will have substantial impact.

Appendices

APPENDIX 11-1
TAX RESOURCES

HOW TO GET IRS FORMS AND PUBLICATIONS

Order federal tax forms and publications from the IRS Forms Distribution Center for your state. If you prefer, photocopy tax forms from reproducible copies kept at many public libraries. In addition, many libraries have reference sets of IRS publications that you can read or copy.

SMALL BUSINESS TAX WORKSHOPS

The Internal Revenue Service offers tax workshops applicable to small businesses and professional practices. These workshops are designed to provide an understanding of federal taxes, explain business taxes, tax benefits, and employer tax responsibilities. As soon as federal tax reforms are enacted, these workshops include discussion of the changes and their impact on various forms of business (IRS Pub. No. 1057).

APPENDIX 11–2
TAX CALENDAR*

Some federal taxes for which a sole proprietor, a corporation, or a partnership may be liable are listed below.

Organizational Structure	Form of Taxation	IRS Form	Due Date
Sole proprietor	Income tax	1040 (Schedule C)	Same day as Form 1040
Individual who is a partner or Sub-chapter S corporation shareholder		1040	15th day of 4th month after end of tax year
Corporation		1120	15th day of 3rd month after end of tax year
Sub-chapter S corporation		1120S	15th day of 3rd month after end of tax year
Sole proprietor, or individual who is a partner	Self-employment tax	1040 (Schedule SE)	Same day as Form 1040
Sole proprietor, or individual who is a partner or Sub-chapter S corporation shareholder	Estimated tax	1040 (Schedule ES)	15th day of 4th, 6th, and 9th month of tax year, and 15th day of the 1st month after the end of the tax year
Corporation	Estimated tax	1120W	15th day of 4th, 6th, 9th, and 12th month of tax year
Partnership	Annual return of income	1065	15th day of 4th month after end of tax year

*From *Your Private Practice*, Marshall, Lord, & Johnston, 1982, and IRS Publication No. 509, 1984.

Organizational Structure	Form of Taxation	IRS Form	Due Date
Sole proprietor, corporation, Subchapter S corporation, or partnership	FICA tax and withholding of income tax	941 501 (to make deposits)	January 31 April 30 July 31 October 31
	Providing information on FICA tax and the withholding of income tax	W-2 (to employee)	January 31
		W-3 (to the Social Security Administration)	Last day of February
Sole proprietor, corporation, Subchapter S corporation, or partnership	FUTA tax	940	January 31
		508 (to make deposits)	April 30 July 31 October 31 January 31 (But only if the liability for unpaid tax is more than $100)

Chapter 12

Responsibility and Liability

LEGAL AND ETHICAL PROFESSIONAL ISSUES

It is clear to most members of a profession that they are charged to uphold their professional code of ethics and to offer information about those who fail to do so. Less clear are the distinctions between ethical behavior and prudence and between ethical behavior and observing rules of conventional propriety. All are guidelines for regulating behavior; an *ethical code*, however, is a guideline specifically relating to professional activity. Unethical behavior usually is considered to be that behavior which causes harm or violates some principle without being justifiable on the basis of doing good or upholding another principle. Ethical behavior is based on ethical reasoning which involves the application of one's principles to one's actions in consideration of the consequences of those actions (Haas, 1983, p. 320). *Prudence* is sensible, sane, judicious behavior, but one who is prudent need not give consideration to the consequences that one's behavior may have for others. *Conventional behavior*, or *politeness*, only accounts for those consequences to others that are of a social nature, rather than for consequences for the welfare of others. As Haas (1983) indicates, it is possible for an act to be ethical, prudent, and polite, all at the same time; for an act to be ethical but both impolite and imprudent; and for an act to be unethical, yet prudent and polite (pp. 320–321).

It is easier to describe the differences between unethical behavior and illegal behavior. For example, negligence, malpractice, and fraud are legal issues, resulting in legal investigation and penalties. While illegal behavior may also be unethical, certain unethical issues are not illegal in the eyes of the courts. Violations of the law can involve fines, financial settlements, imprisonment, and other penalties. Violations of the code of ethics that is established by professions apply only to members of those professions who voluntarily subscribe to that code.

Technical Versus Ethical Issues

One way professional actions can be judged ethical or unethical is on technical grounds. For example, suppose a clinician attempted a certain kind of approach designed to change speech or language behavior. Should this approach fail, it could be said that the professional made a mistake, although the professional would not necessarily have acted unethically. Ethical questions more often concern questions about the goal itself, rather than whether the goal was accomplished. Each professional providing services is an autonomous individual who also is a member of the profession. This fact adds another dimension to ethical considerations. The actions of any professional affect not only that professional, but other holders of the same professional role. Actions of a professional are based on an explicit promise to clients as well as to society. Many of the benefits bestowed upon professionals, such as respect and prestige, are based upon certain expectations from society and from colleagues that they will use whatever power, knowledge, and skill they possess for the benefit of their clients and society in general.

Professional Morality

Inherent to understanding the spirit underlying ethical regulations are certain aspects of professional morality. These include *professional responsibility, integrity,* and *competence.* Professional responsibility assumes that each professional is the creator of his or her own actions and is a causal agent in the results of those actions. Professionals, regardless of work setting, cannot hide behind the fact that they were instructed to act in certain ways or paid to perform certain actions. Any services delivered must be provided with consideration for the impact of those services on the client. Professional morality assumes a value system that controls professional behavior and includes professional honesty and values. Professional values must center on a total concern for enhancement of the client's well-being and the extension of every effort on behalf of the client. Any exploitation of the client for personal gain on the part of the professional is unethical. The principle of ''let the buyer beware,'' fairly common to the open market place, is not permissible in professional services, where clients are incapable of accurately evaluating the knowledge, skill, product, or promises of the professional.

An important aspect of professional responsibility is the provision of competent service. Assessment of competence is one not easily made, although professional associations and agencies, as well as professional preparation programs, spend a great deal of time pursuing the issue and writing guidelines for its achievement. All self-regulating professions have criteria for the professional qualifications necessary for certification and/or licensing. When a professional delegates duties that are unethical or irresponsible in nature to a nonlicensed or noncertified employee, responsibility for the unethical action remains that of the licensed professional.

Delivery of human services has many features that distinguish it from most other human relationships. Because the entire interaction is designed and executed with the intention of advancing the well being of the client, there are numerous aspects of the relationship that are ethically prescribed and/or legally regulated. Many, but not all, of the prescriptions and regulations are designed to protect the consumer. Some critical dimensions within human services professions that have potential legal implications are informed consent, privileged communication, the duty to warn, and professional malpractice. It is the professional's responsibility to understand these dimensions and to act appropriately with that understanding.

Informed Consent

The consent to receive human services creates a composite of diverse legal issues. For example, court decisions have upheld an individual's *right to refuse treatment* as a constitutional right. Because many issues are interpreted in the light of circumstances and without definitive legal guidelines, professionals delivering human services frequently are left with their good intentions as the only safeguard against legal liability.

The principle of informed consent traditionally is defined in terms of the physician–patient relationship, which is ''one in which the patient has received sufficient information from his physician concerning the health care proposed, its incumbent risks, and acceptable alternatives to that care in order that the patient can participate and make an intelligent, rational decision about himself'' (Hemelt & Mackert, 1978, p. 94). This principle is designed to honor an individual's ''right to know when you're sick, what is happening to you, how it is happening, by whom, and under what conditions of risk'' (Parry, 1981, p. 537). The giving of consent becomes an essential condition for advancement in many therapeutic interactions. The patient or client takes responsibility for his well-being, even though he may be under the care and control of a professional.

In some situations, professionals object to the principle of informed consent on the basis that clients need not have access to all information and are not prepared to be involved in choice of treatment. In most professions, however, it seems prudent to ensure that the recipient of services understands and consents to treatment. Any professional who acts without informed consent of the client must understand the potential for disciplinary action for unethical and/or illegal conduct.

Margolin (1982, p. 794) provides a set of guidelines for obtaining informed consent. The potential client should be informed of the following:

1. Recommended procedures and their purpose;
2. The role of the person who is providing treatment and the personal qualifications of that person;
3. The expected or predicted discomforts or risks associated with treatment;
4. Projected and associated benefits of treatment;
5. Alternatives to treatment that might be of similar benefit;
6. The fact that any questions about procedures will be answered to the best of the professional's ability;
7. The fact that the person can withdraw consent, pursue other treatment, or discontinue participation at any time.

In most situations, the professionals in speech-language pathology/audiology need only discuss the issues and recommendations inherent to the proposed intervention. Discussion should be recorded and a statement of informed consent obtained from the client. In the event of significant modifications in the course of intervention, the client should again be informed of the necessary changes. Certainly, the professional should be aware of the amount of influence exerted over a client, particularly in times of crisis when the client is not likely to remember or understand what the professional is saying. The professional should make sure the client has been properly safeguarded in the eyes of the law and appropriate measures of self-protection have been exercised before proceeding with intervention.

Confidentiality and Privileged Communication

Confidentiality and privileged communication are inherent in any human services interaction. Inappropriate disclosure of confidential information could be the basis for professional disciplinary or legal action (Woody, 1984). *Confidentiality* is endorsed by the constitutional right to privacy and is an ordinary expectation in professional–client interaction. Confidentiality covers the legal and ethical responsibility of a professional not to volunteer any information about a client without the client's specific consent. Confidentiality, with its expectancy for privacy, does not always attain the level of privileged communication. *Privileged communication* is a statutory declaration of a right to keep certain information from legal proceedings as long as that information conforms to the reasonable basis of privacy and confidentiality (Woody, 1984). It should be noted that the professional does not have privileged communication; the client is the one with that privilege. The primary holder of privileged communication is the one whose immediate interests are harmed if disclosure occurs (Haas, 1983). The client is the communicator, and it is the communicator that the law seeks to protect and encourage. If the client is suing the professional, the privileged communication surrounding the relationship disappears. The professional is free to communicate anything to a source relevant to legal action (Woody, 1984). The professional is also free to set aside privileged communication if there is a substantial threat to the safety and welfare of the client and/or others. This responsibility of setting aside privileged communication in the light of dangerous circumstances is called the *"duty to warn."*

Duty to Warn

Some statutes specify that professionals must notify health or law enforcement authorities of clients who have contagious diseases, who are drug dependent, or who are involved in child abuse. Those statutes usually include a stated immunity from legal action for any professional who breaches confidentiality in order to comply with them. Some statutes include a penalty for those who do not comply with the reporting requirement. If a professional provides information because of statutory requirement or court order, then that professional is removed from any kind of liability for alleged breach of confidentiality that otherwise might be brought against him or her in terms of suits charging defamation, invasion of privacy, and so forth. In slander or liable suits, defamatory language (language that blemishes the client's honesty, integrity, virtues, sanity, or other personal characteristics and that could potentially create damage) is sometimes alleged (Woody, 1984). The defamatory statement must go to a third person (known as "publication") and be made either intentionally or negligently. Usually a defamation suit must establish that the person suffered damages, and sometimes these damages have to be computed as out-of-pocket loss. Damage to reputation, standing in the community, and so forth may be viewed by the court as damages and transposed into a dollar figure. In addition to legal distinctions regarding breach of confidence that results in defamation, codes of ethics for many human services professionals include numerous restrictions regarding such statements. The best rule of thumb is never talk about clients except in those situations or contexts associated with professional services and with helpful intent. Professionals are expected to exercise a reasonable degree of skill, knowledge, and care ordinarily exercised by members of that profession under similar circumstances. Therapists are not required to disclose a confidence unless such disclosure is necessary to avert danger to someone.

When third-party payments for health services become a factor, the client has little reason to expect privacy. When a client submits a bill for services to an insurance company, there is an implicit or explicit waiver of confidentiality and privileged communication. Some insurance companies require explicit waiver of confidentiality; some employers also require such waivers by virtue of their paying all or part of health insurance costs, requiring a right to information that otherwise would be privileged.

Confidentiality and Written Records

The professional should record any information about a client with full knowledge that records may be open to inspection by others, including those in a court of law. Statements that are potentially damaging should be avoided in any kind of record keeping. Current trend in public policy is that justice supercedes personal privacy. The professional may have to yield any information considered appropriate by a court, whether through a waiver signed by a client, subpoena issued to the professional through a court order, or various others means (Woody, 1984). A professional usually cannot refuse to cooperate with a subpoena on the grounds that the intervention process will be interrupted or affected destructively by any statement from the therapist. If a professional issues a reasoned request to withhold certain information in a client's best interest, and the court rules in opposition to this request, then the professional who does not finally yield requested information is potentially in contempt of court. Although some professionals have succeeded in deliberately withholding confidential information against court requests, it seems advisable for a professional to be prudent in maintaining any written information regarding a client. It would also be wise to engage an attorney when one's choice seems to be between contempt of court or a violation of confidence.

Some courts have held that if a client wants all records destroyed (in order to avoid providing information to an opponent in approaching legal action), the professional does not have to comply with the demand. In fact, the professional could be charged with purposefully destroying evidence and could incur personal liability, (i.e., if the records were later needed as defense in a malpractice action brought by the client against another professional).

When a court subpoenas records, they become part of the court record. Any professional called for deposition or court appearance should have at least one set of duplicates of all materials for the court. The professional keeps all original records to avoid having to copy them later from court records. The admission of duplicates requires only that the professional certify that the duplicates are, in fact, true copies of the originals (Woody, 1984).

Each release of information obtained from a client in the course of a professional–client relationship should be preceded by a signed document specifying the information that is to be released and the recipient of that information. Even when written consent is obtained, disclosure of any confidential information with which a client entrusts a professional should be done judiciously. Confidential information to which professionals have access, frequently is associated with strong emotions including shame, guilt, or feelings of stigma at receiving professional services. Every client has the right to expect protection from invasion of privacy in any professional interaction. Sometimes professionals are tempted to bend professional and personal ethics by mentioning important clients or discussing intriguing disorders in social situations. The professional should remember that potential repercussions of such conversations can be more powerful than any positive affects. As Flower points out (1984, p. 253) our tendency in the profession to use individuals with communication disorders in research and teaching, our tolerance for inadequately trained personnel, and other earmarks of a profession so immature, sometimes lead to the neglect of our clients' best interests. Based on the basic human rights of clients receiving services, Flower suggests a Client Bill of Rights for consumers of speech-language pathology/audiology services (see Appendix 12–2).

Invasion of Privacy

A court action that alleges invasion of privacy may be brought against a person if a picture of a client is used for commercial advantage without expressed permission from that person or if the use of the client's picture or name intrudes into the client's personal affairs, makes public disclosures of private facts about the client, and so forth.

A license to practice could be revoked if a breach of confidentiality is proven to be willful or malicious in a court of law. Professional associations can impose sanctions such as a censure made before the total membership, or the removal of certification, licensure, membership, and so forth. In most situations loss of credibility suffered by the professional is by far the most damaging. When this professional's credibility has been questioned, even when innocent of any legal wrong doing, he or she may be required to engage in a costly defense of his or her professional position.

Professional Malpractice

Professionals, regardless of discipline, are to be held accountable for the quality of their services. Professional liability, or malpractice, may be held against a practitioner if negligent or otherwise improper or unacceptable professional actions result in harmful or damaging effects and may encompass inferior skill or immoral conduct by the professional. It is typical to claim the use of ''customary practices'' or ''standard of care'' of the profession as sufficient to determine appropriateness of behavior. Usually in order for malpractice to be proven, a professional relationship must have existed. In other words direct delivery of services must have occurred from professional to client, and the professional must have acted in an inappropriate manner, and damages from that inappropriate action must have resulted (Wright, 1981). A court may hold a professional to be negligent when that professional ''fails to do something a reasonable and prudent professional would do, or when that professional does something that a reasonable and prudent professional would not do'' (Flower, 1984, p. 261).

Malpractice is a breach of professional responsibility; the foundation for legal action is a violation of an established standard of care for the particular professional service with resulting damage to a client (Woody, 1984). The responsibility, discussed by Woody, is the ''duty of care.'' In both professional and private life, creation of reasonable risk of injury to another person is not permissible. In professional affairs, as in personal matters, the basic question is ''what would a reasonable person do in this situation?'' (Woody, 1984, p. 393). The practitioner is not expected to be superior, but to exercise the same judgment and same level of skills and knowledge as would another professional of the same discipline who is in good standing. Although many of the standards for conduct for professional practice come from analyses of the medical profession, many principles governing professional actions may apply with similar force to malpractice claims alleged against any other professional.

According to Woody, some professionals hold that if they practice within a discrete theoretical framework (i.e., Gestalt therapy), only *that* theory and its tenets should determine what is acceptable, not the theory or tenets of another school. A ''school'' is one recognized with definite principles that represents a line of thought of (at least) a respectable minority of the profession. Although many professionals seek legal protection behind the postulates of a particular theory or school, Woody (1984), Prosser (1971), and others are of the current opinion that it is unlikely that a professional dealing in human services would be able to use that as the higher solitary defense for an action that was considered to be inferior, unnecessary, or injurious.

Over time, the standard of care for practitioners has been based on what other practitioners in the same professional and geographical community would do under the same circumstances. This is still an important frame of reference, although nationwide certification and licensing programs tend to be moving toward a national standard, particularly with regard to certain specialties. That is, a professional in a human services area, who claims to be a specialist in a particular area, is more likely to have national standards imposed on his or her practice than one who is not declared to be a specialist in a particular discipline. This seems to be the case regardless of whether the professional is a member of the association that promulgates those standards.

According to Woody (1984), informed consent is the best defense against charges of malpractice. If the client has been adequately informed of procedures and has knowingly consented to those procedures, which have been properly administered, the professional is protected.

Malpractice accusations do not occur only when there is malicious abuse of the client. Certainly there are some malpractice actions that are brought before the public by the media because of the nature of the danger or abuse that was inflicted on the client. But other instances of malpractice have arisen from a client's misunderstanding and/or distortion of information, advice, or recommendations from the therapist. Psychologists and psychiatrists are most vulnerable to such accusations because of the personal and intimate level of interaction with their clients. However, many speech-language pathologists/audiologists are in frequent and close contact with small children, and a few words from a child to a parent about ''what happened'' in therapy could lead to damaging accusations. Allegations of sexual misconduct, fondling, and other impugning of a professional's behavior with a client have resulted in public investigations or lawsuits against professionals in almost every child-related health care service.

The professional should realize his or her vulnerability to being sued, regardless of the setting, and take measures against such possibilities. Woody (1984) advises that the prudent human services professional should

1. Have a clear delineation of the standard of care applicable to his or her services;
2. Adopt procedures to ensure that services are reasonably tailored to the needs of each client and are consonant with the standards of care;
3. Maintain a system by which clients are informed about and consent to professional intervention;
4. Consistently exercise safeguards against any knowing or inadvertent deviations from any real or imagined breaches of established standards of care.

Human services professionals must function with the endorsement of society and public policy that imposes legal sanctions. Regardless of the extent of professional self-regulation, public policy and legal sanction will continue to be justified by the court and applied by the public to professional conduct. Content of professional conduct is far ranging and encompasses every facet of service delivery.

Referrals

Most malpractice claims involving speech-language pathologists/audiologists also involve members of other professions. Clearly it is the responsibility of any non-medical service provider to refer any client for medical attention when it is appropriate. When a client is referred by a physician, it is the responsibility of the professional receiving the referral to maintain communication with the physician, apprising him or her of the condition of the client. Malpractice actions may depend on whether the nonphysician, the physician, or the health care facility has liability for the act involved. Some malpractice cases against physicians concentrate on the fact that the physician may have failed to refer the patient to a specialist or to advise the patient that such a specialist was available (Downey, 1982). In the instance of any referral from a speech-language pathologist/audiologist to another professional, the client should be fully apprised of the reason for referral and the relationship of the referring professional to the other professional. The credentials of the therapist or professional to whom the client is referred should be discussed. For example, if a practitioner hired a professional of another discipline and referred a client, the referring professional may incur problems with the client, if that client has not been made aware of the reason for referral. If a practitioner gives clients to an employee who is not licensed or who is a paraprofessional without first informing the client of this fact, problems could also ensue.

If a professional becomes involved in allegations against another professional, it is necessary to provide evidence that is accurate and objective. Flower (1984, p. 263) suggests guidelines for appropriate behavior in such situations, including the following:

1. Never criticize another professional in the presence of a client. When differences of opinion are obvious, they should be clearly identified as differences of opinion, not as reflections on the competence of another professional.
2. When a client seems to be receiving or to have received services that may reflect on the competence of another professional, encourage the client to seek a second opinion from another member of the same profession. Enter the recommendation in the client's record. In the final analysis, the competence of any professional is best assessed by a member of that same profession.
3. When reporting, either orally or in writing, about clients or other professionals in litigenous circumstances, include only factual material and observations that are clearly within areas of primary professional expertise. Be particularly wary of attributing causes to observed behaviors unless there is unequivocal evidence of direct cause–effect relationships.
4. Be wary of becoming a client's advocate in instances of alleged malpractice. A professional should be dedicated to ensuring that all salient facts are available that may facilitate a just disposition of whatever is at issue. However, his or her participation must always be as an impartial expert, rather than as an advocate.

Advertising and Public Information

Professionals usually seek to promote public image and awareness of the profession, as well as to increase public understanding of problems served by that profession. In questions regarding ethics of advertising, however, the issue usually involves specific marketing efforts by professionals wishing to encourage more people to seek their services. Advertising, in many senses, is permissible and even acceptable, although some states still impose restrictions on solicitation by professionals. Because of the public's inability to evaluate the quality of professional services or products, potential consumers do expect different conduct from professionals than they do from other advertising enterprises. Many professionals are indicating a tendency to avoid referring to other professionals who market their practices too vigorously. Whatever the effort is in promotion or marketing, any professional should adhere strictly to the highest standards of professional conduct. More directly, this involves the avoidance of misrepresentation of training, professional competence, and professional services and products. It also requires that the professional not promote commercial enterprises that mislead or limit services to persons who might be served professionally (Code of Ethics, ASHA, 1981). Litigation currently involves controversies over appropriate use of titles. For example, use of the term *audiologist* is continuing to be a matter of appeal before the United States Patent and Trade Mark Board of Appeals. The National Hearing-Aid Society is continuing its efforts to use the term *audiologist*; part of the audiologists' contention, as in other cases respecting the use of professional titles, is the extent to which the public may be mislead regarding qualifications of the advertiser using the term (Downy, 1982, pp. 13–14).

Any marketing effort that in the judgment of other professionals, as well as the public, provides accurate information representative of quality professional services or products will not be the target of malpractice allegations.

Fees

It is not public practice to sue professionals for exhorbitant fees—were that the case, there might be a dearth of doctors and lawyers. There are numerous instances, however, of bad feelings and threatened lawsuits when fees and fee arrangements were misunderstood, misrepresented, or third-party reimbursement did not proceed as expected by any of the parties involved. Allegations of fraud have been made against professionals who have misrepresented a product or a service, or have guaranteed results based on payment of fees. Other disputes over fees have arisen between client and professionals where an enforceable contract did not exist from the outset of the service provision or in situations in which the client failed to pay for services they agreed to receive for payment. Some malpractice claims involve allegations of breach of contract when the client feels that a specific offer or promise of accomplishment has been presented by a professional following which the client pays or agrees to pay for the promised service.

It is almost impossible to make a legal claim against third-party insurers if they refuse to pay for certain kinds of intervention or if they refuse to pay full fees-for-services. The practitioner usually has no contract with third-party insurers and, therefore, no right to bring claims against them. The provider has the contract with the client for fees; in which case, legal action against the client is possible. The exception is when the provider has signed an agreement with an agency or program to accept their reimbursement as full fee. In those situations the provider is bound by rules and interpretations of the paying agency. Many practitioners charge insurance companies, as well as the clients, for missed sessions and extended telephone consultations. There is no legal reason not to do this, although some insurance companies will not reimburse for these claims.

Fee splitting is one area in which professionals find it remarkably easy to stumble into trouble. For example, some clinicians have reimbursed their supervisors for overseeing their work as practitioner in a new practice or as an interning practitioner. The form that reimbursement often takes is a percentage of fees collected for supervised work. This practice is convenient, although unacceptable. It is considered fee splitting, just as it is considered fee splitting when practitioners give referral sources a certain percentage of income realized from referrals.

Price fixing, a violation of the Sherman Anti-Trust Act, usually refers to an agreement among competitors establishing a common price or system for setting the price of their products. This term can also encompass agreements among competitors regarding prices that they will pay for products which they all must purchase. In the human services area, accusations of price fixing have been directed toward Relative Value Scales, in which various professional associations have provided suggested charges for various services. Relative value scales could influence pricing mechanisms and actual cost of services, forcing conformity to the relative charges suggested by the schedules. Most attempts by associations to develop relative value scales have been discouraged on legal grounds, although many such efforts to establish relative value scales have been for the purpose of enhancing the professional's interaction with insurance companies. Professionals should seek legal advice when any issues regarding relative value scales or other possible price fixing arrangements occur.

Dispensing

When a professional engages in the dispensing of products, legal and ethical scrutiny sharpens. The professional who dispenses products becomes, in the eyes of the law, a retailer and is subject to commercial regulations. This dilemma is not new for many professionals. Veterinarians, physicians, dentists, physical therapists, and occupational therapists have been involved for years in dispensing various aids, appliances, and pharmaceuticals as part of their professional services. The dispensing of hearing aids by members of the profession, as well as the expanding number of marketed books, tests, augmentative communication devices, intervention programs, and test materials, now place speech-language pathologists/audiologists in the same role as any other professional who provides services that are related to sale of products.

The Federal Trade Commission, as well as the Food and Drug Administration, have been involved in the development of regulations relating to dispensing and sale of hearing aids. Specific FDA regulations regarding hearing-aid sales pertain to conditions of sale and labeling requirements. Instructional information also is required with sale of the aid regarding its use, care, repair, and its association with a rehabilitative program.

Self-Regulated or Self-Interested

One criticism levied at professionals by the public is that self-regulation in terms of licensing and certification are usually monitored and enforced by boards composed of members of the same profession. These board members are faced with potential conflicts of interest. The regulations they enforce and interpret could serve in their own professional interests. In the opinion of some (Bierig, 1983), professions do not rigorously maintain self-regulation and do not eliminate professionals from practice who abuse, neglect, or otherwise do gross disservice to their clients.

Allegations that self-regulation efforts are self-serving and not in the public interest have caused some federal agencies to be involved in certain aspects of professional regulation. For example, certain activities of the Federal Trade Commission address issues related to raising professional standards, thus reducing competition among professionals. Some states require public representation on licensing boards, and some state have removed disciplinary authority from licensure boards, although the licensure boards remain responsible for investigating complaints and for making recommendations. Many in the legal system continue to endorse professional self-regulation and permit professionals to confront inferior, unnecessary, or injurious practices within their own profession without fear of imposition of antitrust liability. Clearly professionals need to be unrelenting in the regulation of their own professional practices.

All practitioners, whether in public or private practice, should be well acquainted with the law, as well as with the profession's code of ethics. Codes of ethics and legal requirements change from time to time. Practitioners must stay as current with ethical and legal principles as they do with professional content and technology.

Part of the responsibility of a self-regulating, autonomous profession is not just safeguarding client welfare, but safeguarding the welfare of the profession against inappropriate professional behaviors. Among these inappropriate behaviors are the following:

1. Failure to maintain professional propriety in one's own practice;
2. Failure to inform appropriate regulating bodies of the profession of ethical or legal violations by other members of the profession; and
3. Failure to maintain professional expertise.

Staying Abreast Professionally

Whether or not professional regulations at state or national levels require continuing education, professional propriety demands continuation of professional knowledge and development. Technological changes, medical findings, and shifts in theory and practice within the field force even the least conscientious professional to seek current information.

Each member of the profession must decide for himself or herself what is the most efficient and preferred means of keeping abreast of professional advances. Some of the methods include reading professional journals, attending professional meetings, buying books, renting or buying audiotapes or videotapes, pursuing personally-designed study programs, and so forth. It is no longer necessary to leave one's home to become current in the profession. Some journals are designed specifically for independent and small group study, and computer software programs and terminal hookups provide excellent means of supplementing traditional lecture presentations. Sometimes professionals prefer to combine continuing education study with travel in various countries, visiting professional institutions, clinics, and other service delivery facilities. In addition to fulfilling one's professional responsibilities, many continuing education projects can be deducted from income tax.

RECOMMENDATIONS FOR AVOIDING TROUBLE

Whatever the basis for professional conduct, the best way to minimize allegations of unethical or illegal practice is to avoid having them occur in the first place. A major concern of professionals is what defensive steps can be taken to minimize exposure to such allegations. Some recommendations for avoiding trouble summarized from Flower (1984), Foonberg (1984), Haas (1983), and Woody (1984) include the following:

1. Know the law. Read regulations governing practice in the state where you see clients. Remember that state laws vary widely, and laws within states vary from legislative session to legislative session. Part of keeping up with the law is keeping up with important court judgements. Many laws are written very broadly, and the impact derives from judges' rulings in court cases.
2. Know the code of ethics in your professional association. Not only does a code of ethics usually provide a guide for professional behavior, but it also provides information about legal boundaries. Many state's codes of ethics are tied to the licensing law.

3. Know your own values.
4. Develop clear contracts. This pertains to consultations, employment, and service delivery to clients. All parties involved have an understanding in writing of the arrangement, including fees, fee schedules, and other important agreements regarding the service delivery process.
5. Maintain communication with the client and the family. Inform them of recommendations and changes in the original intervention program. Be sure to obtain written permission from clients and/or families for any information sent regarding them.
6. Maintain communication with referral sources. Acknowledge referrals and contact them occasionally by letter or telephone regarding referrals. When possible, make referrals back to them.
7. Never promise recovery or guarantee results to a referring agent, to a family, or to a client. Don't depend on legal privilege. Remember the distinction between confidentiality and privilege. Privilege is the client's right to keep a court from requiring testimony by a professional. Since it is the client's right, the client can waive it. Confidentiality is the requirement that a therapist not divulge information without the client's release.
8. Inform clients of their rights. In some states clients have the right of access to their personal records in public facilities. This has yet to be tested in some states in terms of private facilities. In some states the clinician must release information to parents if the child is below a certain age.
9. Know which clients not to accept, as well as which clients to accept. For example, if you are the second, third, or fourth professional who has been consulted about a client's problem, or asked to ''give *real* help this time,'' the problem could be with the client or family attitude. The problem could be irreversible, the clients could be nonpayers, the family may be extremely difficult to work with or may tend to refute or fail to take professional advice.

   Some clients are high risks for suing a professional and can be identified by their constant expression of dissatisfaction, resistance to intervention, nonpayment of bills, notes of dissatisfaction to the professional, and word of mouth from other professionals about dissatisfaction expressed by a client.

   A high risk client also is one who has been extremely critical of previous treatment and previous services from other professionals, and has unrealistically high expectations of therapeutic gain. If the professional suspects that the high-risk client is indeed at hand, then steps should be taken to alter the situation, either by changing the conditions under which the client is seen, referring the client to another professional, contacting a lawyer, or selecting other options before litigation is indeed put into action by the client.

10. Know which times not to give advice. For example, beware of the potential client who will not come into the office for an appointment but pumps for advice or opinion over the telephone. Some unseen potential clients, and some old clients who refuse to come in and pay for a face to face discussion, have a tendency to request free advice about an unseen client. In addition to economic reasons for not doing a telephone sight-unseen conference are the reasons of ethical and legal responsibility of the practitioner. When a professional has not seen a client for a long time, has not seen the client at all, or responds to ''theoretical'' questions, the outcome can be disastrous. Be firm in these

situations, and indicate that the client must be seen and an appropriate conference held before decisions and recommendations can be made.

11. Do not give professional advice in social situations. Remember that professional talk is not cocktail conversation. In social situations it is not unusual for professionals to be approached regarding their specialty and asked to ''tell me about my speech.'' When, and if, this happens, the only appropriate response is for the professional to say, ''If you're serious, we can talk about this in my office. Call me, and we'll set up an appointment.'' The reasons for this approach are numerous and probably obvious. But the situation is tempting, particularly when one's professional and social appearance can be enhanced by showing professional expertise to social acquaintances.

12. Do not practice beyond your professional competence. Any professional who holds himself as an expert in a specialty incurs greater ethical and legal obligations.

13. Practice office safety. Some charges of malpractice result from the use of faulty instruments, materials, or carelessness in the intervention process, particularly with young children. Maintain the office, equipment, and furniture to a reasonable degree, leaving nothing out that might pose a hazard to clients. Do not allow children to be alone in the waiting room. Make sure dangerous objects are not within reach of children.

14. Only treat minors with parental consent. In treatment of minors, waiver of privilege must come from the parent or guardian.

15. Keep careful records. Document contacts with and on behalf of the client, even if the notes are summaries. Keep all records as though they were about to be subpoenaed.

16. Follow through with each client. In some instances a professional may not accept a client for treatment, or a client may be unable to accept treatment. There are many reasons for not accepting a client for treatment, but once intervention is begun, the client should not be abandoned by the practitioner. If the practitioner makes a referral of the client to another professional in lieu of seeing that client, a follow-up should be done in order to insure that contact was made and that the client is now in other professional's hands.

17. Keep a record of client termination of therapy against the recommendations of the professional. When a client terminates therapy abruptly, it is important to schedule a conference with the client, discuss reasons for the termination, record the session and notes if appropriate, and suggest continued therapy with another therapist. If a conference is not possible, send a letter to the client's last known address stating that you understand he is terminating therapy and that you recommend this be pursued either with you or another clinician.

18. Be careful about substitute therapists, paraprofessionals, and ''giving away'' clients to employee clinicians. Make certain that the client understands reasons for substitutions of clinicians, qualifications of employees, and referrals to other professionals. Many clients become quite unhappy, as do referral sources, if a practitioner abruptly and without explanation places another clinician in charge of the client's intervention program. Some clients go to a particular practice because of a particular practitioner and expect that that practitioner

will be the one seeing the client for the duration of the intervention program. If for some reason this is not to be the case, whether on a temporary or permanent basis, clear explanation should be given to the client and to the referral source and consent obtained for the change of practitioner.

Malpractice risks are slight if a professional is reasonable. ''Best professional judgment'' and ''common and appropriate practice'' are usually the best guidelines in the face of any decision regarding professional conduct. Courts rarely award damages for honest mistakes. Courts are aware that dealing with human beings and their problems is a variable and complex task that requires the best available judgement of a competent professional.

Demands for preparing students on the highest level must be met in order to establish the profession as one that beyond a doubt has the highest quality professionals who can rely upon their decisions, act with authority, and interact on an equal basis with other human service professionals. Recent legislation indicates that the trend is clearly to expansion of nonphysician health care. In light of that fact and the general public's growing awareness of available services, our responsibility increases for preparing the highest quality professional.

Appendices

APPENDIX 12–1
ISSUES IN ETHICS STATEMENT

GENERAL PRINCIPLE

Public statements or announcements of services attributable to individuals* should serve to provide accurate and adequate information to aid the consumer public in making informed choices in matters concerning the profession and the services rendered by its practitioners. This principle must be observed as an affirmative ethical obligation of all individuals, whether acting on an independent basis or in representing an institution, agency, or organization.

GENERAL GUIDELINES

I.   Announcement of Services

    A. Generally individuals may use as a guide the type of announcement customarily used by other professionals in their local communities. Individuals are encouraged, however, to include a simple listing of such of the following items as they consider appropriate:
       1. Identification, using appropriate titles. "Speech-Language Pathologist" and "Audiologist" are the official titles of professionals in the field of Speech-Language Pathology/Audiology.
       2. Fees, listing fixed prices or a stated range of prices for specified professional services. When additional charges may be incurred for an integral part of the overall service, it shall be so stated.
       3. Qualifications, including certification; licensure; educational, experimental, and biographical data.
       4. Services, including specialties or restrictions.
       5. Location, hours, and telephone number.
       6. Staff or associates' names and qualifications.
    B. In making information available to the consumer public, individuals have the responsibility of fairly and accurately representing their services and the profession so that the public is not misled that competence exists in areas in which it does not. It is thus appropriate to list such items as certification, licensure, honorary awards, and accreditation at a service facility or training program by the Professional Services Board or the Education and Training Board, but not to describe any particular expertise which supposedly results from any of those matters. Additionally, individuals should
       1. Avoid misrepresentation of the nature or extent of services provided.
       2. Ensure that when fees and services are listed they are listed in a manner that is not misleading. For example, one level of service (diagnostic) may not be offered at a specified fee when in fact a lower level of service (screening) is provided for that fee.
       3. Not use laudatory comments or testimonials by implication or quotation of persons served professionally.
       4. Not state or imply claims of unusual professional skills.
       5. Not use comparisons of abilities with those of other individuals.

---

6. Describe services, qualifications, facilities, staff, products dispensed, etc., in a factual, nonevaluative manner.
7. Use appropriate and accurate terminology, such as speech-language pathologist, audiologist, professional/clinical services, clinical management, and diagnosis and treatment.
8. Avoid "blind" listings in the classified section of newspapers or other periodicals. "Blind" listings are announcements which omit the name of the individual or agency offering services.

II. Promotional Activities

A. In representing their services or professional products to the general public, individuals accept the obligation of presenting information objectively and accurately, avoiding misleading the public by misrepresentation through implication, deception, exaggeration, half-truths, or superficiality.
B. Individuals offering free speech and/or hearing screening should provide those who need further services with a choice of referral sources. Individuals should avoid participation in any activities recommending to the general public the use of any single source of product or service.
C. Individuals shall not use their affiliation with the American Speech-Language-Hearing Association to endorse the marketing and promotion of products, whether related or unrelated to the profession.

III. Other Constraints on Advertising

The rules set out in this statement are offered only as general guidelines for application of the Code of Ethics of the Association with regard to public statements and announcements. In addition, individuals may be subject to various state laws such as licensure laws. Individuals may be subject also to the regulations of the Federal Trade Commission governing the use of endorsements and testimonials in advertising. Individuals must be aware therefore that there are other restraints in the area of professional advertising and indeed they may be greater than those set forth in this statement. If ASHA guidelines should prove less restrictive in any respect, individuals must adhere to any higher standards that might be applicable. This statement does not purport to give legal advice in this regard.

DEFINITIONS

Public Statement. Any direct or indirect statement, suggestion or implication, including but not limited to one that is made orally, in writing, pictorially, or by any other audio or visual means, or by any combination thereof.

Announcement of Services. Any written or oral statement, illustrations, sign, notice or depiction which is designed to inform the public about professional services or products related to the field.

APPENDIX 12-2
A CLIENT BILL OF RIGHTS

As you become a client of this program/department, agency, it is our duty to remind you that the services you receive are a cooperative effort between you as the client and the members of our professional staff. While you are receiving our services, someone will always be available to assist you in the decisions you must make and to help you understand your rights as a client. The following is a list of your rights. You should always advise us of any questions or concerns about any of these rights.

1. A potential client has the right to complete and accurate information regarding services available and procedures employed.
2. A client has the right to informed participation in all decisions regarding his or her care.
3. A client has the right to a clear, complete, and accurate evaluation of his or her condition and prognosis before being asked to consent to any procedure.
4. A client has the right to a clear, concise explanation, in layperson's terms, of all proposed procedures and their probability of success and will not be subjected to any procedure without his or her voluntary, competent, and understanding consent.
5. A client has the right to know the identity and professional status of all those providing services.
6. A client has the right to know when he or she is participating in teaching or research programs and to be informed of what alternatives are available in the community.
7. A client has the right not to be subjected to any test or procedure designed for educational purposes rather than for his or her direct personal benefit.
8. A client has the right to refuse any particular test or procedure.
9. A client has the right to privacy of both person and information with respect to the professional staff, other professionals, students, and other clients.
10. A client has the right to discuss his or her condition and care with a consultant specialist, at the client's request and expense.
11. A client has the right to all information contained in his or her record and to examine the record on request.
12. A client has the right not to be transferred or referred to another facility unless he or she has received a complete examination of the desirability and need for the transfer or referral, and the client has agreed.
13. A client has the right, regardless of the source of payment, to examine and receive an itemized and detailed explanation of all bills for services rendered.
14. A client has the right to competent counseling to help in obtaining financial assistance from public or private sources to meet the expense or services.
15. A client has the right to timely prior notice of termination of eligibility for services or eligibility for third-party payment for those services or of any other circumstances that will influence the client's financial liability.

From *Delivery of Speech-Language Pathology and Audiology Services* by R. M. Flower, 1984, Baltimore: Williams & Wilkins. Copyright 1984. Reprinted by permission.

Chapter 13

Personal Finances

When considering personal financial planning, it is not necessary to think in big numbers, nor is it necessary to think in terms of tax-advantaged investment plans that double or triple investments. Many of us need to begin with basic personal financial planning before advancing to the consideration of investment realignment.

Basic financial planning on a personal level requires dealing with day-to-day, week-to-week, and month-to-month income and expenditures, specifically household and family budgets. Frequently, people do not budget on a systematic basis, but spend until the checkbook balance is zero, then begin using credit cards. This nonsystem obviously does not allow for emergencies nor for the realization of any personal financial goals.

Everyone in the family who is involved in utilizing the family's income needs to be involved in planning how it will be spent. The initial step is to define individual and family goals designed to meet both short- and long-term needs and desires. Next, the family should prioritize its goals in order to allocate existing funds to the more important short-term goals and to develop plans for accumulating funds to meet long-term goals. Time and circumstance can change or modify goals and priorities. Therefore, the family should understand that over time fund allocation may have to be adjusted as well.

In order to identify funds from which allocations may be made, it is necessary to establish a means for predicting or estimating income. If salary is the major source of revenue, estimation of income is predictable which simplifies the process of creating a budget. Income from investments that depend on market variables or other fluctuating sources is harder to predict. Estimates must be made from the experiences of previous years and from current economic information. When estimating income, it is generally wiser to err on the conservative side. Allocations in one's budget for revenue to meet anticipated expenditures are based on estimations of such expenses. Some are obvious and predictable and vary only from year-to-year rather than from month-to-month. Such expenses include rent or mortgage payments, taxes, insurance, loan payments, and routine health care. Expenses that have a wider variation include clothing, food, transportation, entertainment and recreation, accident and severe illness, and other special needs.

A good personal accounting system offers a family a way of projecting expenditures and then comparing actual costs with budgeted figures to determine variations and what accounted for these variations. Without good record keeping, it is impossible to track expenditures and to determine if budget figures have indeed been met. It is part of good record keeping to develop a financial statement and to update this statement yearly. A financial statement describes all of one's assets in comparison with all of one's liabilities to arrive at a figure of net worth. Producing yearly financial statements is a good way to chart one's progress toward financial goals.

Some practitioners use their office bookkeeping systems to track their personal accounts and use their office accounting consultants for personal financial record keeping. The accounts are kept separate, of course, but the organization already in place for the office makes an easily adaptable system for home or personal accounting records.

If you prefer to do your own personal financial planning, ask yourself these questions to determine which direction to choose. For example, consider the following points:

1. Do you have higher than needed balances in no-interest checking accounts?
2. Should you move funds from passbook savings accounts to certificates of deposit (C.D.s), which earn higher interest rates?
3. Is your tax-sheltered retirement fund growing fast enough? If you do not have a fund, do you have another way of deferring tax on income while saving money for retirement?
4. Should you reconsider those depressed stocks and mutual fund shares in your safety deposit box?
5. Can the cash value of life insurance be better used in other investments or to pay future premiums? This is one way to cut the cost of insurance.
6. Have you checked your high-interest charge accounts and credit card balances to see how much you owe? How much have you paid in interest to those accounts this past year? Is that out of hand?

Your answers to these questions may suggest that you need to take steps to bring your investment program, and your finances in general, under control. Some alternatives for being assertive with your money include the following:

1. Get rid of stocks, mutual funds, or other investments that are not carrying their weight in comparison with the alternatives. What you paid for an investment is not important. What the investment is worth now and how much it is earning is what counts. Periods of high inflation are not good times to concentrate on the stock market or on bonds.
2. Gold, as an investment, is difficult even for the most sophisticated investor. (See Annotated Bibliography for related newsletters and literature.) Gold is a commodity that earns no return and may even cost you money to hold. It earns no interest while it is stable, and your investment decreases as the price of

gold drops. If you want to own some gold, invest in a form that is easy to buy and sell, such as gold certificates offered by banks or metal brokers.

3. An effective anti-inflation investment is to own your own home. If you don't own a home, you should seriously consider buying one, in spite of high down payments and interest rates. (At the time of this writing, interest rates are falling, and long-term home owners' mortgages are less expensive then they have been in the past 5 years.) If you already own your home, consider other real estate investments to take advantage of their inflation-fighting and tax-shelter features.

4. Adjust your insurance program so that it adequately covers the increased amounts of potential loss. Be sure that home insurance is high enough to cover at least 80 percent of the replacement value. Be sure that you have adequate coverage on contents. Many home insurance policies cover only the structure with a very small amount allowed for contents. If you have valuable paintings, antiques, or other fine collectibles *be sure* they are appraised and placed on a coverage rider to your home owner's policy. If you must save money on insurance, it is better to take a higher deductible rate than to skimp on coverage you would need in the event of a catastrophe. Life insurance should be a term policy. Term insurance allows you to buy greater face value at lower cost. The savings you might realize on regular life insurance are worth even less during rapid inflation.

5. Look at your tax savings program. Rapid inflation tends to drive up your income, as well as your expenses. When your income rises, you also enter a higher tax bracket, and saving on taxes becomes even more important. Here are some steps to consider (Ridgewood Financial Institute, 1984):

    a. Make your contributions to tax-sheltered retirement plans—IRA, Keogh, corporate—as high as you can afford. Not only does this cut your taxes in the year of contributions, but it keeps more money working for you, since investment profits are not taxed each year.

    b. Investigate municipal bond funds and other tax-free investments. The closer you get to the 50 percent income tax limit on earned income, the more attractive these bonds and bond funds are. Many therapists with working spouses are likely to be in the 50 percent bracket.

    c. Write down all professional expenses. The best way to do this is to keep accurate day-to-day records in an expense diary.

Individuals and families without a working knowledge of accounting, income tax, insurance, investments, other taxes, law, and banking, may utilize professionals who do have this knowledge and are prepared to guide their clients in the implementation of personal financial goals. Some professional corporations offer services for personal financial planning, including computer programs which can recap all of the disbursement transactions from a family checkbook for the prior year to provide a basis for planning the next year's finances. Many brokerage firms and other legitimate investment advisors will help analyze investment opportunities designed to produce maximum returns. They can also provide information on the benefits you can derive from existing tax structures and help you prepare for changes in tax laws and tax structures.

Portfolio advisors frequently suggest that maximum benefit from investments comes from diversification. No investment is forever; not stocks, precious metals, or even real estate. Flexibility is the overriding criterion in planning your portfolio. The first goal of every investor should be preservation of capital. This requires that one not allow money to remain dormant without incremental changes that keep abreast of the cost of living and inflation. The second goal should be to generate a positive real return on investments.

PLANNING YOUR PORTFOLIO

Your portfolio is your investment plan. You should begin planning your portfolio now, even if you think your holdings are too insignificant to deserve a plan. Some investment managers advise against putting money in an IRA or Keogh Plan as an initial step but, instead, putting small amounts yearly in other forms of managed long-term and tax-sheltered investments. Many investors currently are recommending that a quarter to a third of one's investment should be in cash, such as T-bills or short-dated treasury papers. Such a move provides a way of receiving a fairly decent return, that is, about 8.5 percent with little or no risk. This could be a comfortable way to ride things out until the economy is more predictable. Other investment managers are recommending U.S. Government Bonds with 2-year maturity for the same reason.

Investment Managers

If you decide to consult a money manager, be sure your expectations are not unrealistic. Even the best money managers have good times and bad times. Investors should try to keep as much of the total portfolio under their own control as possible.

There are some general criteria investors should keep in mind when looking for a money manager. The most important criterion is a successful track record over time (Ridgewood Financial Institute, 1984). Obviously past performance doesn't guarantee future performance, but it does provide valuable information. Investors should avoid programs that show wide swings in performance, such as dramatic gains followed by dramatic losses, quarter after quarter. The best track records show good consistency over a period of years. Make sure that the portfolio planner or ''money manager'' has been in business for at least 5 years. A money manager handles assets and the stock or bond markets for individuals, pensions, corporations, or institutions. For this, he or she usually receives a management fee, but not commissions or a share of the profits.

Whether you decide to manage your own investments or consult a money manager, you need to be clear about your own investment objectives. You must decide if you are interested primarily in growth—that is, in building your net worth—or in real income.

An investment manager is not a salesman or broker but an advisor who works to provide you with investment advice relevant to your needs. As your assets grow, you may decide to risk more for the chance of a larger return on your investment than that provided by money market funds, C.D.s, and other easy-to-manage investments. You may want to consider a professional investment firm. If your personal investment is worth $100,000 or more, or if you have full judiciary responsibility for pension accounts of several employees, then you should consult an investment firm for investment fund management. Such a firm can provide you with published information describing how their accounts have been managed and what their performance has been over the past 5 years. If you do place sizable funds with an investment firm, you will need to consider the following (Ridgewood Financial Institute, 1984; Seidman and Seidman, 1984):

1. Is the manager accessible?
2. Do you have as much control as you want?
   You may have to choose between a discretionary or advisory account. A discretionary account permits the investment manager to purchase or sell securities in your portfolio without consulting you. With an advisory account, the manager recommends which stocks and bonds to buy or sell, but you make the final decision.
3. Is the fee worth the help?
   A minimum management fee is $1,000 or 1 percent of the assets. If you want to cut down on commission costs, you can arrange to do the actual trading of securities through a discount broker. With some investment companies, particularly when you do not have a long-term contact with your broker you must watch for over-activity or ''churning.'' This is a situation in which much buying and selling occurs, but little positive change is realized in investment growth. This device is employed to increase commissions for brokers. The average turnover rate for a pension plan's portfolio is about 50 percent a year. If you have the time and knowledge to supervise and execute this kind of activity with investment improvement, you should elect to do it and save yourself the brokerage and advisor fee.
4. What is the investment manager's philosophy about risk tolerance and investment goals? Is it similar to yours?
   Pension fund investors are looking for new ways to squeeze extra return out of liquid assets in portfolios, such as buying bank C.D.s through brokerage houses. Their reasons include the following:
   a. *Higher Returns:* Broker C.D.s usually are sold for a 4-year period; because of their purchasing power brokers can get a 0.5 to 1 percent higher rate than an individual can.
   b. *Flexibility:* Because major brokers usually maintain secondary markets in these C.D.s, you can sell before maturity without getting the bank's permission or paying the interest penalty.
   c. *Safety:* These C.D.s receive the same federal insurance as regular C.D.s (up to $100,000 cash). If you sell your C.D. before maturity, the broker will probably give you less than the nominal value of the C.D., and when you sell a C.D. before maturity its value is determined by what has happened to interest rates since you bought it. (If rates have gone up, your C.D. will be worth less; if rates have gone down, your C.D. will be worth more.)

Sometimes it is difficult to match your investment or pension plan's needs with a brokerage house that has an investment management program. Some larger brokerage houses, such as E. F. Hutton, Paine-Webber, and Shearson-American

Express, will match independent investment advisors with your portfolio size and investment goals. This approach, of course, is available for a nominal fee. See the Annotated Bibliography for contacts regarding this approach.

When one decides to invest part of an individual pension or portfolio in speculative ventures, the safety factor diminishes. As the risk of loss increases, the amount of possible return on investment grows, but it is not always parallel to the risk. There are very few specific legal limits on that in which individual pension plans or company pension plans can invest. Options, futures contracts, and speculative real estate are possibilities, as are oil and gas limited partnerships.

Oil and Gas

Oil and gas limited partnerships aim at income rather than at tax deductions, which is the usual goal of the tax-sheltered drilling partnerships. Oil and gas income partnerships offer higher rates of return than investors could obtain with a money market fund (Ridgewood Financial Institute, 1984). In some instances, limited partnerships offer low risk and high yields, which make them fairly attractive for IRA and Keogh investments. It is usually better to follow ratings of experts when selecting specific investments in oil and gas partnerships. This includes staying with ''public'' oil and gas programs. A note of caution when considering investment in a low-risk with high-yield partnership: the money you put into the partnership has no liquidity, thus the money you invest is unattainable for the period of time the partnership agreement specifies. General partners of the income partnership will charge a fee for management and expenses of the program, and this should be specified in the legal agreement. When investing in an oil and gas partnership, look at the revenue-sharing ratio between general partners and limited partners. You will be a limited partner. Look also at the terms of the agreement. Who pays for what? Who shares the risks? How are revenues shared to compensate for risk? (See Reference and Resource section under Finances.)

Bonds

At the time of this writing, yield on bonds is fairly high, particularly considering inflation rate. If you are interested in bonds, the most convenient way to buy them is through bond funds. They can be obtained in all amounts and offer greater diversity and greater liquidity than when you buy several separate bonds. There are generally two types of funds:

1. *Open-Ended Funds:* Similar to stock mutual funds in which shares can be purchased and sold at any time. The fund managers buy bonds on the open market and trade when they see a chance to improve earnings or increase safety.
2. *Closed-End Funds:* A fixed portfolio of bonds is set up by the management firm, and investors buy a share of it. Interest is passed along to investors each year. Principal is returned as bonds mature.

Sometimes there are differences in returns between funds that invest in government bonds and those that buy corporate issues.

TAXES AND PERSONAL FINANCES

Tax changes are always in the legislative mill, either at the state level, the federal level, or both. At this writing, proposed changes in federal tax plans will affect tax rates, interest income, net long-term capital gains, employer-provided health and accident insurance, group term life insurance, IRAs, employer contributions to pension and profit-sharing plans, business meals and entertainment expenses, state and local income taxes, real estate taxes, sales taxes, cash contributions, and other items. When these and other tax changes are passed, consult your accountant or other business consultant regarding ways these changes affect both your professional and personal finances and plans. For example, if sales taxes are disregarded as tax deductions at some future date, it would be to your benefit to make large purchases the year prior to the time the change becomes effective. Certainly changes will be made in the near future regarding net long-term capital gains and the way they are taxed. This will have an important effect on your investment plans and the way you execute them. The new law requiring explicit records for travel, entertainment, and business expenses is already in effect. Even if these laws are relaxed, it would be to your tax advantage to keep receipts, records, and documents that verify deduction claims and their pertinence to business-related activities.

No one knows *how* tax laws will change, only *that* they will change. It is likely that any tax legislation will allow existing investments to receive the tax treatment in effect at the time they were transacted. This is a primary reason one should continue to invest in propositions that receive tax-sheltered treatment under existing laws.

Real Estate

It is generally unwise to consider investments in which the only return is from tax breaks. Look for true investments in which tax savings are but one component. Consider limited partnerships and their potential tax advantages. The investor, who is one of the limited partners, has no management responsibility nor any financial liability beyond the cash investment and any cash calls specified in the legal partnership agreement. Losses and tax credits can be passed on to limited partners; profits, when they do occur, are taxed only once at the investor level. This type of arrangement is in contrast to corporate profits, which are subject to both corporate income tax and dividend taxes. Limited partnership arrangements are available through most brokerages in real estate, oil and gas, and cable TV systems. Such partnerships are analogous to buying stock that is not necessarily available in the general stock market.

At this writing, real estate and real estate limited partnerships are providing many people the opportunity to take advantage of a healthy economy. Making a decision about how and with whom to invest in a limited partnership is a problem. Proceeding cautiously is advisable. The best way to choose a general partner in an investment is to select someone who has a history of making money from investments with limited partnership arrangements. One disadvantage of any limited partnership is the sizable up-front cash required. Another can be the amount of total obligation to which the limited partner agrees that may be evoked through cash calls to support the project.

Most limited partnerships are arranged in the following way:

A *general partner* can be anyone from a publicly held brokerage to an entrepreneur who puts together an investment package by collecting funds from the public or from associates. Property purchased with these funds usually includes apartment houses, office buildings, shopping centers, or other carefully selected packages. Partnerships of this type do not usually hold the property for more than 4 years.

With publicly sold shares, a price per unit is determined and usually a declared minimum purchase of a specified number of units is required. Sometimes for IRA or Keogh Plans, smaller purchases are allowed. The individuals who purchase these units become *limited partners*. The general partner buys and manages the property and its financing for a nominal fee. Rents are passed through to the partnership.

When the properties are sold, capital gain is divided according to an agreed-upon formula, which was part of the original arrangement among the partners. Limited partners usually pay a commission to buy into the investment. The general partner is the controlling partner, and also bears the liability for the investment. Liability of the limited partners is confined to the amount of money originally invested and specifically agreed to in the investment contract.

Another way of participating in real estate investment without entering a limited partnership is to buy stock in a real estate investment trust (REIT). Real estate investment trusts are like mutual funds on the stock market, except one buys shares in the ownership of properties instead of in industrial enterprises. Operating and investment decisions are made by the REITs trustees. A REIT is not a corporation and must pay at least 95 percent of its profits to shareholders to maintain a tax-free status. Like limited partnerships, REITs have more than one form: those involved with equity, which are best for taxable shareholders; and those that are mortgage-oriented, which are preferable for pension plans (See *Agencies and Institutions* in References).

Some Myths about Real Estate

1. *Quick Profits Are Typical.*
   Real estate investment is often a longer term proposition than stocks, bonds, or currency investments.

2. *Buying Land Pays Big Dividends.*
   Location and timing are the keys to profit; not all land will increase in value. Ultimate use for the land is the factor that determines its value and appreciation.

3. *Investing in Properties Is Always Wise.*
   Not every home, office, or apartment building is a sure thing. ''Over-improved'' properties and unique properties often are hard to sell. Do not invest in property just because you ''fall in love with it.''

4. *Buying in Boom Areas Always Pays Off.*

   The time to buy is when property values look the worst. Boom times are times to sell.

5. *Do Not Buy When Supply Exceeds Demand.*

   Under a ''supply exceeds demand'' situation, the buyer can make the best deal. If the investor can afford to hold the property long term, when the market improves, his or her profit margin will be high. Buy when there is an abundance of unrented office space or resort area property; then sit back and wait.

Tax-Sheltered Life Insurance

Tax-sheltered life insurance may be a good tax-sheltered investment vehicle. In the 1984 tax-reform law, Congress defined a *life insurance policy.* Under that definition a life insurance policy is ''a policy whose ratio of cash value to death benefits falls within the guidelines in the new law, regardless of the interest rate that is being credited'' (Phillips, 1985, p. 44). The older the individual, the less insurance he or she needs to purchase in order to maintain the policy's tax free status. For example, a 40-year-old client who wishes to deposit $100,000 in a new plan must purchase a $350,000 insurance policy to act as the vehicle to which the $100,000 deposit can be made while still maintaining its tax free status. A 65-year-old person making the same $100,000 deposit needs only a $120,000 policy. A 75-year-old needs only a $105,000 policy (Phillips, 1985).

The *Unscheduled Premium Account* (UPA) is an example of one way you can accumulate ''tax sheltered'' wealth while earning high-interest rates, but also pay insurance premiums with nontax dollars, if you choose. The Unscheduled Premium Account is a financial instrument that could net 12 percent untaxed (a large difference when compared to 12 percent in a taxed investment such as C.D.s and money market funds). With new clarification of an insurance policy, nontaxed premium payments are available to anyone who wants them. Suppose an individual wants to buy a $500,000 permanent policy for spousal income and estate liquidity for an annual premium of $4,800 until a specified age at which the policy would be paid up and no further premiums would be required. This individual elects to transfer a $100,000 C.D. into the UPA of this new policy, giving the plan an instant cash value of $100,000. Because of certain sections of the Internal Revenue Code and the 1984 tax reform act, this UPA would accumulate tax free under the guise of a life insurance contract. As interest accumulates each year, the owner can withdraw money from his UPA to pay the $4,800 premium due on the $500,000 policy. Because this withdrawal is classified as a withdrawal of principal, not interest, the money is not taxed. Not only does the UPA continue to compound but so does the cash value of the life insurance policy. Other benefits include

1. As the UPA grows, so does the death benefit increase.
2. Because every premium paid increases the principal each year by equal proportions, there is no chance of violating the new definition of insurance.
3. One does not need to make deposits into the UPA unless one wishes to do so. Generally, a UPA can begin with an initial deposit of $1,500, adding additional funds as they become available.

4. Money borrowed from the cash value is not subject to income taxes (Phillips, 1985).

Spouse on the Payroll

There are many reasons to have a spouse on the payroll if he or she actually performs work for your business. Take, for example, the following reasons:

1. *Additional IRA*: At this writing, a $2,000 IRA is available to any person with at least $2,000 of earned income. With only one wage earner in the family, the maximum is $2,500. If there are two wage earners, $4,000 may be contributed. This is beyond, over, and above any pension contribution.
2. *Reducing Social Security Taxes*: For a sole proprietor netting less than $39,600 (maximum subject of FICA—at least at the time of this writing), a spouse on the payroll saves on self-employment taxes. This is possible because payments by an unincorporated proprietor to a family member are FICA-exempt, yet deductible as salaries. The payments are, however, subject to income tax. It should also be noted that this tax break is available only to the sole proprietor. If a spouse works for a spouse's partnership or corporation, wages are subject to all payroll taxes.
3. *Travel and Entertainment*: Deductions for a spouse's expenses for travel, entertainment, meetings, and courses are easier to justify if the spouse is a necessary company employee, familiar with work and requirements of the office.
4. *Child Care Credit*: If the spouse works, one may be eligible for a tax credit of at least 20 percent of eligible child care expenses.
5. *Deductions for Married Couples*: Their wages are subject to a 10 percent deduction when both work.

Planned Annual Gifts to Children

One way to utilize personal tax planning is to establish custodial accounts for minor children. Each year an individual can give each child up to $10,000 (up to $20,000 if both spouses consent) free of gift tax. Interest on money earned in the custodial account may escape taxes altogether, or may be taxed at a significantly lower rate than if it were earned by the giver. Opening custodial accounts is uncomplicated and involves little or no cost. However, the funds are transferred to the child irrevocably. If the parent dies before the child reaches maturity, custody of the account is administered by the parent's estate unless the parent has named another custodian.

IRA—As a Savings Account

At this writing, any wage earner is entitled to invest $2,000 in an IRA—or total wages if less than $2,000—and deduct that amount from gross income as reported on his or her tax return. In addition, any earnings generated by the IRA are tax-deferred until the date of withdrawal at age 59½ or later. The significant amounts that can be accumulated over an average working career have been well publicized. Many tax-payers do not choose to take advantage of an IRA because of the 10 percent penalty levied by the IRS on withdrawals made before retirement age. If $5,000 is withdrawn early, the penalty is $500 in addition to the regular income tax applicable to that amount of income. People become worried that funds held in IRAs will be needed to meet unanticipated expenses, thus causing any potential benefits to be offset by early withdrawal penalties. This fear is not necessarily well-founded because future earnings are also tax-deferred in an IRA. After a number of years, even early withdrawal will result in a net benefit. This is, of course, dependent on actual tax bracket and rate of return on the IRA.

If one feels that his or her income will remain high at retirement, it is better to put one's money in investments that are tax-exempt. They provide better long-term growth.

There are both managed and self-directed IRAs. In a managed IRA, your investment—usually mutual fund or annuity—is in the hands of professional managers. The self-directed IRA allows you to make all investment decisions.

Receiving Lump-Sum Money

One may receive a distribution from a company as the result of retirement, job change, and so forth. When this occurs, there are financial decisions to be made involving the best use of dollars with the least tax consequences. When this happens, the individual needs to answer some immediate questions, such as the following:

1. What tax options are available?
2. What investments would best meet investment objectives?
3. Are liquid investments needed to provide easy access to funds?
4. Is investment income needed to supplement present income?

Brokerage firms, savings and loans, and banks have instructional brochures or pamphlets regarding management of retirement plans and their tax implications.

Borrowing Against Investments

Some brokerage firms lend money for personal loans at fairly low rates for short time periods. If an individual has stocks or bonds to put up against the loan as collateral, a loan can be obtained without having to sell shares (which might incur substantial short-term capital income taxation) and without having to borrow at higher rates from a bank or savings and loan.

Wills and Estate Planning

In many states, if one dies without a will (intestate), the court system will decide who gets the assets. Sometimes the beneficiary is a total stranger to the deceased. Sometimes the state gets the possessions. For example, Texas is a community property state. When one dies without a will, 50 percent of the community property belonging to the deceased goes to the children of the deceased or to grandchildren of the deceased. The remaining 50 percent of the deceased's community property goes to the surviving spouse. It is estimated that in Texas 83 percent of adults and 68 percent of parents with minor children do not have a will. However, the process of probating an estate of a person who dies intestate can be a prolonged affair. During this time, all property belonging to the deceased is held in suspension. Since much of this property is community and therefore affected by what the surviving spouse does with his or her property, most transactions are halted until the estate is settled. It behooves one to write a will, rather than subject his or her family to the restriction, delay, and cost of settling an estate where no will provides for its disposition.

In some states, a do-it-yourself family will kit is designed so that anyone may learn the legal requirements for a valid will. This kit provides formats for printed wills and samples of wills; describes the property law of the state and how it affects the will; indicates whether a holographic will is applicable; describes how one appoints an executor, how one changes or revokes a will, and how one customizes a will (for example, how to give money to a distant relative or forgive a debt); lists requirements for witnessing a will and setting up a living will; and describes how to list assets. Will kits are legal and, if followed carefully, can save a great deal of money and time and still be valid.

Whether one writes a do-it-yourself will or pays an attorney to draw up a will, it is important that contesting the will be discouraged by the language of the will, that provisions be made for guardians for minor children, that simultaneous death of a person and his or her spouse be covered, and that provision be made for an executor and for his or her right to function with maximum flexibility and minimal interference from the courts.

If you have a will, review it at least once a year (income tax deadlines provide a good reminder). Ask yourself questions that could affect your will, such as the following list (Ridgewood Financial Institute, 1984):

1. Has your marital status changed? If so, you must revise your will, or be certain that you have protected the rights of children after divorce or remarriage.
2. Have you reviewed your list of beneficiaries recently? Update it.
3. Is the executor of your will still available?
4. Have you named guardians to look after your children? Are they still available?
5. Will your estate be as liquid as it should be? If your assets are difficult to obtain at a moment's notice, your spouse may have difficulty covering living expenses until the estate is settled, or, your executor could have trouble with taxes. Either change some investments or add insurance to cover these possibilities. Many life insurance policies provide for the family to have cash available to cover estate taxes.
6. Is your tax-sheltered retirement plan bigger than expected? If most of your assets are in a pension fund, you may want to change the way in which the remainder of your assets are handled.
7. Do you have property in other states? Get legal advice, particularly if the other state has a community property law.
8. Are your lump-sum bequests still as substantial as you intended them to be? What was generous 5 years ago may not be so generous today.

9. Are you acquainted with current tax laws that affect inheritance taxes on many estates?

Regardless of the condition of your will, it will be important to your heirs to have some notes of instruction regarding the handling of small details and information that include the location of important papers, such as insurance policies, family records, and so forth, that will be needed to simplify settlement of the estate (see *Answers*, 1984, outlined and referenced in Appendix 13–1).

At this writing, some of the most dramatic changes in tax laws have occurred in estate and gift tax laws. Amendments passed in 1981 affected the amount of estate and gift monies one could transfer to another person, either during one's lifetime or after death, without estate liability. Anyone with an estate equal to or less than $325,000 in 1982 and no greater than $600,000 in 1987 may be able to dispose of assets without tax consequences (Ridgewood Financial Institute, 1984).

A Living Trust

Set up a living trust while you are still alive. Put all or most of your assets in this living trust. The trust then owns your real estate, stocks, and so forth, but you retain complete control of the assets during your lifetime. You can change the trustee, perform any transactions with the assets you wish, change beneficiaries, and even liquidate the trust anytime you want to.

The advantage is to your heirs after you die. The living trust automatically converts to a post-mortem trust, which carries out major provisions of your will but without the probate process. There is no savings on estate taxes, but the living trust will save your spouse or heirs money and energy. Someone is there to manage the trust (for example, a trust department of a bank or an investment advisor) after your death and before the terms of your will go into effect. The courts cannot interfere. The living trust is very flexible with few tax regulations, since it is not a tax-savings program.

ECONOMIC PHASES AND INVESTING

The economy and its cycles are closely related to struggles for political domination of our country. The struggle for power affects every aspect of the economy. Of course, the state of the economy and the business climate affect the political scene. These interactions are intricate and somewhat cyclical in nature. For example, the political party in power feels that it is important to maintain the illusion of economic strength, particularly as election time nears. American voters are strongly influenced by money in their bank accounts when they vote. The appearance of a healthy economy creates a sense of well-being, and a sense of well-being creates a healthy economy.

How does the party in power create a feeling of economic soundness and governmental stability when throughout our lifetimes the national debt has continuously grown? By manipulating the money supply, the Federal Reserve Board (FRB) can make an administration look good, or bad. The FRB usually cooperates happily with the President. It pumps currency—makes more paper bills and circulates them—into the economy. This usually occurs about 2 years before presidential elections. Interest rates fall, business borrows heavily and expands operations, and more people go to work. Competition increases and prices fall temporarily. Consumers borrow more money, travel, and begin their own businesses. All is well.

However, unrestrained growth in the money supply eventually results in increases in the prices of items and services. If left unrestrained, we would experience extreme hyperinflation. Immediately after an election, the FRB turns to restrictive money supply policies that drive interest rates higher and prevent a wild inflationary spiral from destroying the dollar. Inflation is controlled, but the price is high. Businesses have more difficulty borrowing money to maintain their level of operation or to start up new phases. Consumers begin to delay purchases and elective surgery, and unemployment soars. Small businesses go bankrupt and the recession comes.

Midterm congressional elections are also crucial. The economy must show some signs of recovery before the majority party's candidates arrive at the polls. The cycle of inflation is set into motion again; interest rates go down, the stock market responds as the value of stocks go up, and investors buy (a bull market). With some minor adjustments, the easy money cycle continues until the next presidential election. With uncanny timing, interest rates reach their lowest point a few months before November.

The cycle continues with an important effect. Each recession comes nearer to depression; each inflation more closely approaches hyperinflation. With this cycle in mind, it is easier to understand how an investment in one economic environment flourishes, while it withers in another environment.

Using the State of the Economy for Investing

Recession. Recession is induced by restrictions of the money supply through higher reserve requirements, higher discount rates, and restrictive open market policies. Sometimes new money is minted. It is done to control inflation. In a recession, the business environment is poor, the stock market is down (a bear market), and conventional investments do not work. Good investments in times of recession are bonds, T-bills, money market funds, real estate. Do not borrow money at these times, at least from conventional sources. Rates soar.

Growth. Growth begins as the Federal Reserve releases more money into the economy to curb recession. Interest rates go down as the stock market goes up. The beginning phase of this cycle is the time to invest in the stock market, not a "little later," because often a sudden correction will occur in the market, and the market can drop without warning. The best investments are securities, penny stocks, growth stocks, mutual funds, and business investments.

Inflation. The expansion that halted recession begins showing a steady increase in prices. The bull market fluctuates, then stops. Frightened investors sell at a loss, erasing their momentary profits. The best investments in inflation are antiques and rare coins, foreign currency, gold and silver, and mining stocks.

Because there are so many factors that affect each moment of the economy, the best financial planning is done with the aid of someone who is informed and alert to changes that influence investments. The best financial plan for long-term profits is to have a diversification of investments. You can usually talk about one of your successes if your investments are diversified. Do not mention those that are not doing well at the moment.

Appendices

APPENDIX 13–1
TABLE OF CONTENTS AND SELECTED ITEMS
FROM *ANSWERS*

CONTENTS

INTRODUCTION

Family

Household Answers
Household Special Instructions
Consent for Emergency Treatment
  and/or Surgery
Personal History
Living Will
Funeral and Burial Instructions
Pallbearers
Persons to Notify
Letter of Instruction
Copy of Will
Copy of Trust
Military Papers
Marriage Certificate
Birth Certificates
Divorce/Separation Papers

Finances

Advisors
Bank Accounts
Safe Deposit Box
Credit Cards
Stocks and Bonds
Other Assets
Social Security

Retirement Plan
Loan Information
Accounts, Loans, and Notes Receivable
Loan Agreements and Information
Income Tax Returns
Financial Statement

Properties

Real Estate
Real Estate Papers
Major Improvement Receipts
Auto/Boat Information
Auto Ownership Papers/License Receipts
Boat Ownership Papers/License Receipts

Insurance

Life Insurance
Health and Major Medical
Disability Insurance
Property Insurance
Auto/Boat Insurance

Business

Business Information
Employment Contracts/Buy–Sell
  Agreements/Business Papers
Partnership Agreements/Joint Ventures

This book was written by a young widow who identifies specific ways to prepare and organize documents to facilitate difficult decisions and responsibilities that fall to the immediate family in the event of one's severe disablement or death. Selected items from the book are reproduced or adapted here with the permission of Mrs. Barker.

1. *RIGHT TO DIE STATEMENT*

To My Family, My Physician, My Lawyer, and All Others to Whom It May Concern:

If at such a time the situation should arise in which there is no reasonable expectation of my recovery from extreme physical or mental disability, I direct that I be allowed to

---

From *Answers* (rev. ed.) by B. Barker, 1984, Corpus Christi, TX: Author. Copyright 1984 by B. Barker. Reprinted by permission.

die and not be kept alive by extraordinary measures and that medication be mercifully administered to me to alleviate suffering even though this may shorten my remaining life.

Insofar as they are not legally enforceable, I hope that those to whom this will is addressed will regard themselves as morally bound by these provisions.

2. *FUNERAL AND BURIAL DIRECTIONS*

DONOR's CERTIFICATION: I, the undersigned, being of sound mind and over age 18, donate my ______________________ as an anatomical gift at the time of death, under provisions of Art. 6687b VCS [Vernon's Civil Statutes] and in conformity with Art. 4509-a VCS.

3. *OBTAINING SOCIAL SECURITY BENEFITS*

Social Security benefits should be applied for as soon as possible following the death of a wage earner. You will need the following documents when applying:

Death Certificate

Marriage License (to prove next-of-kin)

Previous Divorce Papers of Deceased

Birth Certificate of Deceased, Spouse, Children, including step-children living in the household of the deceased. (When applying for social security benefits, the birth certificates must be originals or certified copies. If the hospital certificate is used, be sure the mother's maiden name is shown.)

Military Discharge Papers

Income Tax Returns—Previous 2 years

Social Security Number of Deceased, Spouse, Children, including step-children living in household of deceased.

APPENDIX 13–2
PERSONAL FINANCIAL STATEMENT

(Date)

Assets

Cash on Hand (Checking and Savings) $ __________
Money Market Funds, Certificates of Deposit   __________
Government Securities   __________
Stocks and Bonds (Current Value)   __________
Accounts, Loans, and Notes Receivable   __________
Retirement Plan or Account (Current
  Retrievable Funds)   __________
Real Estate   __________
Life Insurance (Cash Value)   __________
Valuation of Business Practice   __________
Collectibles (Rare Coins, Art)   __________
Refunds/Rebates   __________
Income (Salary, Bonuses, Dividends)   __________
Other Assets   __________
                          TOTAL ASSETS $ __________

Liabilities

Notes Payable to Banks/Savings & Loans   __________
Accounts and Notes Payable to Others   __________
Credit Card Balances   __________
Mortgages   __________
Taxes Due   __________
Contracts Payable   __________
Other Liabilities   __________
                     TOTAL LIABILITIES $ __________

                         TOTAL ASSETS $ __________

                  less TOTAL LIABILITIES $ __________

                        = NET WORTH $ __________

APPENDIX 13–3
COST OF LIVING—MONTHLY BREAKDOWN

Routine Monthly Payments

Appliances (TV, Microwave) $____________
Car   ____________
Home (Mortgage, Rent)   ____________
Home Improvement   ____________
Insurance (Car, Home,
   Health, Life)   ____________
Loan Payments   ____________
Taxes (Home, Other
   Property)   ____________
Other   ____________
                   Total $____________

Personal Expenses/Month

Clothing (Purchase) $____________
Clothing (Care)   ____________
Dental   ____________
Dues and Subscriptions   ____________
Education (Classes, Books) ____________
Entertainment   ____________
Gifts and Contributions   ____________
Medical Care   ____________
Medication   ____________
Travel   ____________
Spending Money   ____________
Vehicle Maintenance   ____________
Other   ____________
                   Total $____________

Household Operating Expenses/Month

Telephone $____________
Utilities   ____________
Water/Waste Water   ____________
Repairs, Maintenance   ____________
Other   ____________
                   Total $____________

Quarterly/Yearly Taxes by Month

Federal and State
   Income Taxes   ____________
Estimated Income Tax
   Payments   ____________
Other   ____________
                   Total $____________

Food Expenses/Month

At Home   ____________
Away from Home   ____________
                   Total $____________

SUMMARY

Regular Monthly
   Payments   ____________
Household Operating
   Expenses   ____________
Food Expenses   ____________
Income Tax Payments
   by Month   ____________
             MONTHLY TOTAL $____________

References

Alpiner, J. G., Odgen, J. A., & Wiggins, J. E. (1970). The utilization of support personnel in speech correction in the public schools: A pilot project. *ASHA, 12,* 412–417.

Altman, M. A., & Weiler, R. I. (1978). *Managing your accounting and consulting practice.* New York: Matther, Binder, & Co.

American Medical Association. (1981). *Physician's current procedural terminology.* Chicago: Author.

American Psychiatric Association. (1980). *Diagnostic and statistical manual of mental disorder*—III. Washington, DC: Author.

American Psychological Association. (1960). *Media guide.* Public information. Washington, DC: Author.

American Speech-Language–Hearing Association. (1976). *Comprehensive assessment and service evaluation information system.* Rockville, MD: Author.

American Speech-Language–Hearing Association. (1978). *Multidisciplinary quality review: Advanced patient care.* Audit workshop manual. Rockville, MD: Author.

American Speech-Language–Hearing Association. (1981a). Code of ethics of the American Speech-Language–Hearing Association. Reprint. Rockville, MD: Author.

American Speech-Language–Hearing Association. (1981b). Guidelines for supportive personnel. *ASHA, 23*(3), 165–169.

American Speech-Language–Hearing Association. (1981c). Issues and ethics statement, public announcements and public statements. *ASHA, 23*(2), 107–108.

American Speech-Language–Hearing Association. (1981, September). *The prevalence of communicative disorders: A review of literature, final report.* Rockville, MD: Author.

American Speech-Language–Hearing Association. (1982). Definitions—Communication disorders and variations, *ASHA, 24*(11), 949–950.

American Speech-Language–Hearing Association. (1985). *Planning and initiating a private practice in audiology and speech-language pathology.* Rockville, MD: Author.

Balliett, G. (1978). *Getting started in private practice.* Oradell, NJ: Medical Economics Co.

Bank of America. (1980). Understanding financial statements. *Small Business Reporter,* SBA-109. Bank of America, Dept. 3401, P.O. Box 37000, San Francisco, CA 94137.

Bank of America. (1981). Steps to starting a business. *Small Business Reporter, 14*(7). Bank of America, Dept. 3401, P.O. Box 37000, San Francisco, CA 94137.

Barker, B. (1984). *Answers* (rev. ed.). Corpus Christi, TX: Author.

Battin, R. R. (1983). Clinical accountability: Private practice. *Seminars in Speech and Language, 4,* 147–157.

Battistella, R. M., & Rundall, T. G. (Eds.) (1978). *Health care policy in a changing environment.* Berkeley: McCutchan Publishing Corporation.

Baumback, C. M., & Lawyer, K. (1979). *How to organize and operate a small business* (6th ed.). Englewood Cliffs, NJ: Prentice-Hall.

Belew, R. C. (1973). *How to negotiate a business loan.* New York: Van Nostrand Reinhold Co.

Berryman, J., & Johnson, R. (1984). *Planning individualized speech and language intervention programs: Computer software.* Tucson: Communication Skill Builders.

Bierig, J. R. (1983). Whatever happened to professional self-regulation? *American Bar Association Journal, 69,* 616–619.

Blue Cross–Blue Shield Association. (1982, July). *Legal Affairs Bulletin* (No. 478-4). Chicago: Author.

Bouhoutsos, J. C. (1981). *Ethical standards of psychologists.* Washington, DC: American Psychological Association.

Brantman, M. (1973). The status and outlook for commercial health insurance: Coverage of speech and hearing services. *ASHA, 15,* 183–187.

Braverman, J. (1980). *Crisis in health care.* Washington, DC: Acropolis Books, Ltd.

Breen, G. E. (1977). *Do-it-yourself marketing research.* New York: McGraw-Hill Book Co.

Brill, J. E. (1979). *The thrifty fifty.* Houston: Author.

Browning, C. H. (1982). *Private practice handbook* (2nd ed.). Los Alamitos, CA: Duncliffs International.

Bullock, B. (1985, February). Texas comptroller of public accounts. *Texas Fiscal Facts.*

Bureau of Labor Statistics. Cost of living index. *Consumer Price Index.* Monthly publication. Washington, DC: Department of Labor.

Bussman, J. W., & Davidson, S. V. (1981). *PSRO: The promise, perspective, and potential.* Menlo Park, CA: Addison-Wesley.

Caccamo, J. M. (1973). Accountability—A matter of ethics. *ASHA, 15,* 411–412.

Carnell, C. M., Jr. (1976). *Development and management of community speech and hearing centers.* Springfield, IL: Charles C Thomas.

Chapey, R., Chwat, S., Curlans, G., Pieras, G. (1981). Perspectives in private practice: A nationwide analysis. *ASHA, 24(3)L,* 335–342.

Commission on Professional and Hospital Activities. (1978). *International classification of diseases (9th rev. ed.). Clinical modification.* Ann Arbor, MI: U.S. National Center for Health Statistics.

Committee on Private Practice. (1982a). Academic and clinical preparation standards of service delivery. A report of the Committee on Private Practice. Rockville, MD: American Speech-Language–Hearing Association.

Committee on Private Practice. (1982b). Questions and answers on private practice. *ASHA, 24(11),* 953–954.

Committee on Professional Autonomy. (1985). *Paper on professional autonomy.* Report of the Ad Hoc Committee on Professional Autonomy, ASHA.

Cooper, E. (1982). The state of the profession and what to do about it. *ASHA, 24(11),* 931–936.

Cotton, Horace (1985). *Medical Practice Management.* Oradell, NJ: Medical Economics Co.

Cromwell, F. S. (1974, June). *The development of the occupational therapy assistant: History and status report.* Paper presented at the National Conference for Clinical Directors, ASHA, New Orleans.

D'Asaro, M. J. (1971, February). Who is private practice? Reprint from *The California Journal of Communicative Disorders.*

Davis, Kinard & Co. (1984, December). *Financial insights.* Austin, TX: Author.

Dempsey, V. (1976). Planning for health planning. *ASHA, 18,* 348–352.

Dible, D. (1981). *Up your own organization! A handbook on how to start and finance a new business.* Reston, VA: The Entrepreneur Press.

Division of Manpower Development and Training. (1971). *Audiometric assistant: A suggested guide for manpower training.* Washington, DC: U.S. Office of Education.

Downey, M. (1982). Health care without physicians—Recent legal developments relating to non-physician health care providers. *1982 Health Law Update.* Washington, DC: National Health Lawyer's Association.

Dublinske, S., & Healey, W. (1978). PL 94-142: Questions and answers for the speech-language pathologist and audiologist. *ASHA, 20,* 188–205.

Edmonds, S. W. (1982). *Performance measures for growing businesses: A practical guide for small business management.* New York: Van Nostrand Reinhold.

Elliot, L. L., Vegely, A. B., & Falvey, N. Y. (1971). Description of computer-oriented record-keeping system. *ASHA, 13,* 435–443.

Feinstein, A. (1973). The problems of the ''problem oriented medical records.'' *Annals of Internal Medicine, 78,* 751–762.

Feldman, A. S. (1981). The challenge of autonomy. *ASHA, 23,* 941–945.

Flower, R. M. (1984). *Delivery of speech-language pathology and audiology services.* Baltimore: Williams & Wilkins.

Foonberg, J. G. (1984). *How to start and build a law practice* (Career Series). Chicago: American Bar Association.

Fox, D. (1971). *Private practice: Guidelines for speech pathology and audiology.* Danville, IL: Interstate Printers.

Freudenberger, H. J. (1974). Staff burn-out. *Journal of Social Issues, 30,* 159–165.

Gleason, G. (1981). Microcomputers in education, the state of the art. *Educational Technology, 21*(3), 7–8.

Goates, J. S., & Goates, W. A. (1977). Increasing third-party coverage of speech-language pathology and audiology services. *ASHA, 19,* 887–889.

Gorlick, S. H. (1982). *The whys and wherefores of corporate practice* (4th ed.). Oradell, NJ: Medical Economics Books.

Governmental Affairs Department. (1981). Medicare supplement. *Governmental Affairs Review.* Rockville, MD: ASHA.

Governmental Affairs Department. (1982). Serving speech-impaired children under PL 94-142. Rockville, MD: ASHA.

Governmental Affairs Department. (1983). *Governmental Affairs Review, 3*(4).

Governmental Affairs Department. (1985, January). Medicaid speech-language-pathology and audiology coverage. *Governmental Affairs Review.* Rockville, MD: ASHA.

Graham, S. R. (1985). We are money, you are people. *The Independent Practitioner: Bulletin of the Division of Psychologists in Independent Practice, Division 42 of the American Psychological Association, 5*(4), 7–8.

Haas, L. J. (1983). Ethical issues in consultation. In P. Keller & R. Litt (Eds.) *Innovations in clinical practice* (Vol. 2, pp. 319–387). Sarasota, FL: Professional Resource Exchange.

Hall, P. K., & Knutson, C. L. (1978). The use of preprofessional students as communication aides in the schools. *Language, Speech and Hearing Services in Schools, 9,* 162–168.

Halleck, S. L. (1971). *The politics of therapy.* New York: Science House.

Halleck, S. L. (1980). *Law in the practice of psychiatry.* New York: Plenum.

Hayes, R. S. (1980). *Business loans: A guide to money sources and how to approach them successfully.* Boston: CBI Publishing.

Hemelt, M. D., & Mackert, M. D. (1978). *Dynamics of law in nursing care.* Reston, VA: Reston Pub.

Henry, D. L. (1985). *The profitable professional practice.* Englewood Cliffs, NJ: Prentice-Hall.

Hester, E. J. (1981). Health planning agencies and speech-language pathology. *ASHA, 23,* 85–92.

Hickock, R. J. (Ed.) (1982). *Physical therapy administration and management.* Published for the American Physical Therapy Association. Baltimore: Williams & Wilkins.

Hofling, C. K. (1981). *Law and ethics in the practice of psychiatry.* New York: Brunner/Mazel.

Internal Revenue Service. (1983a). *Election by a small business corporation (Sub-Chapter S)* (IRS Publication No. 2553, Rev. May 1983). Washington, DC: Government Printing Office.

Internal Revenue Service. (1983b). *Employment taxes* (IRS Publication No. 539, Rev. Nov. 1983). Washington, DC: Government Printing Office.

Internal Revenue Service. (1983c). *Information for business taxpayers* (IRS Publication No. 583, Rev. Nov. 1983). Washington, DC: Government Printing Office.

Internal Revenue Service. (1983d). *Self-employment tax* (IRS Publication No. 533, Rev. Nov. 1983). Washington, DC: Government Printing Office.

Internal Revenue Service. (1983e). *Small business tax workshop* (IRS Publication No. 1057, Rev. Nov. 1983). Washington, DC: Government Printing Office.

Internal Revenue Service. (1983f). *Tax calendar for 1984* (IRS Publication No. 509, Rev. 1983). Washington, DC: Government Printing Office.

Internal Revenue Service. (1983g). *Tax guide for small business, income excise, and employment taxes for individuals, partnerships, and corporations* (IRS Publication No. 334, Rev. Nov. 1983). Washington, DC: Government Printing Office.

Internal Revenue Service. (1983h). *Tax withholding and estimated tax* (IRS Publication No. 505, Rev. Nov. 1983). Washington, DC: Government Printing Office.

Iowa Speech and Hearing Association. (1977). *Iowa quality assurance program: Manual.* Cedar Rapids, IA: Author.

Irwin, J. V. (1967). Supportive personnel in speech pathology and audiology. *ASHA, 9,* 348–354.

Jelinek, J. A. (1976). A pilot program for training and utilization of paraprofessionals in preschools. *Language, Speech, Hearing Services in Schools, 7,* 119–123.

Joint Commission on Accreditation of Hospitals. (1979). *Accreditation manual for long-term care facilities.* Chicago: Author.

Joslyn-Scherer, M. S. (1980). *Communication in the human services.* Beverly Hills: Sage Publications.

Kamara, C., & Kamara, A. S. (1976). Computer billing, service analysis, and financial reporting in a hearing and speech agency. *ASHA, 18,* 229–331.

Kamaroff, B. (1976). *Small-time operator.* Laytonville, CA: Bell Springs Publishing.

Kansas State Department of Education. (1977). *Guidelines for the training, utilization and supervision of paraprofessionals and aides.* Topeka: Author.

Keith, R. L. (1978). Professional accountability. *Tejas: Texas Journal for Audiology and Speech Pathology, 3*(3), 8.

Keller, P. A., & Ritt, L. G. (1982). *Innovations in clinical practice: A source book* (Vol. 1). Sarasota, FL: Professional Resource Exchange.

Keller, P. A., & Ritt, L. G. (1983). *Innovations in clinical practice: A source book* (Vol. 2). Sarasota, FL: Professional Resource Exchange.

Kelley, P. C., Lawyer, K., & Baumback, C. M. (1973). *How to organize and operate a small business.* Englewood Cliffs, NJ: Prentice-Hall.

Kelley, R. E. (1978). *Consulting: The complete guide to a profitable career.* New York: Matthew, Binder, & Co.

Kent, L. R. (1980). Problem-oriented records in a university speech and hearing clinic. *ASHA, 22,* 151–158.

King, J. H., Jr. (1977). *The law of medical malpractice.* St. Paul: West Publishing.

Kissel, S. (1983). *Private practice for the mental health clinician.* Rockville, MD: Aspens Systems Corp.

Klein, H. E. (1983). How to improve the marketing of therapy services. In P. Keller & L. Ritt (Eds.), *Innovations in clinical practice* (Vol. 2, pp. 233–241). Sarasota, FL: Ridgewood Financial Institute, Professional Resource Exchange.

Knight, P. D. (1968). Private practice in speech pathology. *ASHA, 10,* 436–441.

Kubr, M. (1976). *Management Consulting: A guide to the profession.* Geneva: International Labour Organization.

Landis, P. A. (1973). Training of a paraprofessional in speech pathology: A pilot project in South Vietnam. *ASHA, 15,* 342–350.

Larson, J. G. (1983). *Mandated health insurance review mechanisms: Report to the Bureau of Insurance.* State of Virginia Department of Health Administration. School of Allied Health Professionals. Richmond: Medical College of Virginia, Virginia Commonwealth University.

Lasky, E. Z. (1984). Introduction to microcomputers for specialists in communication disorders. In A. H. Schwartz (Ed.), *Handbook of microcomputer applications in communication disorders* (pp. 1–33). San Diego, CA: College-Hill Press.

Lawrence, C. F. (1966). Communicative disorders and public health. *ASHA, 8,* 35–36.

Lawrence, C. F. (1967). Public Law 89–749. Comprehensive health planning. *ASHA, 9,* 261–266.

Lehrhoff, I., & Koroshec, S. (1981). *Speech and language procedures manual.* Beverly Hills: Irwin Lehrhoff and Associates.

Lewin, M. H. (1978). *Establishing and maintaining a successful private practice.* Rochester, NY: Professional Development Institution.

Loavenbruck, A. M., & Madell, J. R. (1981). *Hearing aid dispensing for audiologists.* New York: Grune and Stratton.

Luvera, P. N. (1976). *How to operate an efficient law office.* Mount Vernon: Paul Luvera.

McCall, R., & Stocking, S. (1982). Between scientists and the public: Communicating psychological research through the mass media. *American Psychologist, 37,* 985–995.

Macfarlane, W. N. (1977). *Principles of small business management.* New York: McGraw-Hill, Inc.

Mancuso, J. R. (1978). *How to start, finance, and manage your own small business.* Englewood Cliffs, NJ: Prentice-Hall.

Mancuso, J. R. (1980). *Small business survival guide.* Englewood Cliffs, NJ: Prentice-Hall.

Mandel, J. (1984, April). *Starting an independent consulting practice.* Management Assistance, Starting Out Series 204. Fort Worth, TX: Small Business Administration.

Margolin, G. (1982). Ethical and legal considerations in marital and family therapy. *American Psychologist, 37,* 788–801.

Marshall, M., Lord, P., & Johnston, B. (1982). *Your private practice; planning and organization.* Lake City, FL: Peter J. Lord & Associates.

Maslach, C. (1976). Burned-out. *Human Behavior, 5,* 177–182.

Meltzer, M. L. (1975). Insurance reimbursement—A mixed blessing. *American Psychologist, 30,* 1150.

Merrill, Lynch, Pierce, Fenner, & Smith, Inc. (1979). *How to read a financial report* (4th ed.). One Liberty Plaza, 165 Broadway, New York, NY 10080.

Michigan Association of Psychotherapy Clinics v. Blue Cross–Blue Shield of Michigan, Michigan App. 301 N.W. 2nd 33 (1980).

Miller, M., & Potter, R. (1982). Professional burn-out among speech-language pathologists. *ASHA, 24*(3), 176–180.

Moll, K. L. (1974). Issues facing us—Supportive personnel. *ASHA, 16,* 357–358.

Monohan, J. (Ed.). (1980). *Who is the client? The ethics of psychological intervention in the criminal justice system.* Washington, DC: American Psychological Association.

Musselman, V. A., & Hughes, E. H. (1981). *Introduction to modern business: Issues and environment.* Englewood Cliffs, NJ: Prentice-Hall.

National Association of Speech and Hearing Action. *Do your health benefits cover speech, language or hearing services?* Series of brochures for the consumer. Available from the Publications Department, NASHA, 10801 Rockville Pike, Rockville, MD 20852.

National Conference of Nomenclature. (1961). *Standard nomenclature of diseases and operations.* New York: McGraw-Hill.

Newman, P. W. (1973). Communication: Its disorders, and professional implications. *ASHA, 15.* 290–293.

Nickerson, Clarence B. (1975). *Accounting handbook for non-accountants.* Boston: Cahners Books/Cahners Pub. Co.

Nicolosi, L., Harryman, E., & Kresheck, J. (1983). *Terminology of communication disor-*

ders: Speech-language-hearing (2nd ed.). Baltimore: Williams & Wilkins.

Norma Morris Enterprise Pub. (1981). *How to set up a business office*. Wilmington, VA: Author.

Orlich, D. C., Clark, B. A., Fagan, N. M., & Rust, G. A. (1975). *Guide to sensible survey research*. Olympia: Coordinating Unit, Washington State Commission for Vocational Education.

Parry, J. K. (1981). Informed consent, for whose benefit? *Social Casework, 62*, 537–542.

Pelissier, R. F. (1984). *Planning and goal setting for small business*. Small Business Administration, Management Assistance Support Services, MA: 20010.

Perkins, W. H. (1971). *Speech-pathology: An applied behavioral science*. St. Louis, MO: C. V. Mosby.

Perrin, K. L. (1979). Personal incomes in the speech-language-hearing profession. *ASHA, 21*, 522–524.

Peterson, H. A. (1977). More about computer-assisted record-keeping. *ASHA, 19*, 617–618.

Phillips, D. V. (1985, Spring). Tax-sheltered life insurance. *Wealth, 41*–45. Metairie, LA.

Pines, A. & Maslach, C. (1978). Characteristics of staff burn-out in mental health settings. *Hospital and Community Psychiatry, 19*, 233–237.

Pines, P. L. (1981). Revised medicare requirements. *ASHA, 23*, 357–358.

Popelka, G. R. (1983). *Computer-assisted hearing-aid evaluation and fitting program*. St. Louis: Publications Department of the Central Institute of the Institute for the Deaf.

Pressman, Robert M. (1984). Microcomputers and the private practitioner. Homewood, IL: Dow Jones-Irwon.

Professional Practices Division. (1985, February). *Determining the cost of speech, language, and hearing services: A guide to developing cost analysis procedures*. Rockville, MD: ASHA.

Professional Services Board. (1983). *Standards for PSB Accreditation. ASHA, 25*, 51–58.

Prosser, W. L. (1971). *Handbook of the law of torts* (4th Ed.). St. Paul, MN: West.

Punch, J. (1982). *ASHA Survey, salary and employment characteristics*. Rockville, MD: Research Division, American Speech-Language Hearing Association.

Rappoport, P. S. (1983). *Value for value psychotherapy—the economics of therapeutic barter*. NY: Praeger.

Rees, N. S. (1979). President's page. *ASHA, 21*, 990–991.

Research Institute of America. (1978). *Executive Wealth Accumulation*. Special Report, Research Institute Recommendations. New York: Author.

Research Institute of America. (1984, February). *Business deductions: Staff recommendations*. New York: Author.

Research Institute of America. (1984). *Wealth plan tax experts use*. New York: Author.

Ridgewood Financial Institute. (1984). Collection policies. *Guide to private practice*. Ho-Ho-Kus, New Jersey: Author.

Ridgewood Financial Institute. (1984). Estate planning. *Guide to private practice*. Ho-Ho-Kus, NJ: Author.

Ridgewood Financial Institute. (1984). Realistic investing. *Guide to private practice*. Ho-Ho-Kus, NJ: Author.

Right, G. M. (1981). Guidelines for the review of do-it-yourself treatment books. *Contemporary Psychology, 26*, 189–191.

Rushakoff, G. E. (1984). Clinical applications in communication disorders. In A. H. Schwartz (Ed.), *Handbook of micro-computer applications in communication disorders* (pp. 147–171). San Diego: College-Hill Press.

Safeguard Business Systems. (1975). *How to improve medical office financial controls*. East Orange, NJ: Author.

Scalero, A. M., Czkenasi, C., & Lasky, E. Z. (1976). The use of supportive personnel in a public school speech and language program. *Language, Speech, Hearing Services In Schools, 7*, 150–158.

Schultz, M. C., & Carpenter, M. H. (1973). The bases of speech-pathology and audiology: selecting the therapy model. *Journal of Speech and Hearing Disorders, 38,* 395–404.

Schwartz, A. (Ed.). (1984). *Handbook of microcomputer application in communication disorders.* San Diego: College-Hill Press.

Schwartz, A. (1984). Software specification sheet. Peoria, IL: Office for Research and Sponsored Programs, Bradley University.

Seidman and Seidman. (1984, November). *Washington tax report, 1.* New York: Author.

Seidman and Seidman. (1985, February). *Washington tax report, 2.* New York: Author.

Seidman and Seidman. (1985, April). *Washington tax report, 1.* New York: Author.

Seigel, G. M. (1975). The high cost of accountability. *ASHA, 17,* 796–797.

Shimberg, E. (1979). *The handbook of private practice in psychology.* New York: Brunnen/Mazel Publishers.

Sippl, C. J. (1981). *Microcomputer dictionary.* Indianapolis: Howard W. Sams.

Smith, R. A. (1982). *Setting up shop: The do's and don'ts of starting a small business.* New York: McGraw-Hill.

Social Security Administration. (1984, May). *Employer guidelines: Social security and your employees.* (SSA Publication No. 05-10155). Baltimore: Department of Health and Human Services, Social Security Administration.

Steinhoff, D. (1982). *Small business management fundamentals.* New York: McGraw-Hill.

Task force on private health insurance. (1980). A report on third-party reimbursement of speech-language pathology and audiology services. Rockville, MD: ASHA.

Texas Committee of Examiners for Speech-Language Pathology and Audiology. (1985). Rules and regulations governing the practice of speech-language pathology and audiology associates. *The Texas Registry, 10,* 4529–4532.

The Rehabilitation Codes. (1967). *The Rehabilitation Codes.* New York: Author.

Thompson, J. L. (1982, October). *Trends in third-party reimbursement for non-physician health care providers.* Paper presented at the Licensing and Credentialing of Health Care Providers' Conference, American Society of Law and Medicine, Washington, DC.

U.S. Office of Education. (1970). *Standard terminology for curriculum and instruction in local and state school systems.* Washington, DC: Government Printing Office.

Vernon's Civil Statutes (1983). St. Paul, MN: West.

Virginia Academy of Clinical Psychologists versus Blue Shield of Virginia. [649 F. Supp. 552 (E. D. Va. 1979)]. affim/revd. in part F 2d (4th Cir., June 16, 1980).

Weed, L. (1970). *Medical records, medical education, and patient care.* Chicago: Year Book Medical Publishers.

Weiner, S. M. (1980). Health care policy and politics. Does the past tell us anything about the future? *American Journal of Law and Medicine, 5(4),* 331–341.

Woody, R. H. (1984). Professional responsibilities and liabilities. In R. H. Woody and associates, *The law and practice of human services* (pp. 373–401). San Francisco: Jossey-Bass Pub.

Wright, R. H. (1981). Psychologists and professional liability (malpractice) insurance: A retrospective review. *American Psychologist, 36,* 1483–1484.

Yoder, D. (1984). Presidential Address. *ASHA, 26: 9,* 37–38.

Ziskin, J. (1975). *Coping with psychiatric and psychological testimony* (2nd ed.). Marina del Rey, CA: Law and Psychology Press.

Annotated Bibliography and Source List

Administration and Finances

American Speech-Language-Hearing Association. (1985). *Determining the cost of speech, language and hearing services*. Rockville, MD: Author.

Provides methods of determining costs of services and establishing fees for services.

American Speech-Language-Hearing Association. (1985). *Planning and initiating a private practice in audiology and speech-language pathology*. Rockville, MD: Author.

Includes sections on locating and equipping an office for private practice, financial planning, promoting services, and choosing an organizational structure.

American Speech-Language-Hearing Association. *Governmental Affairs Review*. (Published Quarterly).

Cost varies with membership status. Contents range from federal legislation to state regulations pertaining to speech-language-hearing delivery of services.

Bank of America (1981). Steps to starting a business. *Small Business Reporter, 14(7)*. Department 3401, P.O. Box 37000, San Francisco, CA 94137. (415) 622-2491.

Provides steps for translating the basic idea of the entrepreneur into a concrete plan. Describes business forms (organizational structures), financing, selecting a location, federal, state, and local regulations regarding various permits and licenses, taxes, setting up books, and promotion.

Bank of America. (1980). Understanding financial statements. *Small Business Reporter, 109*, Department 3401, P.O. Box 37000, San Francisco, CA 94137.

Analyzes financial reports and describes problem detection techniques. Includes basic definitions of financial terms. One of 25 issues in the *Small Business Reporter* series. Free listings are available.

Chapey, R., Chwat, S., Gurlans, G. and Pieras, G. (1981). Perspectives in private practice, a nationwide analysis *ASHA, 24(3)* 335, 342.

Represents the results of a survey of private practitioners in 48 states (1,134 individuals) listed by ASHA as full-time practitioners in speech-language pathology and or audiology.

Davis, Kinard & Co. (1984, December). Where work day earnings go. *Financial Insights.*

Estimates expenditures of the average U.S. wage earner in 1984, based on an 8-hour day. Includes other items such as personal business, private education, savings, and investments.

Department of Health and Human Services. (1984). *Employer guidelines: Social security and your employees.* SSA Publication No. 05-10155. Baltimore: Social Security Administration.

Tells employers some of the responsibilities involving social security, including record keeping, forms, and deadlines.

Fund Raising School, P.O. Box 3237, San Rafael, CA 94912.

Applies principles and techniques of fund-raising particularly applicable to not-for-profit executives and fund-raisers in training courses.

Keller, P. A., & Ritt, L. G. (1982–1985). *Innovations in clinical practice: A source book.* Vols. 1–4. The Professional Resource Exchange, Dept. M, P.O. Box 15560, Sarasota, FL 34277-1560.

Provides information related to clinical practice. It is complemented by an examination module, which may be used to earn continuing education credits. Designed primarily for psychologists. Pertains to financial and organizational aspects of private practice; many of the sections in Volume II are related to clinical issues of the psychologist in practice.

Mandel, J. K. (1984, April). *Starting an independent consulting practice.* Starting Out Series, #204, Small Business Administration, Management Assistance, P.O. Box 15434, Fort Worth, TX 76119.

Defines *consultant*, discusses consulting opportunities, how consultants may avoid failure, how consultants can market skills, and fee proposals. Fairly cursory treatment of subject, with some tips and information sources.

Merrill, Lynch, Pierce, Fenner & Smith. (1979). *How to read a financial report.* One Liberty Plaza, 165 Broadway, New York, NY 10080.

Explains income statement and balance sheet for hypothetical company's annual report. Defines terms and provides examples of definitions.

Pelissier, R. F. (1978). *Planning and goal setting for small business.* Management Aids, #2.010. Arlington, VA: International Consulting Associates, Small Business Administration, Management Assistance Support Services.

Identifies and discusses functions of management: planning, organizing, directing, and coordinating. Written for owner/manager of small business; offers suggestions for strengthening management through goal setting.

Small Business Administration. (1983). *The ABC's of borrowing.* Management Aids #1.001. Small Business Administration, Management Assistance Support Services. P.O. Box 15434, Fort Worth, TX 76119.

Summarizes fundamentals of borrowing, including credit worthiness, kinds of loans, amount of money needed, collateral, loan restrictions and limitations, the loan application, and standards that lenders may use in evaluating loan applications.

Small Business Administration. (1973). *Business plan for small services firms*. Management Aids #2.022. Small Business Administration, Management Assistance Support Services, Education Division, Office of Management Assistance. P.O. Box 15434, Fort Worth, Texas 76119.

Provides specific suggestions for owner/manager of small service firm in designing a business plan. Covers areas such as marketing, equipment and furniture, organizational charts, and using profit/loss statements as feedback for the business.

Small Business Administration. (1984). *Management assistance publications*, Pub. #115A. Office of Management Assistance, P.O. Box 15434, Fort Worth, TX 76119.

Superintendent of Documents. (1984). *Management assistance publications*, Pub. #115B, SBA. Washington, DC: Government Printing Office.

Both leaflets list Small Business Administration produced brochures on various aspects of business initiation, management, and business basics.

COMPUTERS

Compu-Psych, Inc., One Liberty Plaza, Liberty, MO 64068.

Hardware and software systems for administration, scoring, and interpretation of various assessment tools.

Psychological Assessment Resources, Inc., P.O. Box 98, Odessa, FL 35556.

A source of administrative, scoring, and interpretive software for various assessment devices, including the WISC-R, WAIS-R, Bender, Gestalt, Rorschach.

Psych Systems, 600 Reisterstown Road, Baltimore, MD 21028.

Hardware and software systems for administration, scoring, and interpretation of various assessment tools.

Pressman, R. (1984). *Microcomputers and the private practitioner*. Homewood, IL: Down Jones-Irwin.

Includes samples of computer written reports, an annotated bibliography, and glossary of terms. The book is designed for the novice as well as for the practitioner who has some knowledge of computer science. Describes a ''do-it-yourself turn-key operation'' from beginning searches through catalogs to the acquisition of computer software, and supplies.

Schwartz, A. Acting Director, Office for Research and Sponsored Programs. Bradley University, Peoria, IL 61625. Referenced by Computer Conference, American Speech-Language-Hearing Foundation, 10801 Rockville Pike, Rockville, MD.

Software Specification Sheet. Encompasses a range of information for the software user to obtain in determining usefulness and applicability of software programs. Included are program characteristics, equipment, peripheral devices, software design, and validation.

Schwartz, A. (Ed.). (1984). *Handbook of microcomputer application in communication disorders*. San Diego: College-Hill Press.

Contains information on microcomputer systems that may be pertinent to communication disorder specialists and communication scientists. Sections of the book include a review of critical concepts regarding microcomputers, information to assist the professional in decision-making about computer systems, current and future applications for computers, and the use of microcomputers in the office. The last section contains more than 400 definitions of computer-related terms.

INSURANCE

American Speech-Language-Hearing Association. (1984). *Who would care?* Videotape. Rockville, MD: Author.

A 7-minute videotape that describes communication disorders, their effect on the average American family, and how to get insurance coverage. American Speech-Language-Hearing Association, 10801 Rockville Pike, Rockville, MD 20852.

American Speech-Language-Hearing Association. (1983). Medicare legislative and regulatory changes: Impact for speech-language pathologists and audiologists. Rockville, MD: Author.

Contains information crucial to hospital-based practices. Information on Medicare prospective payment system, Medicare regulations governing physician reimbursement, and proposals from the Joint Committee on Accreditation of Hospitals (JCAH) is included (48 pages).

American Speech-Language-Hearing Association. (1982). *The medicare supplement*. Rockville, MD: Author.

A collection of Medicare-related materials; includes legislative history of PL 96-499, new articles on professional independence, and necessary steps in improving Medicare coverage for speech-language pathologists/audiologists (58 pages).

National Association of Speech and Hearing Action. (1984). *Do your health benefits cover speech, language or hearing services?* Rockville, MD: Author.

Contains basic information to assist consumers in finding out whether coverage exists in their present health plans; gives an example of a communication disorder benefit. Guidance for what consumers should do if they think that coverage is not included is also provided.

TAXES AND TAX DEDUCTIONS

Home Financial Education Services, 836 Franklin Court, Box 105627, Atlanta, GA 30348.

Provides booklets and articles on various real estate investments and tax changes affecting real estate. Price lists on booklets and articles are available from the company.

Internal Revenue Service. (1983). *Information for business taxpayers*. Internal Revenue Service Pub. #583, Rev. Ed.

Gives basic information for both new and existing businesses, covering (a) kinds of federal taxes businesses have to pay; (b) identification numbers used by businesses, including information on how numbers are used, how to apply for a number, and when a business may have to get a new number; and (c) kinds of records a small business may find it helpful to keep.

Internal Revenue Service. (1983). *Tax calendars*. Internal Revenue Service Publication Stat. Rev. Washington, DC: Government Printing Office.

Includes a general tax calendar, and two specialized calendars: An employer's tax calendar and an excise calendar. These calendars explain when to file tax returns, pay estimated tax, apply for extensions, send in information returns, and meet other schedules required by federal tax laws.

Research Institute of America. (1984). *Business deductions, staff recommendations.* 589 Fifth Avenue, New York, NY 10017.

Provides a reference guide as to what was tax deductible in 1984. Discusses in detail the back-up records to maintain in order to substantiate claims for deductions.

Research Institute of America. (1984, February). *The wealth plan tax experts use.* Special Report. 589 Fifth Avenue, New York, NY 10017.

Provides information for executives regarding deductions, investments, and other financial advice related to federal and state income tax.

AGENCIES AND INSTITUTIONS*

American Association of Minority Enterprise
Small Business Investment Companies
92 New Street
Newark, NJ 07012

American Institute of Certified Public Accountants
1211 Avenue of the Americas
New York, NY 10036

Department of Economic and Business Development
Office of Small Business Development
Sacramento, CA 95814

Farmers Home Administration
U.S. Department of Agriculture
Washington, DC 20250

Minority Business Development Agency
U.S. Department of Commerce
Washington, DC 20230

Monarch Office Systems
Division of Dennison Monarch Systems, Inc.
P.O. Box 4081
New Windsor, NY 12550

National Association of Independent Insurance Adjustors
222 West Adams Street
Chicago, IL 60606

---

*Several brokerage firms, including E. F. Hutton, Paine-Webber, and Shearson/American Express, will search out independent investment advisors who specialize in small accounts. They try to match individual accounts with advisors according to portfolio size and investment goals. Costs vary widely.

National Association of Public Insurance Adjustors
131 E. Redwood Street
Suite 210
Baltimore, MD 21202

National Association of Real Estate Investment Trusts
1101 17th Street, N.W.
Suite 700
Washington, DC 10036

National Association of Women Business Owners
200 O Street, N.W.
Washington, DC 20036

National Venture Capital Association
10 South LaSalle Street
Chicago, IL 60603

Office of Minority Business Enterprise
U.S. Department of Commerce
Washington, DC 20230

Records Management Systems
10304 Brockwood Road
Dallas, TX 75238

The Resort Timesharing Council
1000 16th Street, N.W., Suite 604
Washington, DC 20036

Small Business Administration
Washington, DC 20416

Superintendent of Documents
Government Printing Office
Washington, DC 20402

U.S. Securities and Exchange Commission (Headquarters)
500 North Capitol Street
Washington, DC 20549

Business Forms

The Clowell Company
201 Kenyon Road
Champaign, IL 61820

Emicke Co.
P.O. Box 160
Brownsville, NY 10708

The Physicians Record Company
3000 S. Ridgeland Avenue
Berwyn, IL 60402

The Drawing Board, Inc.
Box 505
256 Regal Road
Dallas, TX 75521

Directories

Directory of Operating Small Business Investment Companies (Annual)
U.S. Small Business Administration
Washington, DC 20416

Guide to Venture Capital Sources (3rd Ed., 1974)
Capital Publishing Corporation
10 South LaSalle Street
Chicago, IL 60603

OMBE Funded Organizations Directory (Biannual)
Office of Minority Business Enterprise
Washington, DC 20230

Western Association of Venture Capitalists
Directory of Members (Annual)
244 California Street, Room 500
San Francisco, Ca 94111

References and Resources for Further Information

FINANCES

American Institute of Certified Public Accountants. *CPA Client Bulletin.* 1211 Avenue of the Americas, New York, NY 10036.
Bank of America. *Small Business Reporter.* Box 37000, San Francisco, CA 94137.
Davis, Kinard & Co., 323 Congress Avenue, Austin, TX 78701.
Dun and Bradstreet, Business Economics Division, 99 Church, New York, NY 10007.

> *The business failure record*
> *Cost of doing business (corporations)*
> *Cost of doing business (proprietorships/partnerships)*
> *Key business ratios*

Home Financial Education Services, 835 Franklin Court, Box 105627, Atlanta, GA 30348.
Kiplinger Washington Editors. *Kiplinger Washington Letter.* 1729 H Street, N.W., Washington, DC 20066.
Paine-Webber. *Money Notes (formerly Money Matters).* Monthly Publication for Paine-Webber clients. 1285 6th Avenue, New York, NY 10019.
Paine-Webber. Investment Advisor Research, 55 W. Monroe, Chicago, IL 60603. (312) 580-8310.
Personal Finance: The Inflation Survival Letter. 1300 North 17th Street, Suite 1660, Arlington, VA 22209.
Resorts Condominiums, Int., 9333 N. Meridian, Indianapolis, IN 46260-1814.
Ridgewood Financial Institute. *Psychotherapy Finances.* 500 Barnett Place, Ho-Ho-Kus, NJ 07423.
Rotan Mosle Portfolio Strategy Group. *Viewpoint.* Rotan Mosle, 1500 South Tower, Penzoil Place, Houston, TX 77022.
Seidman and Seidman, BDO. 110 Union Bank Building, Grand Rapids, MI 49503.
Small Business Administration (1985). *Guides for profit planning.* SBA Series No. 25, Stock #045-000-000-00137-7). Washington, DC: Government Printing Office.
United Business Services. *United Business and Investment Report.* 210 Newbury, Boston, MA 02116. (617) 267-8855.

INSURANCE

Bradford National Life Insurance, 475 85th Road, A215, Sausalito, CA 94965.
Crown Life, 3101 N. Central Avenue, Suite 435, Phoenix, AZ 85012.

Consumer and Professional Relations Division. *Allied Health Relations.* Health Insurance Association of America, 1750 K Street, N.W., Suite 600, Washington, DC 20006. (202) 331-1336.
Old Line Life, 620 East Canyon Rim Road, Suite 208D, Anaheim, CA 92087.

MARKETING

Small Business Administration (1980). *Marketing Strategy.* SBA Basics Series, No. 1009, Stock #045-000-00188-1. Washington, DC: Government Printing Office.

STARTING A BUSINESS

Small Business Administration. *Business plan for small services firms.* MA. 2.022. Fort Worth, TX: SBA Publications.
Small Business Administration. *Feasibility checklist for starting a small business of your own.* MA 2.026. Fort Worth, TX: SBA Publications.
Small Business Administration. (1982). *Starting and managing a small business of your own.* Starting and Managing Series No. 1, Stock #045-000-00212-8. Washington, DC: Government Printing Office.
Small Business Administration. (1983). *Incorporating a small business.* MA 6.003. Fort Worth, TX: SBA Publications.
Small Business Administration. (1983). *Selecting the legal structure for your business.* MA 6.004. Ft. Worth, TX: SBA Publications.
Small Business Administration. (1983). *Women's handbook.* Publication No. 518. Fort Worth, TX: SBA Publications.
Small Business Administration. (1985). *Starting and managing a small service firm.* Starting and Managing Series No. 101, Stock #145-000-00207-1. Washington, DC: Government Printing Office.

TAXES

How to get trouble free travel and entertainment expense deductions under the latest 1985 tax rules. Englewood Cliffs, NJ: Prentice-Hall.
Internal Revenue Service. (1983). *Employment taxes.* IRS Publication No. 539 (Rev. 1983). Washington, DC: Government Printing Office.
Internal Revenue Service. (1983). *Information for business taxpayers.* IRS Publication No. 583. Washington, DC: Government Printing Office.
Internal Revenue Service. (1983). *Self-employment tax.* IRS Publication No. 533. Washington, DC: Government Printing Office.
Internal Revenue Service. (1985). *Small business tax workshop.* IRS Publication No. 1057. Washington, DC: Government Printing Office.
Internal Revenue Service. (1986). *Tax calendar for 1986.* IRS Publication No. 509. Washington, DC: Government Printing Office.
Internal Revenue Service. (1983). *Tax guide for small business, income, excise, and employment taxes for individuals, partnerships, and corporations.* IRS Publication No. 334. Washington, DC: Government Printing Office.
Internal Revenue Service. (1983). *Tax withholding and estimated tax.* IRS Publication No. 505. Washington, DC: Government Printing Office.
Seidman & Seidman. (1985). *Tax Letter: Publication Devoted to Current Tax Matters.* BDO New York Office, 15 Columbus Circle, NY 10023.
Seidman & Seidman. *Washington Tax Report, Nov. 1984.* No. 1, BDO, Special Edition, New York Office, 15 Columbus Circle, NY 10023.

Index

Italic page numbers refer to figures and
tables.

A